Gastroenterology Yesterday – Today – Tomorrow: A Review and Preview

FALK SYMPOSIUM 144

Gastroenterology Yesterday – Today – Tomorrow: A Review and Preview

Edited by

G. Adler
*Ulm,
Germany*

A.L. Blum
*Romainmôtier
Switzerland*

H.E. Blum
*Freiburg
Germany*

U. Leuschner
*Frankfurt
Germany*

M.P. Manns
*Hannover
Germany*

J. Mössner
*Leipzig
Germany*

R.B. Sartor
*Chapel Hill,
USA*

J. Schölmerich
*Regensburg
Germany*

*Proceedings of the Falk Symposium 144 held in Freiburg, Germany,
October 16–17, 2004
Presidents of the Conference: J.L. Boyer, M. Classen, G.N.J. Tytgat*

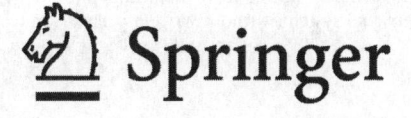

Springer

Library of Congress Cataloging-in-Publication Data is available.

ISBN-10 1-4020-2896-2
ISBN-13 978-1-4020-2896-0

Published by Springer,
PO Box 17, 3300 AA Dordrecht, The Netherlands

Sold and distributed in North, Central and South America
by Springer,
101 Philip Drive, Norwell, MA 02061 USA

In all other countries, sold and distributed
by Springer,
PO Box 322, 3300 AH Dordrecht, The Netherlands

Printed on acid-free paper

All Rights Reserved
© 2005 Springer and Falk Foundation e.V.

No part of the material protected by this copyright notice may be reproduced or utilized in any form or by any means, electronic, mechanical, including photocopying, recording or by any information storage and retrieval system, without written permission from the copyright owners.

Contents

List of principal contributors	ix
List of chairpersons	xiii
Preface	xv

SECTION I: ESOPHAGUS
Chair: R Arnold, AL Blum

1   Treatment of uncomplicated reflux disease
J Labenz   3

2   Management of Barrett's oesophagus, dysplasia and early adenocarcinoma
C Ell, O Pech   22

3   Selective COX-2 inhibitors – safety and side-effects
CJ Hawkey   39

SECTION II: STOMACH
Chair: J Mössner, EO Riecken

4   Pathogenesis of peptic ulcer and distal gastric cancer
A Axon   57

5   Vaccination against *Helicobacter pylori* revisited
P Michetti   67

6   Mucosa-associated lymphoid tissue lymphoma: lessons from Germany
W Fischbach   76

7   Who gets gastric cancer – predisposition or bad luck?
KEL McColl   84

CONTENTS

8   Future of endoscopic imaging
GNJ Tytgat   91

SECTION III: LIVER I
Chair: R Schmid, R Williams

9   Portal hypertension: diagnosis and treatment
D Lebrec   99

10   Current therapy of hepatitis C
SW Schalm   109

11   The role of mutation in drug resistance and pathogenesis of hepatitis B and hepatitis C
T Shaw, SA Locarnini   115

SECTION IV: LIVER II
Chair: W Gerok, MP Manns

12   Aetiology, pathogenesis and treatment of haemochromatosis
LW Powell   135

13   Wilson disease: from gene to patient
DW Cox   148

14   Hepatic stem cells and hepatocyte transplantation: future therapeutic applications
S Gupta, M Inada   158

SECTION V: BILIARY TRACT
Chair: AF Hofmann, U Leuschner

15   Pathomechanisms of cholestasis: targets for medical treatment
G Paumgartner   175

16   Adaptive regulation of bile salt transporters in cholestasis
JL Boyer, WS Chen, SY Cai, G Denk, A Bohan, C Soroka, L Denson   186

17   Treatment of primary biliary cirrhosis: current standards
R Poupon, C Corpechot, F Carrat, Y Chrétien, RE Poupon   189

18   Primary sclerosing cholangitis: neoplastic potential and chemopreventive effect of ursodeoxycholic acid
A Stiehl, D Rost   196

CONTENTS

19   The pruritus of cholestasis: treatment options
NV Bergasa   203

SECTION VI: PANCREAS
Chair: G Adler, RW Ammann

20   Stages and course of chronic pancreatitis
RW Ammann   213

21   Basis and future of enzyme replacement therapy
P Layer, H Panter, J Keller   226

22   Hedgehog signalling in pancreatic cancer
M Hebrok   234

SECTION VII: INTESTINAL DISORDERS I
Chair: DP Jewell, F Guarner

23   Does JC virus initiate chromosomal instability in colorectal cancer?
CR Boland, A Goel, L Laghi, L Ricciardiello   247

24   Testing the gut and its function – faecal samples – breath tests and more?
I Bjarnason, L Maiden, K Takeuchi   253

SECTION VIII: INTESTINAL DISORDERS II
Chair: RB Sartor, J Schölmerich

25   Regulatory T cells in animal models: therapeutic potential
CO Elson, Y Cong, A Konrad, N Iqbal, CT Weaver   269

26   Imaging of the small and large bowel – from ultrasound to virtual endoscopy
JF Riemann, U Damian   276

27   Colorectal carcinoma – primary prevention and screening
C Pox, W Schmiegel   284

28   Treatment of inflammatory bowel disease: 'early hit' or stepwise escalation
WJ Sandborn   299

29   Clinical impact of mesalazine for research and therapy in inflammatory bowel diseases
U Klotz   305

CONTENTS

30   Gastroenterology: history of the future
     DK Podolsky   314

     Index   323

List of principal contributors

RW Ammann
Division of Gastroenterology and Hepatology
University Hospital Zurich
Rämistrasse 100
CH-8091 Zurich
Switzerland

A Axon
Department of Gastroenterology
The General Infirmary at Leeds
Great George Street
Leeds, LS1 3EX
UK

NV Bergasa
Division of Hepatology
State University of New York at Downstate
450 Clarkson Avenue, Box 50
Brooklyn, NY 11203
USA

I Bjarnason
King's College School of Medicine
Dept of Clinical Biochemistry
Bessemer Road
London, SE5 9PJ
UK

CR Boland
Baylor University Medical Center
3500 Gaston Avenue (Hoblitzelle 250)
Dallas, TX 75246
USA

JL Boyer
Yale University, School of Medicine
Liver Research Center, LMP 1080
333 Cedar Street
New Haven, CT 06520
USA

DW Cox
Department of Medical Genetics
8-39 Medical Sciences Building
University of Alberta
Edmonton, Alberta
Canada

C Ell
Innere Medizin II
HSK Wiesbaden
Ludwig-Erhard-Str. 100
D-65199 Wiesbaden
Germany

CO Elson
The University of Alabama at Birmingham
Division of Gastroenterology and Hepatology
703 19th Street South, ZRB 633
Birmingham, AL 35294-0007
USA

W Fischbach
Medizinische Klinik II
Klinikum Aschaffenburg
Am Hasenkopf
D-63739 Aschaffenburg
Germany

S Gupta
Albert Einstein College of Medicine
Ullmann Building, Room 625
1300 Morris Park Avenue
Bronx, NY 10461
USA

CJ Hawkey
Wolfson Digestive Diseases Centre
Institute of Clinical Research
University Hospital
Nottingham, NG7 2UH
UK

LIST OF PRINCIPAL CONTRIBUTORS

M Hebrok
Diabetes Center
Department of Medicine
University of California, San Francisco
San Francisco, CA 94143
USA

U Klotz
Dr. Margarete Fischer Bosch Institut für Klinische Pharmakologie
Auerbachstr. 112
D-70376 Stuttgart
Germany

J Labenz
Department of Medicine
Jung-Stilling Hospital
Academic Teaching Hospital
University of Bonn
Wichernstr. 40
D-57074 Siegen
Germany

P Layer
Department of Medicine
Israelitic Hospital
Orchideenstieg 14
D-22297 Hamburg
Germany

D Lebrec
INSERM U-481
Hôpital Beaujon
100 Bd du General Leclerc
F-92110 Clichy
France

KEL McColl
Department of Medicine and Therapeutics
Western Infirmary
Gardiner Institute
Glasgow, G11 6NT
UK

P Michetti
Division of Gastroenterology and Hepatology
Lausanne University Medical Center
CH-1011 Lausanne
Switzerland

G Paumgartner
Klinikum der Universität München-Grosshadern
Marchioninistr. 15
D-81377 München
Germany

DK Podolsky
Massachusetts General Hospital
Gastrointestinal Unit GRJ 719
32 Fruit Street
Boston, MA 02114-2696
USA

R Poupon
Hopital Saint-Antoine
184 rue du Faubourg Saint-Antoine
F-75571 Paris Cedex 1e
France

LW Powell
Teaching and Research Unit, Rm 6556A
Level 6, Ned Hanlon Building
Royal Brisbane and Women's Hospital
Butterfield Street
Herston, Queensland 4029
Australia

C Pox
Ruhr-Universität Bochum
Medizinische Klinik
Knappschaftskrankenhaus
In der Schornau 23-25
D-44892 Bochum
Germany

JF Riemann
Medizinische Klinik C
Klinikum der Stadt Ludwigshafen
Bremserstr. 79
D-67063 Ludwigshafen am Rhein
Germany

WJ Sandborn
Mayo Clinic
Division of Gastroenterology
West 19A
200 First Street SW
Rochester
MN 55905
USA

LIST OF PRINCIPAL CONTRIBUTORS

SW Schalm
Department of
 Hepatogastroenterology
Erasmus MC University Medical
 Center
Dr Molewaterplein 40
NL-3015 GD Rotterdam
The Netherlands

T Shaw
Research and Molecular
 Development Division
Victorian Infectious Diseases
 Reference Laboratory
10 Wreckyn Street
North Melbourne, Victoria 3051
Australia

A Stiehl
Medizinische Universitätsklinik
Im Neuenheimer Feld 410
D-69120 Heidelberg
Germany

GNJ Tytgat
Department of Gastroenterology
Academic Medical Center
Meibergdreef 9
NL-1105 AZ Amsterdam
The Netherlands

List of chairpersons

G Adler
Innere Medizin I
Universitätsklinikum Ulm
Robert-Koch-Str. 8
D-89081 Ulm
Germany

RW Ammann
Division of Gastroenterology and
  Hepatology
University Hospital Zurich
Rämistrasse 100
CH-8091 Zurich
Switzerland

R Arnold
Innere Medizin
Klinikum der Universität
Baldingerstr.
D-35043 Marburg
Germany

AL Blum
Rue du Collège
CH-1323 Romainmôtier
Switzerland

W Gerok
Innere Medizin
Universitätsklinikum Freiburg
Hugstetter Str. 55
D-79106 Frieburg
Germany

F Guarner
Hospital General Vall d'Hebron
Servicio de Patologia Digestiva
Pso. Vall d'Hebron 119
E-08035 Barcelona
Spain

AF Hofmann
University of California, San Diego
Department of Medicine (0813)
Division of Gastroenterology
9500 Gilman Drive
La Jolla, CA 92093
USA

DP Jewell
The Radcliffe Infirmary
Gastroenterology Unit
Nuffield Department of Medicine
Woodstock Road
Oxford, OX2 6HE
UK

U Leuschner
Internistisches Facharztzentrum
Stresemannallee 3
D-60596 Frankfurt
Germany

MP Manns
Gastroenterologie/Hepatologie/
  Endokrinologie
Medizinische Hochschule Hannover
Carl-Neuberg-Str. 1
D-30625 Hannover
Germany

J Mössner
Innere Medizin II
Universitätsklinikum Leipzig
Philipp-Rosenthal-Str. 27
D-04103 Leipzig
Germany

EO Riecken
Weddigenweg 17
D-12205 Berlin
Germany

LIST OF CHAIRPERSONS

RB Sartor
University of North Carolina
School of Medicine
Microbiology and Immunology
778 Burnett Womack Building
Chapel Hill, NC 27599-7080
USA

R Schmid
University of California
School of Medicine
San Francisco, CA 94143
USA

J Schölmerich
Innere Medizin I
Klinikum der Universität Regensburg
D-93042 Regensburg
Germany

R Williams
University College Hospital
Medical School
Institute of Hepatology
69-75 Chenies Mews
London, WC1E 6HX
UK

Preface

On the occasion of the 80th birthday of Dr. Dr. Herbert Falk an international symposium was held. The aim of the meeting was to look back, to assess progress made and to look forward speculating on the development of the field of gastroenterology and hepatology.

The symposium was divided into four parts: oesophagus and stomach, liver, pancreaticobiliary tract, and small/large bowel. Internationally renowned speakers contributed to the symposium, many of them as well to this book. The organisers of the symposium hope that this volume will maintain the memory of a remarkable meeting in honour of an even more remarkable person

The Editors

Section I
Oesophagus

Chair: R. ARNOLD and A.L. BLUM

1
Treatment of uncomplicated reflux disease

J. LABENZ

INTRODUCTION

Gastro-oesophageal reflux disease (GORD) is a common condition affecting approximately 10–20% of the adult population of industrialized countries[1]. The great majority of these cases are uncomplicated, i.e. some 50–70% of patients in primary care with troublesome reflux symptoms have no endoscopically recognizable lesions of the oesophageal mucosa, 35% have erosive oesophagitis (75% of which are mild, corresponding to Los Angeles A/B, and 25% severe, corresponding to Los Angeles C/D). In about 5% of patients, complications, in particular Barrett's oesophagus – must be expected (Figure 1)[2]. Epidemiological data support the hypothesis that GORD is not a spectrum disease with occasional reflux symptoms but no lesions at the one end, and

NERD:	Non-erosive reflux disease
ERD:	Erosive reflux disease
CRD:	Complicated reflux disease (Ulcer, stricture, Barrett´s, cancer)

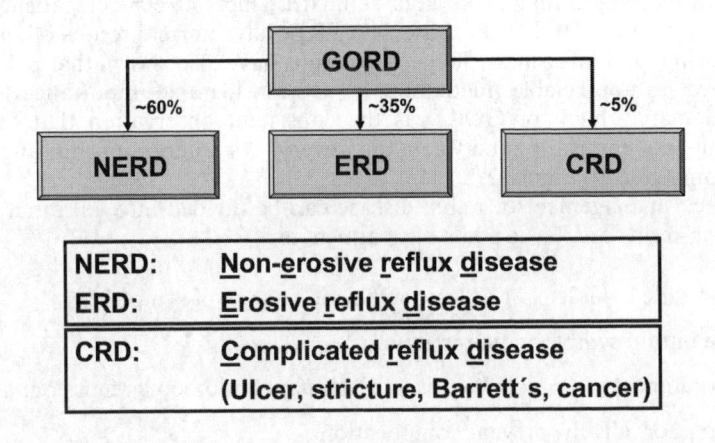

Figure 1 GORD – a categorial disease with three distinct entities (after refs 2 and 3)

severe complications at the other, but can instead be classified into three distinct categories – non-erosive reflux disease (NERD) – erosive reflux disease (ERD), and Barrett's oesophagus – in each of which categories the respective patient remains; that is, progression of the disease over time is, overall, very rare[3]. This category model of GORD is supported by the latest data from a large prospective European study (ProGERD) involving more than 3500 patients with NERD and ERD: the rate of progression (to severe oesophagitis or Barrett's) for patients with NERD and mild erosive oesophagitis (Los Angeles A/B) was less than 1% per year (Labenz et al., unpublished data).

INITIAL MANAGEMENT OF GORD

Uncomplicated reflux disease comprises the non-erosive form; that is, symptoms that impact negatively on the patient's quality of life, but which are not associated with endoscopic evidence of mucosal breaks in the oesophagus, and erosive reflux oesophagitis of varying degrees of severity, e.g. grades A–D in the Los Angeles classification[4].

Contrary to commonly held beliefs, symptom evaluation is the most important assessment for the initial phase of GORD management[5], although an evidence-based analysis of symptoms is hardly possible[6]. Characteristic symptoms are heartburn and acid regurgitation[6]; however, these symptoms are predictive in only 70% of patients, even in cases with an unequivocal history[7], but it must be emphasized that there is no diagnostic gold standard for GORD: endoscopy has a sensitivity of only 30–40%, microscopic features such as dilated intracellular spaces and regenerative changes in the absence of endoscopically visible mucosal breaks of the squamous epithelium in the distal oesophagus are currently not sufficiently validated, and pH monitoring is far from being a diagnostic gold standard, since 30–60% of patients with NERD, as well as 10–20% of those with ERD, have normal results of 24-h pH monitoring, and intra-individual comparisons have also shown that pH-metry is subject to appreciable fluctuations[4,8]. Of considerable importance for the clinical management of GORD is the consistent observation that there is virtually no correlation between the severity of endoscopic findings and symptom severity (Figure 2)[9].

Clinical management of reflux disease can be divided into an initial phase and long-term care. Basic goals of treatment are:

1. to provide complete, or at least sufficient, control of symptoms;

2. to maintain symptomatic remission;

3. to heal underlying oesophagitis and maintain endoscopic remission; and

4. to treat or, ideally, prevent complications.

Adequate control of symptoms is considered to have been achieved when mild reflux symptoms occur at most once a week – more frequent or more

TREATMENT OF UNCOMPLICATED REFLUX DISEASE

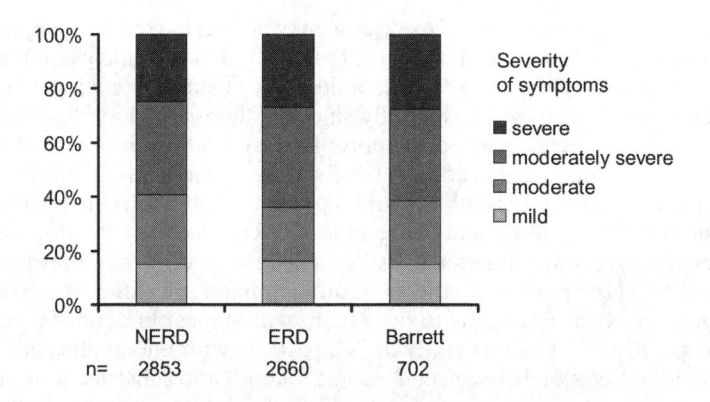

Figure 2 No correlation between endoscopic findings and symptom severity in patients with GORD[9]

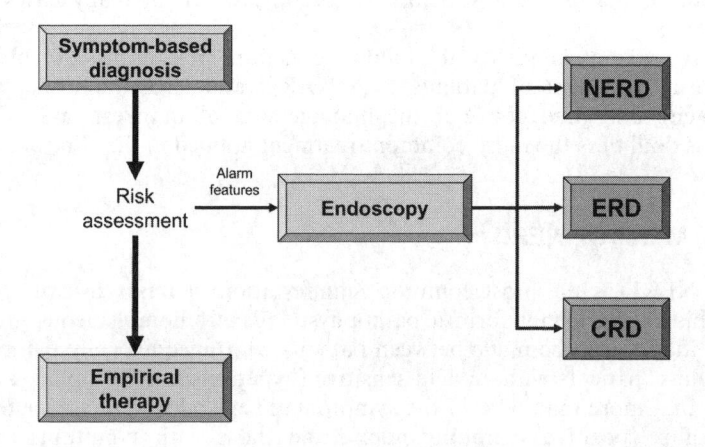

Figure 3 Initial management of patients with symptoms suggestive of GORD

pronounced complaints are not accepted as satisfactory by the patient[10]. Initially, a symptom-based diagnosis is established, and an individual risk assessment made (Figure 3). If such alarm symptoms as dysphagia, unintended weight loss and/or signs of bleeding are present, an endoscopic examination is mandatory, with further management dictated by the endoscopic findings. Other indications for endoscopy at this point in time may include, for example, a family history of upper gastrointestinal tract malignancies, a long prior history of severe complaints, age over 50 years, use of NSAID, and a positive *Helicobater pylori* status[11]. Otherwise, empirical therapy can be offered (Figure 3). Withholding endoscopy in the initial phase is, of course, associated with the theoretical risk that serious complications of GORD or other significant pathologies in the upper gastrointestinal tract mimicking the symptoms of reflux disease may be overlooked or recognized too late. On the other hand, given the facts that GORD is extremely common, and that complications are generally rare, endoscopic evaluation of all patients with GORD is hardly justifiable, especially since an endoscopy-based management strategy has not been subjected to appropriate evaluation. In a cross-sectional study from Finland the detection rate of serious complications of GORD did not differ between regions with low and those with high referral to endoscopy[12]. Considering that most patients have mild GORD, and that the disease is not progressive over time, restricted use of endoscopy does not appear to put patients at risk. However, the economic impact of different diagnostic strategies on expense remains to be established, at least in countries with low endoscopy costs[13]. A recent study in 742 patients with uncomplicated GORD showed no correlation between endoscopic findings and subsequent therapeutic decisions[14]. Further arguments for a primarily symptom-driven strategy are that the ultimate benchmark for the clinical efficacy of treatment of GORD is patient satisfaction, and that accurate determination of oesophagitis requires the withholding of therapy before endoscopy, which in many cases is not possible[15].

For the sake of simplicity, the following sections first discuss the initial and long-term treatment of patients with NERD and ERD (endoscopy-based approach), and then consider the management of uninvestigated GORD, which is doubtless the more common treatment applied in the clinical setting.

TREATMENT OF NERD

While NERD is the most common manifestation of reflux disease, patients with this entity do not form a pathophysiologically homogeneous group. A differentiation can be made between patients with unequivocally pathological acid reflux; patients with an acid-sensitive (hypersensitive) oesophagus, which means that more than 50% of the symptomatic episodes were associated with acid reflux (positive symptom index); and those with symptoms that are independent of acid-reflux events (functional heartburn)[8,16]. This latter category explains the observation that patients with NERD did not respond as well to acid suppressants as did patients with erosive oesophagitis[17,18]. Possible pathophysiological causes of functional heartburn include non-acid reflux (liquid, gas, mixed), minute changes in the oesophageal acidity above a pH of 4, motility disorders such as sustained contractions of the longitudinal musculature, visceral hypersensitivity, and emotional and psychological abnormalities[19].

Initial therapy of NERD

Initially, patients should receive a proton pump inhibitor (PPI) for 2–4 weeks (Figure 4). The effect of other substances such as H_2 blockers or prokinetic drugs is little better than that of placebo[20]. In a large, placebo-controlled study, a dose–response relationship was established for omeprazole: omeprazole 20 mg proved to be more effective than omeprazole 10 mg[21]. In a further

TREATMENT OF UNCOMPLICATED REFLUX DISEASE

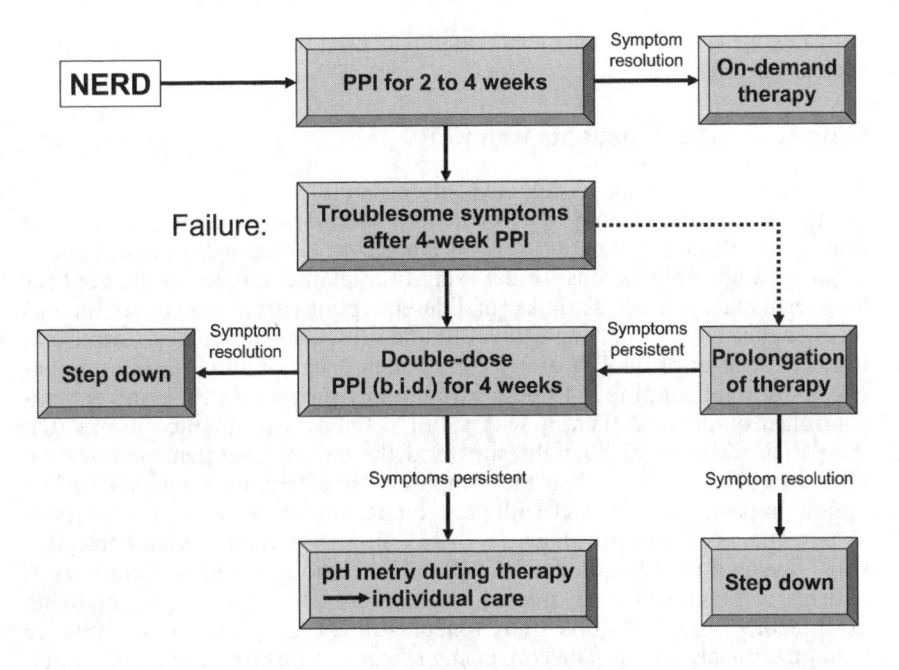

Figure 4 Initial therapy and long-term care of patients with NERD

controlled study, lansoprazole 30 mg was no more effective than lansoprazole 15 mg[22]. The S-isomer of omeprazole, esomeprazole, was investigated in two large, double-blind, multicentre studies involving patients with NERD[23]. Esomeprazole at a dose of 20 mg and 40 mg per day proved more effective than placebo, but a dose–response effect could not be shown. Three further randomized, double-blind, multicentre studies involving a total of more than 2600 patients with NERD treated for 4 weeks with omeprazole 20 mg, and esomeprazole 20 mg or 40 mg, revealed comparable success rates (resolution of symptoms in 60–70% of patients)[24]. Assessment of the response to treatment in studies such as these are greatly influenced by the target criterion (e.g. complete elimination of symptoms, satisfactory symptom control), so that the studies cannot really be compared. From the above remarks it may be concluded that appropriately dosed PPI treatment can achieve a satisfactory initial response in some two-thirds of patients. If initial treatment with 4 weeks of PPI fails to elicit adequate symptom control (Figure 4), increasing the PPI dose (e.g. standard dose PPI twice daily) is recommended, since studies have shown that patients with acid-sensitive oesophagus respond better to a high PPI dose[25–27]. In non-responders to appropriate PPI treatment, it is recommended that oesophageal pH-monitoring be performed during PPI therapy and, if symptomatic acid reflux can be excluded, to discontinue PPI therapy and initiate a trial with a low-dose tricyclic antidepressant at bedtime[28]. Potential therapeutic options for the future might be serotonin reuptake inhibitors, kappa agonists and substances with an impact on transient sphincter relaxation such as baclofen.

Long-term care of patients with NERD

If initial treatment is successful, medication should be discontinued, since 25% (or more) of patients may remain in remission over prolonged periods of time[29], and this clinical entity does not appear to necessitate measures aimed at preventing complications. In the event of a relapse, indicating the need for long-term management, a number of different options are available: continuous maintenance therapy starting with a PPI and subsequent attempts to step down to lower dosages of the PPI or even less potent drugs (Figure 5)[5], intermittent courses of treatment for 2–4 weeks with initially successful PPI[30], and patient-controlled on-demand therapy with a PPI[11]. On-demand therapy means that the patient determines both the start and the end of treatment. Medication should be discontinued when the symptoms have been eliminated. This last option, in particular, has met with great interest in recent years on account of its potential economic advantages[31,32]. In a first large randomized, controlled study lasting 6 months, Lind et al. were able to show that more than 80% of patients were satisfactorily treated with an on-demand strategy employing omeprazole 20 mg[33] In this study omeprazole 20 mg proved more effective than omeprazole 10 mg. The convincing efficacy of this new treatment option was then confirmed with esomeprazole 20 mg[34,35]. All these studies also showed that roughly one-half of these patients were satisfactorily treatable with placebo medication and the use of antacids as required. In a recently

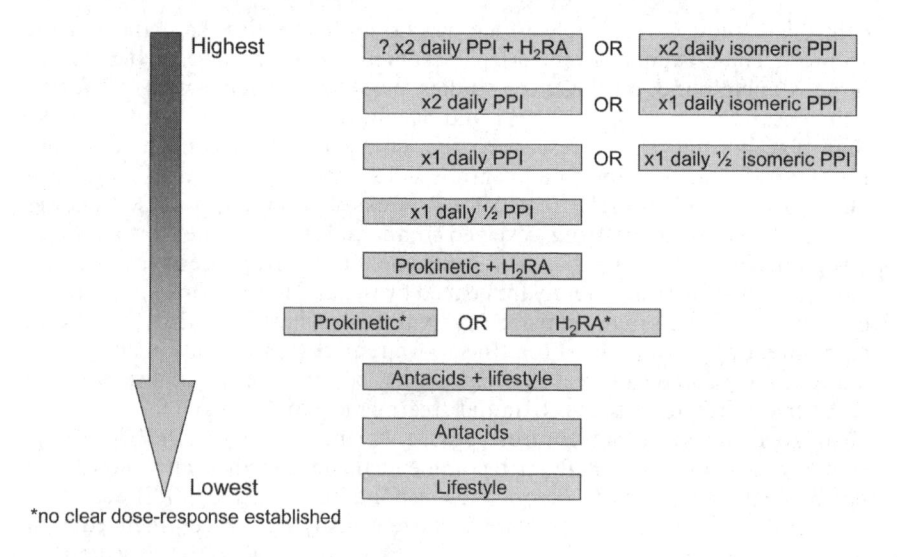

Highest
? x2 daily PPI + H₂RA   OR   x2 daily isomeric PPI
x2 daily PPI   OR   x1 daily isomeric PPI
x1 daily PPI   OR   x1 daily ½ isomeric PPI
x1 daily ½ PPI
Prokinetic + H₂RA
Prokinetic*   OR   H₂RA*
Antacids + lifestyle
Antacids
Lowest   Lifestyle

*no clear dose-response established

Figure 5 Hierarchy of the efficacy of options in the non-invasive treatment of GORD (H₂RA: H₂-receptor antagonist) (modified after refs 4 and 5)

presented randomized, open international multicentre study involving 598 patients, on-demand treatment with esomeprazole 20 mg was compared with continuous treatment with esomeprazole 20 mg o.d. in patients with NERD[36]. The vast majority of patients in both treatment groups were satisfied with the regimen, and medication consumption was considerably lower in the on-demand therapy arm (average consumption: 0.41 vs. 0.91 tablet per day). However, the final endoscopic examination revealed mild erosive oesophagitis (Los Angeles A: $n = 14$; Los Angeles B; $n = 1$) in 5% of the patients receiving on-demand treatment, while none of the patients on continuous treatment had this finding. From the viewpoint of a clinician this observation occasions no major concern, since alternation between the categories NERD and mild ERD (corresponding to Los Angeles A and B) often occurs during the spontaneous course of the disease (Labenz, unpublished data). Other PPIs (lansoprazole, pantoprazole, rabeprazole) have also proven their superiority to placebo in on-demand treatment in individual studies[11]. Head-to-head comparisons between various PPIs are, however, lacking, so that a comparative assessment is not possible.

TREATMENT OF ERD

Erosive reflux oesophagitis can be found in about 30–40% of GORD patients[2]. Endoscopically, reflux oesophagitis is categorized into various degrees of severity. In recent years, and especially in therapeutic studies, the Los Angeles classification in particular has been applied[37,38]. This distinguishes the four degrees of severity A–D (A: mucosal breaks of less than 5 mm on the top of folds; B: mucosal breaks >5 mm in extent on mucosal folds; C: circumferential spreading of mucosal breaks involving less than 75% of the circumference; D: mucosal breaks involving more than 75% of the circumference). The gradings A and B correspond to mild to moderate oesophagitis, and C and D to moderate to severe oesophagitis. One-fourth of patients with erosive oesophagitis are categorized in grade C or D[39–41].

Numerous controlled studies have investigated the efficacy of a variety of medications in the healing of oesophagitis and the elimination of symptoms. In a meta-analysis Chiba et al.[42] showed that PPIs (omeprazole, lansoprazole, pantoprazole) heal the oesophagitis within 8 weeks in 83.6% of patients, with a symptom-resolution rate of 77.4%. All other medications (H_2-receptor antagonists, cisapride, sucralfate) were appreciably less effective. A placebo-related healing rate of 28.2% documents the fluctuating nature of the course of reflux disease in some patients, with spontaneous remissions and exacerbations. When using highly potent PPIs, elimination of symptoms after 8 weeks is predictive for healing of the oesophagitis[40,41].

Initial therapy of ERD

In patients with erosive reflux oesophagitis, treatment with a standard dose of a PPI is always recommended (Figure 6)[4]. Mild cases (Los Angeles grade A/B) usually heal within 4 weeks, while severe cases (Los Angeles C/D) often require

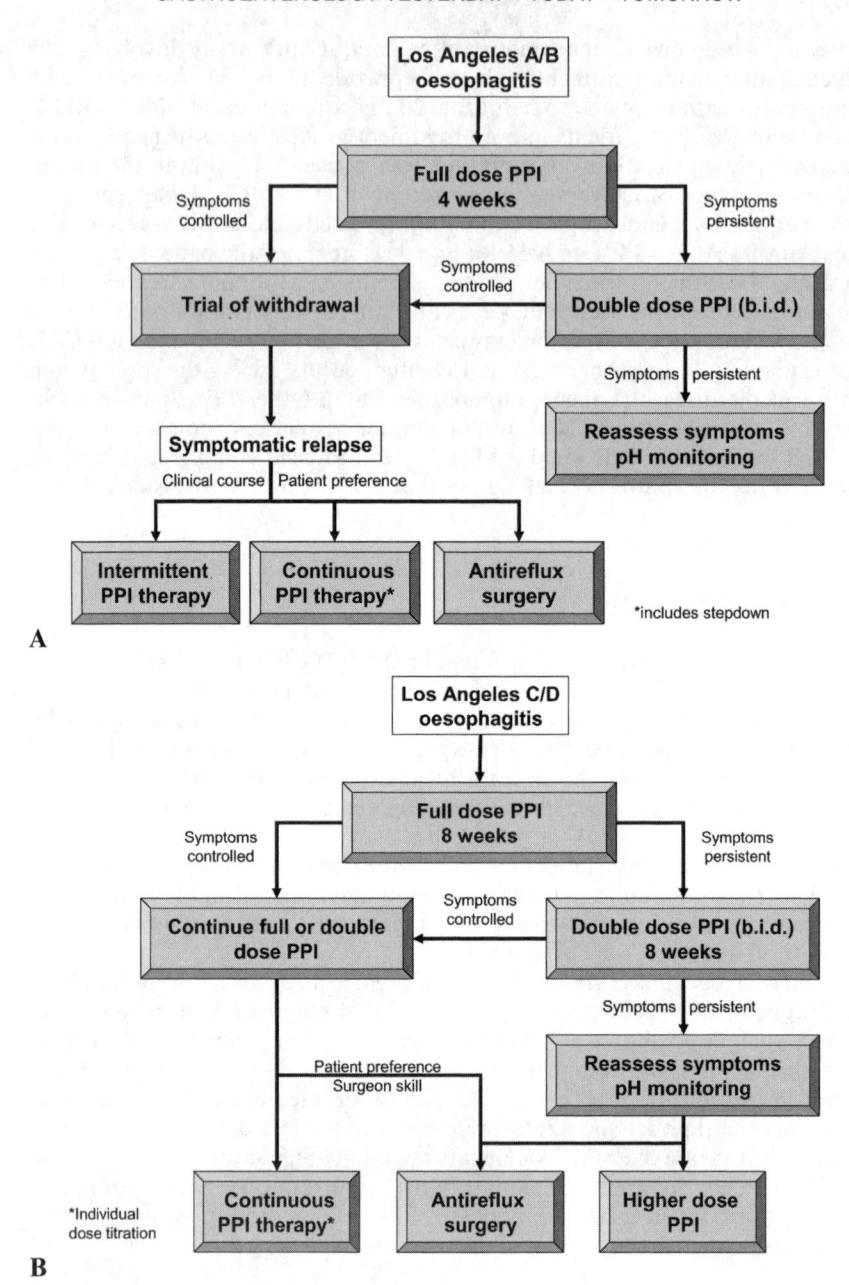

Figure 6 Management of patients with mild to moderate erosive oesophagitis (**A**) and moderate to severe oesophagitis (**B**) (after refs 4 and 5)

longer treatment – 8 or, in some cases more, weeks. Resolution of symptoms in those responding to therapy is achieved appreciably more quickly (median time to sustained symptom resolution 5–10 days). The major predictive factor for the healing rate is the severity of the erosive oesophagitis, but also of significance are concomitant Barrett's metaplasia in the lower oesophagus, which reduces the healing rate, and infection with *H. pylori*, which enhances the efficacy of the PPI[43,44].

Is there any clinically relevant difference between the PPIs available on the market? Racemic PPIs (omeprazole, lansoprazole, pantoprazole, rabeprazole) differ in such pharmacokinetic characteristics as bioavailability and the rapidity with which an effect occurs. This, however, is irrelevant for the healing of oesophagitis at 4 and 8 weeks[45,46], although the substances do differ in terms of the time required to eliminate symptoms. In a large randomized, controlled study involving more than 3500 patients with erosive oesophagitis, lansoprazole 30 mg o.d. relieved heartburn significantly faster than did omeprazole 20 mg o.d.[47]. There is a linear relationship between the degree of acid suppression measured by the time per day that gastric pH is higher than 4, and the healing kinetics of oesophagitis[48]. With regard to the healing rates of reflux oesophagitis after 4 and 8 weeks, no differences are to be seen between the standard doses of the racemic PPIs (omeprazole 20 mg, lansoprazole 30 mg, pantoprazole 40 mg, rabeprazole 20 mg)[45,46]. Nor did doubling the individual dose (e.g. lansoprazole 60 mg, pantoprazole 80 mg) increase efficacy. Of significance for the healing rates and symptom elimination, however, is cytochrome 2C19 polymorphism. Thus, it has recently been shown that the response to treatment with lansoprazole 30 mg o. d. is poorer in extensive metabolisers than in intermediate and poor metabolisers[49].

Cross-over pH-monitoring studies in healthy volunteers and patients with GORD have shown that esomeprazole is more effective than corresponding doses of the racemic PPIs omeprazole, lansoprazole, pantoprazole and rabeprazole[50,51]. Significant differences were seen between half the standard doses and the full standard doses of the respective drugs; for example, esomeprazole 20 mg is more effective than pantoprazole 20 mg, and esomeprazole 40 mg is more effective than pantoprazole 40 mg (Figure 5). In large controlled studies, significantly higher healing rates were achieved with esomeprazole at a dose of 40 mg o.d. than with omeprazole 20 mg o.d., lansoprazole 30 mg o.d., and pantoprazole 40 mg o.d. (Figure 7)[39–41,52,53]. The therapeutic advantage of esomeprazole over the other PPIs increased with increasing severity of the oesophagitis as defined by the Los Angeles classification[54]. These studies also showed a significant superiority of esomeprazole in terms of the time to first, and time to sustained, symptom (heartburn) resolution. Small studies reporting other results (equivalence of esomeprazole and pantoprazole) are scientifically flawed as they did not have the statistical power to detect a difference between the PPIs of the magnitude that has been firmly established by the large-scale studies mentioned above[55–57].

In the event of inadequate efficacy (insufficient control of symptoms or healing of the oesophagitis), doubling the individual dose of PPI does not reliably improve clinical efficacy, but switching from a less potent drug to

Healing of oesophagitis

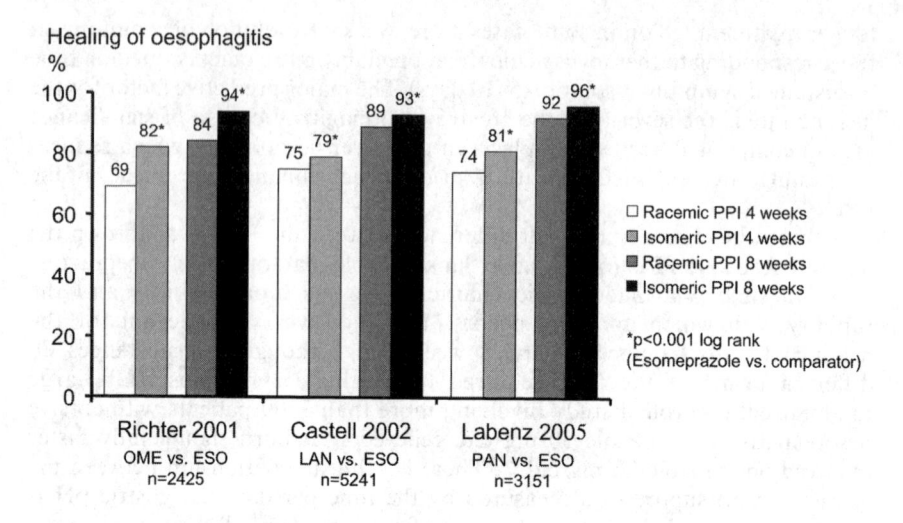

Figure 7 Randomized, controlled studies comparing the 4- and 8-week healing rates of erosive oesophagitis in patients treated with a racemic PPI (OME: omeprazole 20 mg o.d.; LAN: lansoprazole 30 mg o.d.; PAN: pantoprazole 40 mg o.d.) or esomeprazole 40 mg o.d. (ESO) (after refs 39–41)

esomeprazole, or shortening the interval between doses (e.g. twice daily) might increase the response to treatment (Figure 6)[58]. In recent years there has been intense discussion on the clinical relevance of nocturnal acid breakthrough (NABT) in difficult-to-treat cases[59,60]. NABT is defined as a decrease in gastric pH to <4 for more than 1 h during the course of the night. The clinical relevance of this phenomenon has not yet been established. H_2-receptor antagonists given at bedtime can prevent this acid breakthrough, but when administered over a longer period of time they rapidly lose this effect[61]. Treatment with combinations of PPI and prokinetic drugs is of unproven value.

Long-term care of patients with ERD

After responding well to initial treatment, ERD shows a tendency to relapse. Up to 90% of patients will relapse within the next 6 months[29]. Patients with mild oesophagitis (Los Angeles A/B) often have a longer relapse-free interval than patients with severe oesophagitis (Los Angeles C/D), who frequently suffer a relapse within days of discontinuing successful initial treatment[62,63]. In the light of these observations it is recommended that, in patients with mild oesophagitis, therapy first be discontinued and the further course of the disease kept under surveillance, while in severe oesophagitis, initial successful therapy should be followed, *a priori*, by maintenance treatment (Figure 6). Established options for long-term management are intermittent treatment for some weeks and continuous maintenance treatment with an attempt to reduce the daily dosage of the PPI (step-down principle)[4,30]. On-demand therapy has, to date, been investigated in only two studies in patients with erosive oesophagitis[64,65]. Satisfactory control of symptoms was achieved in the vast majority of patients, but continuous therapy proved to be superior with respect to maintenance of remission of erosive oesophagitis, so that an evidence-based recommendation is currently not possible. However, since GORD is usually not progressive, attempts to realize on-demand treatment does not appear to harm patients[3].

For the prevention of relapse in patients with healed oesophagitis, PPIs are clearly superior to H_2-receptor antagonists, prokinetic drugs and combinations of these medications[66–68]. The yield between a standard dose of a PPI and one-half of this dose is, in individual studies, often small, although significant, and even probably clinically relevant differences have occasionally been observed[66]. On the basis of a cost-effectiveness analysis using a Markov model designed to simulate the economic and clinical outcomes of GORD in relation to the cost per symptom-free year, a standard dose of a PPI appears to be superior despite the higher drug costs[68]. Nevertheless, In view of the overall high response rates, an initial attempt with half the standard dose of a PPI is recommended in patients with mild erosive oesophagitis, while patients with more severe disease should be kept on the dose of PPI required to induce remission (Figure 6). If this approach proves successful, a dose reduction, or a changeover to a less potent drug, can be attempted[69,70]. If the reduced dose proves unsuccessful the dose must be increased appropriately. Occasionally, a higher-than-standard dose may be necessary to maintain remission[71].

Remission at 6 months %

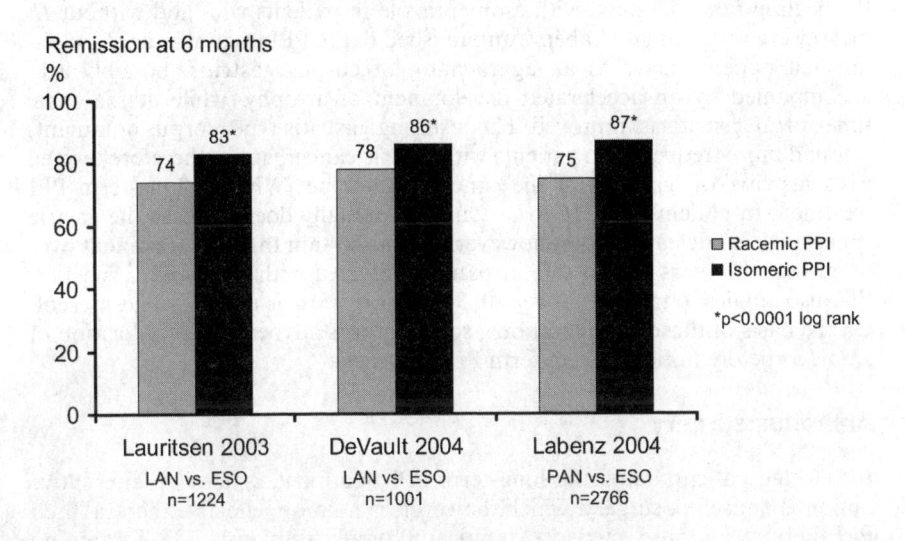

Study	Racemic PPI	Isomeric PPI
Lauritsen 2003 (LAN vs. ESO, n=1224)	74	83*
DeVault 2004 (LAN vs. ESO, n=1001)	78	86*
Labenz 2004 (PAN vs. ESO, n=2766)	75	87*

*p<0.0001 log rank

Figure 8 Randomized, controlled studies comparing the rate of remission after 6-month treatment with the maintenance doses of racemic PPIs (LAN: lansoprazole 15 mg o.d.; PAN: pantoprazole 20 mg o.d.) with esomeprazole 20 mg o.d. (ESO) (after refs 72–74)

With long-term therapy also, differences are found between the isomeric PPI esomeprazole, and the racemic PPIs lansoprazole or pantoprazole. In large double-blind randomized studies in patients with healed oesophagitis, esomeprazole 20 mg o.d. applied over 6 months was significantly more effective than lansoprazole 15 mg o.d., or pantoprazole 20 mg o.d. (Figure 8)[72–74]. As in the case of acute treatment, this superiority was more pronounced with increasing disease severity. Comparative studies showed that the difference between 20 mg and 40 mg esomeprazole was small and not significant[62,63]. Apart from the severity of the baseline oesophagitis, concomitant Barrett's oesophagus (poorer results) and *H. pylori* infections (better results) also have a role as predictors of treatment outcome (Labenz, unpublished data).

Eradication of *H. pylori* in patients with GORD

Whether a concomitant *H. pylori* infection in patients with GORD should be treated or not is still under discussion[75,76]. Since *H. pylori* is probably not involved in the pathogenesis of GORD, it cannot be expected that its eradication can heal this condition[77]. Nor, according to the data of Moayyedi et al., is an aggravation of the spontaneous course of GORD to be expected. *H. pylori* does, however, have an impact on the pH-elevating effect of PPIs, which leads to higher healing rates and faster elimination of symptoms in patients with reflux oesophagitis[44]. It is possible that PPIs differ in this regard: while the EXPO study confirmed the impact of *H. pylori* on the effect of pantoprazole, the healing rates obtained with esomeprazole in patients with and without *H. pylori* were very similar (Labenz, unpublished data). PPI treatment in *H. pylori*-infected patients leads to an aggravation of corpus gastritis, possibly also accompanied by an accelerated development of atrophy, while at the same time antral gastritis is improved. The resulting gastritis type (corpus dominant) is found more frequently in patients with gastric cancer, and is therefore termed 'risk gastritis' or 'gastritis of the cancer phenotype'. Whether long-term PPI treatment in patients with *H. pylori* gastritis actually does increase the gastric cancer risk is unclear. It does, however, appear certain that PPI treatment over more than 10 years is also safe in patients infected with *H. pylori*[71]. Whether this also applies to treatment over 20, 30 or more years is not known at present. On the basis of these considerations, some authors advocate the eradication of *H. pylori* before initiating long-term PPI treatment[78].

Antireflux surgery

In selected patients requiring long-term PPI treatment, a possible alternative option is antireflux surgery, which, however, is no more effective than tailored PPI therapy, and also carries a significant complication risk[79–81]. To date no advantages of surgery in terms of economics have been unequivocally demonstrated[81,82]. The best candidates for fundoplication are probably those with oesophagitis documented by endoscopy, a need for continuous PPI therapy, abnormal pH monitoring studies, normal oesophageal motility studies, and at least partial symptom relief with PPI therapy[83]. Further arguments for surgery are high-volume reflux and young age. Relevant concomitant diseases, in contrast, tend to militate in favour of staying with a conservative approach. A 'treatment-refractory' GORD patient should certainly not be automatically referred for antireflux surgery.

Endoscopic antireflux procedures

In recent years a number of different methods for endoscopic endoluminal treatment of GORD have been investigated (endoscopic gastroplication with differing suturing techniques, application of radiofrequency energy to the lower oesophageal sphincter, endoscopic submucosal or intramuscular injection of inert materials). To date the efficacy of endoluminal therapy for GORD is not supported by a high level of evidence[84]. To date only a single fully published controlled study (radiofrequency energy delivery versus sham procedure) that documented a benefit in terms of symptom relief, but no effect on acid reflux, has been reported[85]. Overall, too few data are currently available on efficacy and safety, so that the use of these methods outside of controlled studies cannot be recommended. In particular, controlled studies comparing endoscopic antireflux procedures with the established options of treatment would be desirable.

UNINVESTIGATED GORD

In patients with troublesome reflux symptoms but no alarm symptoms (e.g. dysphagia, unintended loss of weight, signs of bleeding), empirical PPI therapy is another option for initial management. The goals of empirical therapy are: (a) succeed with initial therapy, (b) determine need for ongoing therapy, (c) maintain satisfactory symptom control, (d) minimize risks from oesophagitis and other consequences of abnormal reflux. These aims should be achieved at the lowest possible cost and minimal risks[86]. Initial therapy should – via rapid relief of symptoms – confirm the symptom-based diagnosis, reassure the patient as to the benign and treatable nature of the reflux disease, and – if present – cure the oesophagitis. For many years patients with GORD received step-up therapy beginning with weakly effective substances, such as antacids and H_2-receptor antagonists, and increasing the intensity of the treatment if the effect was inadequate. With this strategy the above-mentioned aims of empirical treatment cannot be achieved. For this reason, initiation of treatment with a PPI at a standard dose applied for 4 weeks is favoured (step-in approach) (Figure 9). However, few scientific data are available on this approach. In a four-arm controlled double-blind study involving 593 patients and conducted over 20 weeks, the patients initially received lansoprazole 30 mg o.d. or ranitidine 150 mg b.d. over a period of 8 weeks, followed by either continuation of this medication, or a step-down from lansoprazole to ranitidine or a step-up from ranitidine to lansoprazole[87]. The most effective strategy was step-in with a PPI and continuation with this medication. These results were confirmed in another study comparing omeprazole with ranitidine[88].

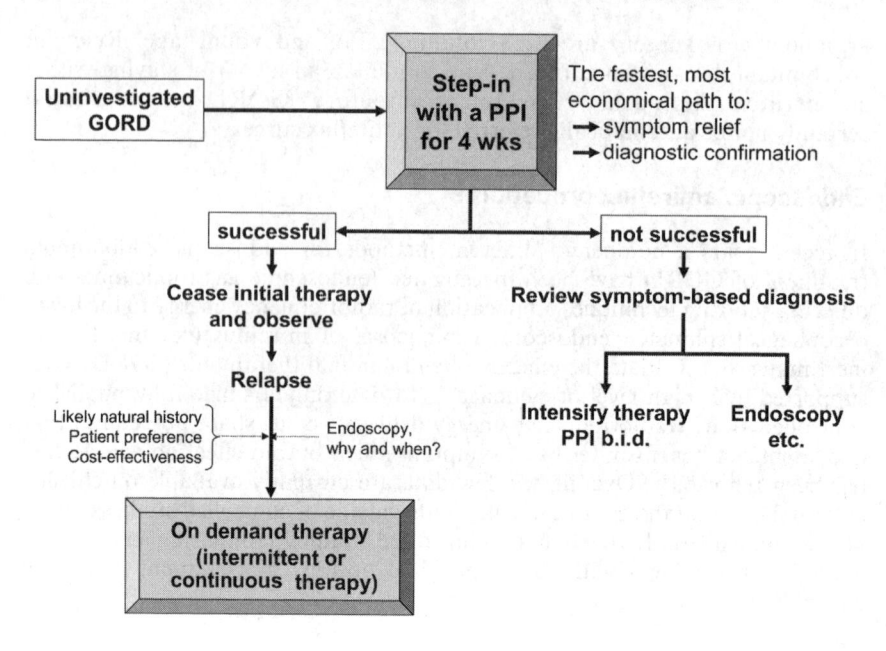

Figure 9 Proposal for the empirical management of patients with uninvestigated GORD (following ref. 86)

Therapy should be withdrawn after initial success. In the case of a relapse the long-term care depends on a careful assessment of the risk and the response to PPI therapy. Potential strategies are on-demand therapy or intermittent treatment. In a controlled three-arm study involving 1357 patients with uninvestigated GORD, Meineche-Schmidt et al.[89] compared on-demand therapy with esomeprazole 20 mg and GP-controlled intermittent strategy with esomeprazole 40 mg o.d. for 2 or 4 weeks applied over 6 months. The direct medical costs were similar in all three arms, but the total costs were substantially higher in patients treated with a GP-controlled intermittent strategy. If continuous maintenance therapy is needed to preserve remission, or if an initial positive response is rapidly followed by relapse, an endoscopic evaluation to exclude/detect severe erosive oesophagitis or complicated reflux disease is recommended. If initial treatment is not successful, and if the clinical data militate against a severe form of GORD, the PPI dose can be increased (standard dose twice daily) or a changeover to a more potent substance implemented[58]; otherwise, in this clinical situation too, endoscopy should be performed[86]. It is not clear whether patients who respond to initial treatment with a PPI and are then well controlled with on-demand therapy need to be submitted to endoscopy at all. Earlier calls for 'once-in-a-lifetime' endoscopy for every patient with reflux disease are no longer considered mandatory. Moreover, the timing of endoscopy is critical: endoscopy off therapy is required to correctly assess the severity of oesophagitis, which is important for the choice of further management, and endoscopy on therapy is needed to assess Barrett's oesophagus which is important with regard to cancer risk and the planning of surveillance.

References

1. Locke GR, Talley J, Fett SL, Zinsmeister AR, Melton LJ. Prevalence and clinical spectrum of gastroesophageal reflux: a population-based study in Olmsted County, Minnesota. Gastroenterology. 1997;112:1448–56.
2. Quigley EM. Non-erosive reflux disease (NERD); part of the spectrum of gastro-oesophageal reflux, a component of functional dyspepsia, or both? Eur J Gastroenterol Hepatol. 2001;13(Suppl. 1):S13–18.
3. Fass R, Ofman JJ. Gastroesophageal reflux disease – should we adopt a new conceptual framework? Am J Gastroenterol. 2002;97;1901–7.
4. Dent J, Brun J, Fendrick AM et al. An evidence-based appraisal of reflux disease management – the Genval Workshop Report. Gut. 1999;44(Suppl. 2):S1–16.
5. Dent J. Management of reflux disease. Gut. 2002;50(Suppl. IV):iv67–71.
6. Dent J, Armstrong D, Delaney B, Moayyedi P, Talley NJ, Vakil N. Symptom evaluation in reflux disease: workshop background, processes, terminology, recommendations, and discussion outputs. Gut. 2004;53(Suppl. IV):iv1–24.
7. Klauser AG, Schindlbeck NE, Müller-Lissner SA. Symptoms in gastro-oesophageal reflux disease. Lancet. 1990;335:205–8.
8. Martinez SD, Malagon IB, Garewal HS, Cui H, Fass R. Non-erosive reflux disease (NERD) – acid reflux and symptom patterns. Aliment Pharmacol Ther. 2003;17:537–45.
9. Kulig M, Nocon M, Vieth M et al. Risk factors of gastroesophageal reflux disease: methodology and first epidemiological results of the ProGERD study. J Clin Epidemiol. 2004;57:580–9.
10. Junghard O, Carlsson R, Lind T. Sufficient control of heartburn in endoscopy-negative gastro-oesophageal reflux disease trials. Scand J Gastroenterol. 2003;38:1197–9.
11. Bytzer P, Blum AL. Personal view: rationale and proposed algorithms for symptom-based proton pump inhibitor therapy for gastro-oesophageal reflux disease. Aliment Pharmacol Ther. 2004;20:389–98.
12. Mäntynen T, Färkkilä M, Kunnamo I, Mecklin JP, Voutilainen M. The impact of upper GI endoscopy referral volume on the diagnosis of gastroesophageal reflux disease and its complications: 1-year cross sectional study in a referral area with 260,000 inhabitants. Am J Gastroenterol. 2002;97:2524–9.
13. Koop H. Gastroesophageal reflux disease and Barrett's esophagus. Endoscopy. 2004; 36:103–9.
14. Blustein PK, Beck PL, Meddings JB et al. The utility of endoscopy in the management of patients with gastroesophageal reflux symptoms. Am J Gastroenterol. 1998;93:2508–12.
15. Jones MP. Acid suppression in gastro-oesophageal reflux disease: Why? How? How much and when? Postgrad Med J. 2002;78:465–8.
16. Fass R, Tougas G. Functional heartburn: the stimulus, the pain, and the brain. Gut. 2002; 51:885–92.
17. Dean BB, Gano Jr AD, Knight K, Ofman JJ, Fass R. Effectiveness of proton pump inhibitors in nonerosive reflux disease. Clin Gastroenterol Hepatol. 2004;2:656–64.
18. Venables TL, Newland RD, Patel AC, Hole J, Wilcock C, Turbitt ML. Omeprazole 10 milligrams once daily, omeprazole 20 mg once daily, or ranitidine 150 milligrams twice daily, evaluated as initital therapy for the relief of symptoms in general practice. Scand J Gastroenterol. 1997;32:965–73.
19. Tack J, Fass R. Review article: Approaches to endoscopic-negative reflux disease: part of the GERD spectrum or a unique acid-related disorder? Aliment Pharmacol Ther. 2004; 19 (Suppl. 1):28–34.
20. Lauritsen K. Management of endoscopy-negative reflux disease: progress with short-term treatment. Aliment Pharmacol Ther. 1997;11(Suppl. 2):87–92.

21. Lind T, Havelund T, Carlsson R et al. Heartburn without oesophagitis: efficacy of omeprazole therapy and features determining therapeutic response. Scand J Gastroenterol. 1997;32:974–9.
22. Richter JE, Kovacs TOG, Greski-Rose PA, Huang B, Fisher R. Lansoprazole in the treatment of heartburn in patients without erosive oesophagitis. Aliment Pharmacol Ther. 1999;13:795–804.
23. Katz PO, Castell DO, Levine D. Esomeprazole resolves chronic heartburn in patients without erosive oesophagitis. Aliment Pharmacol Ther. 2003;18:875–83.
24. Armstrong D, Talley NJ, Lauritsen K et al. The role of acid suppression in patients with endoscopy-negative reflux disease: the effect of treatment with esomeprazole or omeprazole. Aliment Pharmacol Ther. 2004;20:413–21.
25. Bate CM, Riley SA, Chapman RW, Durnin AT, Taylor MD. Evaluation of omeprazole as a cost-effective diagnostic test for gastro-oesophageal reflux disease. Aliment Pharmacol Ther. 1999;13:59–66.
26. Fass R, Ofman JJ, Grainek IM et al. Clinical and economic assessment of the omeprazole test in patients with symptoms suggestive of gastroesophageal reflux disease. Arch Intern Med. 1999;159:2161–8.
27. Watson RG, Tham TC, Johnston BT, McDougall NI. Double blind cross-over study of omeprazole in the treatment of patients with reflux symptoms and physiological levels of acid reflux – the 'sensitive oesophagus'. Gut. 1997;40:587–90.
28. Kahrilas PJ. Refractory heartburn. Gastroenterology. 2003;124:1941–5.
29. Carlsson R, Dent J, Watts R et al. Gastro-oesophageal reflux disease (GORD) in primary care – an international study of different treatment strategies with omeprazole. Eur J Gastroenterol Hepatol. 1998;10:119–24.
30. Bardhan KD, Müller-Lissner S, Bigard MS et al. Symptomatic gastro-oesophageal reflux disease: double-blinded controlled study of intermittent treatment with omeprazole or ranitidine. Br Med J. 1999;318:502–7.
31. Gerson LB, Robbins AS, Garber A, Hornberger J, Triadafilopoulos G. A cost-effectiveness analysis of prescribing strategies in the management of gastroesophageal reflux disease. Am J Gastroenterol. 2000;95:395–407.
32. Wahlqvist P, Junghard O, Higgins A, Green J. Cost effectiveness of proton pump inhibitors in gastro-oesophageal reflux disease without oesophagitis: comparison of on-demand esomeprazole with continuous omeprazole strategies. Pharmacoeconomics. 2002;20:267–77.
33. Lind T, Havelund T, Lundell L et al. On demand therapy with omeprazole for the long-term management of patients with heartburn without oesophagitis – a placebo-controlled randomized trial. Aliment Pharmacol Ther. 1999;13:907–14.
34. Talley NJ, Lauritsen K, Tunturi-Hihnala H et al. Esomeprazole 20 mg maintains symptom control in endoscopy-negative gastro-oseophageal reflux disease: a controlled trial of on-demand therapy for 6 months. Aliment Pharmacol Ther. 2001;15:347–54.
35. Talley NJ, Venables TL, Green JRB et al. Esomeprazole 40 mg and 20 mg is efficacious in the long-term management of patients with endoscopy-negative gastro-oesophageal reflux disease: a placebo-controlled trial of on-demand therapy for 6 months. Eur J Gastroenterol Hepatol. 2002;14:857–63.
36. Bayerdörffer E, Sipponen P, Bigard M et al. Esomeprazole 20 mg continuous versus on demand treatment of patients with endoscopy-negative reflux disease (ENRD). Gut. 2004;53(Suppl. VI):A106.
37. Armstrong D, Bennett JR, Blum AL et al. The endoscopic assessment of esophagitis: a progress report on observer agreement. Gastroenterology. 1996;111:85–92.
38. Lundell LR, Dent J, Bennett JR et al. Endoscopic assessment of oesophagitis: clinical and functional correlates and further validation of the Los Angeles classification. Gut. 1999;45:172–80.
39. Richter JE, Kahrilas PJ, Johanson J et al. Efficacy and safety of esomeprazole compared with omeprazole in GERD patients with erosive esophagitis: a randomized controlled trial. Am J Gastroenterol. 2001;96:656–65.
40. Castell DO, Kahrilas PJ, Richter JE et al. Esomeprazole (40 mg) compared with lansoprazole (30 mg) in the treatment of erosive esophagitis. Am J Gastroenterol. 2002;97:575–83.

41. Labenz J, Armstrong D, Lauritsen K et al. A randomized comparative study of esomeprazole 40 mg versus pantoprazole 40 mg for healing erosive oesophagitis: The EXPO study. Aliment Pharmacol Ther. 2005;21:739–46.
42. Chiba N, De Gara CJ, Wilkinson JM, Hunt RH. Speed of healing and symptom relief in grade II to IV gastroesophageal reflux disease: a meta-analysis. Gastroenterology. 1997;112:1798–810.
43. Malfertheiner P, Lind T, Willich S et al. Prognostic influence of Barrett's oesophagus and of *H. pylori* infection on healing of erosive GORD and symptom resolution in non-erosive GORD. Report from the ProGERD study. Gut. 2005;54:746–51.
44. Holtmann G, Cain C, Malfertheiner P. Gastric *Helicobacter pylori* infection accelerates healing of reflux esophagitis during treatment with the proton pump inhibitor pantoprazole. Gastroenterology. 1999;117:11–16.
45. Edwards SJ, Lind T, Lundell L. Systematic review of proton pump inhibitors for the acute treatment of reflux oesophagitis. Aliment Pharmacol Ther. 2001;15:1729–36.
46. Vakil N, Fennerty MB. Systematic review: Direct comparative trials of the efficacy of proton pump inhibitors in the management of gastro-oesophageal reflux disease and peptic ulcer. Aliment Pharmacol Ther. 2003;18:559–68.
47. Richter JE, Kahrilas PJ, Sontag SJ, Kovacs TO, Huang B, Pencly JL. Comparing lansoprazole and omeprazole in onset of heartburn relief: results of a randomized, controlled trial in erosive esophagitis patients. Am J Gastroenterol. 2001;96:3089–98.
48. Bell NJ, Burget D, Howden CW, Wilkinson J, Hunt RH. Appropriate acid suppression for the management of gastrooesophageal reflux disease. Digestion. 1992;51(Suppl. 1):59–67.
49. Kawamura M, Ohara S, Koike T et al. The effects of lansoprazole on erosive reflux oesophagitis are influenced by CYP2C19 polymorphism. Aliment Pharmacol Ther. 2003; 17:965–73.
50. Miner P Jr, Katz PO, Chen Y, Sostek M. Gastric acid control with esomperazole, lansoprazole, omeprazole, pantoprazole, and rabeprazole: a five-way crossover study. Am J Gastroenterol. 2003;98:2616–20.
51. Röhss K, Wilder-Smith C, Nauclér E, Jansson L. Esomeprazole 20 mg provides more effective intragastric acid control than maintenance-dose rabeprazole, lansoprazole or pantoprazole in healthy volunteers. Clin Drug Invest. 2004;24:1–7.
52. Kahrilas PJ, Falk GW, Johnson DA et al. Esomeprazole improves healing and symptom resolution as compared with omeprazole in reflux oesophagitis patients: a randomized controlled trial. Aliment Pharmacol Ther. 2000;14:1249–58.
53. Fennerty MB, Johanson J, Hwang C, Hoyle P, Sostek M. Esomeprazole 40 mg versus lansoprazole 30 mg in healing and symptom relief in patients with moderate to severe erosive oesophagitis (Los Angeles C & D). Gut. 2004;53(Suppl. VI):A111–12.
54. Labenz J, Armstrong D, Katelaris P, Schmidt S, Nauclér E, Eklund S. Analysis of healing associated with 4 weeks esomperazole 40 mg treatment relative to lansoprazole 30 mg and pantoprazole 40 mg in patients with all grades of erosive esophagitis. Gut. 2004;53(Suppl. VI):A105.
55. Gillessen A, Beil W, Modlin IM, Gatz G, Hole U. 40 mg pantoprazole and 40 mg esomeprazole are equivalent in the healing of esophageal lesions and relief from gastroesophageal reflux disease-related symptoms. J Clin Gastroenterol. 2004;38:332–40.
56. Scholten T, Gatz G, Hole U. Once-daily pantoprazole 40 mg and esomeprazole 40 mg have equivalent overall efficay in relieving GERD-related symptoms. Aliment Pharmacol Ther. 2003;18:587–94.
57. Tinmouth JM, Steele LS, Tomlinson G, Glazier RH. Are claims of equivalency in digestive disease trials supported by the evidence? Gastroenterology. 2004;126:1700–10.
58. Fass R, Thomas S, Traxler B, Sostek M. Patient reported outcome of heartburn improvement: doubling the proton pump inhibitor (PPI) dose in patients who failed standard dose PPI versus switching to a different PPI. Gastroenterology. 2004;126:A36.
59. Hatleback JG, Katz PO, Kuo B, Castell DO. Nocturnal gastric acidity and acid breakthrough on different regimens of omeprazole 40 mg daily. Aliment Pharmacol Ther. 1998; 12:1235–40.
60. Ours TM, Fackler WK, Richter JE, Vaezi MF. Nocturnal acid breakthrough: clinical significance and correlation with esophageal acid exposure. Am J Gastroenterol. 2003;98: 545–50.

61. Fackler WK, Ours TM, Vaezi MF, Richter JE. Long-term effect of H_2RA therapy on nocturnal gastric acid breakthrough. Gastroenterology. 2002;122:625–32.
62. Vakil NB, Shaker R, Johnson DA et al. The new proton pump inhibitor esomeprazole is effective as a maintenance therapy in GERD patients with healed erosive oesophagitis: a 6-month, randomized, double-blind, placebo-controlled study of efficacy and safety. Aliment Pharmacol Ther. 2001;15:927–35.
63. Johnson DA, Benjamin SB, Vakil NB et al. Esomeprazole once daily for 6 months is effective therapy for maintaining healed erosive esophagitis and for controlling gastroesophageal reflux disease symptoms: a randomized, double-blind, placebo-controlled study of efficacy and safety. Am J Gastroenterol. 2001;96:27–34.
64. Johnsson F, Moum B, Vilien M, Grove O, Simren M, Thoring M. On-demand treatment in patients with oesophagitis and reflux symptoms: comparison of lansoprazole and omeprazole. Scand J Gastroenterol. 2002;37:642–7.
65. Sjöstedt S, Befrits R, Sylvan A et al. On demand versus continuous treatment with esomeprazole (ESO) 20 mg once daily in subjects with healed erosive esophagitis (EE) after initial healing with ESO 40 mg once daily. An open, randomised, Swedish multicenter study. Gut. 2004;53(Suppl. VI):A68.
66. Richter JE, Fraga P, Mack M, Sabesin SM, Bochenek W and The Pantoprazole US GERD Study Group. Prevention of erosive esophagitis relapse with pantoprazole. Aliment Pharmacol Ther. 2004;20:1–9.
67. Vigneri S, Termini R, Leandro G et al. A comparison of five maintenance therapies for reflux esophagitis. N Engl J Med. 1995;333:1106–10.
68. You JHS, Lee ACM, Wong SCY, Chan FKL. Low-dose or standard dose proton pump inhibitors for maintenance therapy of gastro-oesophageal reflux disease: a cost-effectiveness analysis. Aliment Pharmacol Ther. 2003;17:785–92.
69. Inadomi JM, Jamal R, Murata GH et al. Step-down management of gastroesophageal reflux disease. Gastroenterology. 2001;121:1095–100.
70. Inadomi JM, McIntyre L, Bernard L, Fendrick AM. Step-down from multiple- to single-dose proton pump inhibitors (PPI): a prospective study of patients with heartburn or acid regurgitation completely relieved with PPI. Am J Gastroenterol. 2003;98:1940–4.
71. Klinkenberg-Knol EC, Nelis F, Dent J et al. Long-term omeprazole treatment in resistant gastroesophageal reflux disease: efficacy, safety, and influence on gastric mucosa. Gastroenterology. 2000;118:661–9.
72. Lauritsen K, Devière J, Bigard M-A et al. Esomeprazole 20 mg and lansoprazole 15 mg in maintaining healed reflux oesophagitis: Metropole study results. Aliment Pharmacol Ther. 2003;17:333–41.
73. DeVault KR, Liu S, Hoyle P, Sostek M. Esomeprazole 20 mg versus lansoprazole 15 mg for maintenance of healing of erosive esophagitis. Gut. 2004;53(Suppl. VI):A111.
74. Labenz J, Armstrong D, Katelaris P, Schmidt S, Adler J, Eklund S. A comparison of esomeprazole and pantoprazole for maintenance treatment of healed erosive esophagitis. Gut. 2004;53(Suppl. VI):A108.
75. Labenz J. Protagonist: should we eradicate *Helicobacter pylori* before long term antireflux therapy? Gut. 2001;49:614–16.
76. Freston JW. Antagonist: should we eradicate *Helicobacter pylori* before long term antireflux therapy? Gut. 2001;49:616–17.
77. Moayyedi P, Bardhan C, Young L, Dixon MF, Brown L, Axon AT. *Helicobacter pylori* eradication does not exacerbate reflux symptoms in gastroesophageal reflux disease. Gastroenterology. 2001;121:1120–6.
78. Malfertheiner P, Megraud F, O'Morain C et al. Current concepts in the management of *Helicobacter pylori* infection – the Maastricht 2-2000 Consensus Report. Aliment Pharmacol Ther. 2002;16:167–80.
79. Lundell L, Miettinen P, Myrvold HE et al. Continued (5-year) follow-up of a randomized clinical study comparing antireflux surgery and omeprazole in gastroesophageal reflux disease. J Am Coll Surg. 2001;192:172–9.
80. Lundell L, Miettinen P, Myrvold HE et al. Long-term management of gastro-oesophageal reflux disease with omeprazole or open antireflux surgery: results of a prospective, randomized clinical trial. Eur J Gastroenterol Hepatol. 2000;12:879–87.

81. Arguedas MR, Heudebert GR, Klapow JC et al. Re-examination of the cost-effectiveness of surgical versus medical therapy in patients with gastroesophageal reflux disease: the value of long-term data collection. Am J Gastroenterol. 2004;99:1023-8.
82. Myrvold HE, Lundell L, Miettinen P et al. The cost of long term therapy for gastro-oesophageal reflux disease: a randomised trial comparing omeprazole and open antireflux surgery. Gut. 2001;49:488-94.
83. Freston JW, Triadafilopoulos G. Review article: Approaches to the long-term management of adults with GERD – proton pump inhibitor therapy, laparoscopic fundoplication or endoscopic therapy? Aliment Pharmacol Ther. 2004;19(Suppl. 1):35-42.
84. Arts J, Tack J, Galmiche JP. Endoscopic antireflux procedures. Gut. 2004;53:1207-14.
85. Corley DA, Katz P, Wo J et al. Improvement of gastroesophageal reflux symptoms after radiofrequency energy: a randomized, sham-controlled trial. Gastroenterology. 2003;125:668-76.
86. Dent J, Talley NJ. Oveview: initial and long-term management of gastro-oesophageal reflux disease. Aliment Pharmacol Ther. 2003;17(Suppl. 1):53-7.
87. Howden CW, Henning JM, Huang B, Lukasik N, Freston JW. Management of heartburn in a large, randomized, community-based study: comparison of four therapeutic strategies. Am J Gastroenterol. 2001;96:1704-10.
88. Armstrong D, Barkun AL, Chiba N et al. 'Start high' – a better acid suppression strategy for heartburn-dominant uninvestigated dyspepsia (DU) in primary care practice (PCP) – the CADET-HR study. Gastroenterology. 2002;122:A472.
89. Meineche-Schmidt V, Hauschildt Juhl H, Ostergaard JE, Luckow A, Hvenegaard A. Costs and efficacy of three different esomeprazole treatment strategies for long-term management of gastro-oesophageal reflux symptoms in primary care. Aliment Pharmacol Ther. 2004;19:907-15.

2
Management of Barrett's oesophagus, dysplasia and early adenocarcinoma

C. ELL and O. PECH

DEFINITION OF BARRETT'S OESOPHAGUS

Barrett's oesophagus represents a complication of reflux disease, and is defined as specialized intestinalized metaplastic columnar epithelium. It needs to be distinguished from complete intestinal metaplasia of the gastric cardiac mucosa, and this has implications for subsequent diagnostic and therapeutic procedures. Complete intestinal metaplasia appears to arise as a sequela of *Helicobacter pylori* infection, and corresponds histologically to type I and II intestinal metaplasia; by contrast, Barrett's mucosa resembles type III intestinal metaplasia.

With regard to the length of Barrett's oesophagus, short-segment Barrett's oesophagus (SSBO), less than 3 cm in length, is distinguished from the classic or long-segment Barrett's oesophagus[1]. The term 'micro-Barrett's' should be reserved for Barrett's mucosa at the Z line that is not identifiable macroscopically. A study published in 1994 demonstrated for the first time that specialized intestinal metaplastic columnar epithelium is found in biopsy material routinely obtained from the oesophagogastric junction in 18% of cases when the endoscopic findings are normal[2]. Independently of the extent of its spread, histological evidence of Barrett's epithelium is sufficient for a diagnosis of Barrett's oesophagus.

CANCER RISK IN BARRETT'S OESOPHAGUS

In the early 1990s there was a sudden increase in the clinical importance of Barrett's oesophagus. This was mainly due to the marked increase in the incidence of adenocarcinoma at the oesophagogastric junction and a growing understanding of the pathophysiological connections between reflux disease, Barrett's metaplasia and adenocarcinoma. Endoscopic technology (above all high-resolution video endoscopy), the training of endoscopists, enthusiasm on the part of pathologists and gastroenterologists, and epidemiological conditions thus all contributed to the current 'Barrett's boom'[3].

The frequency of gastro-oesophageal reflux disease in the general population is estimated at about 10–30%. It is thought that some 10% of patients with endoscopically diagnosed reflux oesophagitis develop Barrett's oesophagus[4].

The prevalence of SSBO reported in the literature, at 2–12%, is much higher than that of traditional Barrett's oesophagus, at 0.3%[5,6]. The risk of developing severe dysplasia or adenocarcinoma in comparison with the normal population is 30–125 times higher in traditional Barrett's oesophagus, and the incidence is reported to be between one in 52 and one in 208 patient-years[7]. The risk of carcinoma appears to correlate with the severity of the reflux symptoms. A Swedish population-based case–control study for the first time demonstrated a direct connection between gastro-oesophageal reflux and the development of oesophageal adenocarcinoma[8]. The study results showed that the risk of developing oesophageal carcinoma was increased by a factor of eight in patients in whom heartburn or regurgitation occurred at least once per week, while with nocturnal reflux symptoms the individual risk was increased 11-fold. Patients with a long history of severe reflux symptoms had a 44-fold increase in the risk of Barrett's carcinoma. However, a surprising finding in this study was that evidence of Barrett's oesophagus only played a minor role in relation to the tumour incidence.

Excess weight also appears to represent an independent risk factor for the development of oesophageal adenocarcinoma. In patients with a body mass index (BMI) over 25.6 kg/m^2 in men, or over 24.2 kg/m^2 in women, the relative risk of oesophageal adenocarcinoma was 7.6. If the BMI was over 30 kg/m^2, the relative risk rose to 16.2[9].

The data linking an increase in the frequency of dysplasia to increasing length of the Barrett's segment are not at present clear. In the study by Weston et al.[10], the prevalence of dysplasia in patients with SSBO at the time of first diagnosis was 8.1%, while in patients with traditional Barrett's oesophagus the figure was 24.4%. During a subsequent follow-up period of 12–24 months, patients with long-segment Barrett's also had dysplasia and carcinoma significantly more often than patients with SSBO. However, Rudolph et al. did not find a clear connection between the frequency of dysplasia and the length of the Barrett's segment. A difference in length of 5 cm was only associated with a 1.7-fold increase in the risk of carcinoma[11].

Although the data are still not conclusive, SSBO must be regarded as a precancerous condition in the same way as traditional Barrett's oesophagus, and endoscopic monitoring is therefore required when the length of the columnar epithelial metaplasia is less than 3 cm, just as it is in long-segment Barrett's oesophagus.

SURVEILLANCE – HOW OFTEN AND HOW MANY BIOPSIES?

During the endoscopic examination the location and extent of Barrett's oesophagus (circular, semicircular, tongue-shaped, length) should be observed and documented. In addition, endoscopic 'mapping' is carried out using four-quadrant biopsies in the form of one excisional biopsy each at the 12-o'clock, 3-o'clock, 6-o'clock and 9-o'clock positions at intervals of 2 cm. Macroscopically abnormal areas of mucosa are also biopsied. High-resolution video endoscopy can be crucially helpful here, and should be regarded as a standard in oesophageal diagnosis. Even during treatment with proton-pump inhibitors, or after fundoplication surgery, regular check-up examinations should be carried out, since treatment of the acid reflux that is the pathophysiological cause does not substantially reduce the risk of carcinoma[12,13].

The obligatory 'random' biopsy is not always representative, and new endoscopic methods using visually guided specialized diagnosis are therefore becoming increasingly important. In addition to video endoscopy, diagnostic procedures such as chromoendoscopy, magnification endoscopy, fluorescence diagnosis and high-frequency miniprobe endosonography are very promising for detection and monitoring purposes.

Chromoendoscopy

Methylene blue staining using a special spraying catheter has been found useful for characterizing specialized columnar epithelium in Barrett's oesophagus, with a sensitivity of about 90%. Methylene blue causes reversible staining of actively absorbant cells, particularly the goblet cells of the intestinal mucosa. Since the segment containing Barrett's epithelium may simultaneously include gastric epithelium (fundus), junctional epithelium (cardia) and intestinal epithelium, vital staining makes it easier to achieve precise biopsy identification of the specialized Barrett's epithelium[14]. In inhomogeneous or more weakly staining and unstained mucosal areas, dysplastic changes may be present, or there may be a focal adenocarcinoma[15,16] (Figure 1).

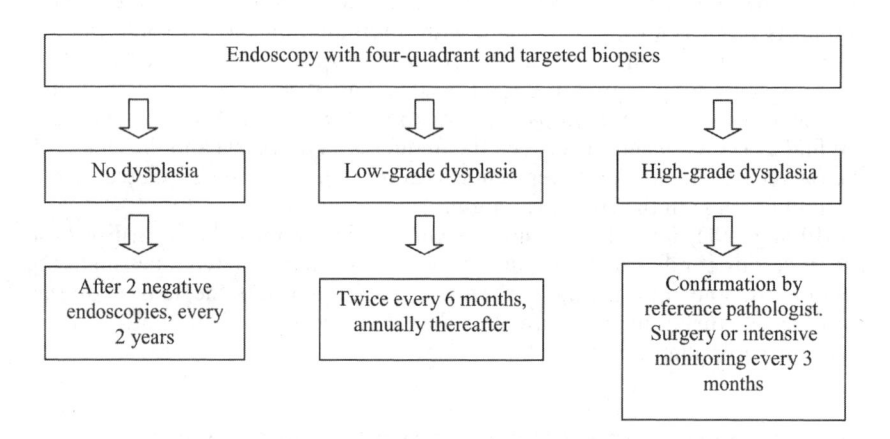

Figure 1 Monitoring strategies recommended in relation to the grade of dysplasia. From Sampliner et al. (1998) (Practice Parameters Committee of the American College of Gastroenterology)

Lugol's stain makes it possible to distinguish with certainty between squamous epithelium and metaplastic columnar epithelium, and to differentiate dysplastic structures[15]. Lugol's solution stains the intracellular glycogen content of squamous epithelium, which is reduced when there is tumour growth. Intestinal metaplasia and dysplastic or tumour-bearing segments do not take up the brown stain.

Spraying indigo carmine in Barrett's oesophagus can lead to more powerful enhancement/raising of dysplastic or tumorous epithelial segments[15].

Magnification endoscopy/high-resolution endoscopy

In low-grade dysplasia, as well as in high-grade dysplasia and focal adenocarcinoma, the macroscopic appearance is often normal. Improvements in endoscopic technology and growing awareness on the part of endoscopists are increasingly allowing the detection of discrete mucosal lesions with minor superficial changes. Discoloration, finely granulated surfaces (resembling orange-peel) and small elevations, hollows and narrow elevations, which give some Barrett's segments a cartographic pattern – particularly in multifocal disease – are just as typical of high-grade dysplasia and early carcinoma as discrete, erosion-like defects. This type of lesion is not always clearly distinguishable from inflammatory tissue. Since active inflammation in the mucosa can contain areas of cellular atypia that may be misinterpreted as dysplasia, patients with fresh reflux-like changes should initially receive treatment with proton-pump inhibitors to allow the mucosa to heal. Samples should only be taken in the interval after resolution of the active inflammation, to ensure that false-positive results are not obtained.

In this type of discrete superficial alteration, additional endoscopic procedures as well as vital staining can be used. The further development of video endoscopy technology, with wide-screen images and 140° lenses (high-resolution endoscopy, e.g. with the Fuji 485-HR) allows more detailed viewing[17]. After indigo carmine staining, magnification endoscopes (e.g. with the Olympus GIF-200Z) allow enlargement up to 35 times, with very considerable improvement in epithelial visualization[18]. In the future it may therefore be possible to make dysplastic areas accessible to endoscopic diagnosis.

Miniprobe endosonography

While endoscopy can delineate the intraluminal spread of the tumour, endosonography serves to assess the depth of tumour invasion into the surrounding area, including the lymph-node status. Endosonography is superior to computed tomography for classic tumour staging, as it allows depiction of the individual wall layers and can therefore precisely describe the extent of tumour spread into the surrounding area. Staining using endosonographic techniques is adapted to the TNM classification[19,20]. The endoscopic ultrasound devices with a 360° sector with a frequency between 7.5 MHz and 12 MHz has a penetration depth of 10 cm and is used for the detection of paraoesophageal lymph nodes. Small ultrasound probes with a frequency from 15 to 20 MHz (miniprobes manufactured by Fujinon, Olympus, Aloka, Machida and Toshiba) are thin and can be introduced through prograde endoscopes; they have recently also made it possible to carry out fine diagnosis in the mucosal and submucosal areas. They are used for specialized description of early oesophageal carcinoma with submucosal assessment (mucosal (uT1m) versus submucosal involvement (uT1sm))[21-24]. Accuracy rates of up to 90% for T staging and up to 80% for lymph-node status have been reported when pretherapeutic tumour staging is correctly conducted. Despite the very good sensitivity of 80% for lymph-node involvement, the specificity is still low at 40%; however, there is still a lack of reliable endosonographic criteria for lymph-node metastases. Incipient invasion of the submucosa also appears to be problematic, and cannot be detected with absolute certainty.

Fluorescence detection

Endoscopic monitoring of Barrett's oesophagus using four-quadrant biopsies to allow endoscopic mapping must be regarded as unsatisfactory, since it involves 'blind' biopsy sampling, with the biopsies being taken at random from an area of the mucosa. Particularly in severe dysplasia that cannot be recognized macroscopically, as well as in small early carcinomas, it would be desirable to have a specialized technique allowing an area to be marked for subsequent biopsy removal. Photodynamic diagnosis after exogenous administration of 5-aminolaevulinic acid might prove useful here in the future. The technique leads to excitation using a 'relatively inexpensive' incoherent light source (xenon gas lamp) with excitation in the blue range. In areas of dysplasia and carcinoma, marked red fluorescence caused by positive porphyrin fluorescence is typically detected[25-28].

WHICH MONITORING STRATEGY IS BEST?

The rationale underlying the use of monitoring strategies in patients with Barrett's oesophagus is that the condition is clearly precancerous, involving an increased risk of carcinoma, and that advanced adenocarcinoma of the oesophagus has a very poor prognosis. Initial studies have shown that regular monitoring identifies early carcinomas more frequently, and that it consequently allows marked improvements in the prognosis in relation to survival time[29]. On the other hand, the low incidence of the disease, and the fact that Barrett's oesophagus represents an 'uncommon cause of death', suggest arguments against excessive use of monitoring[30]. Since the risk of carcinoma also correlates with the length of the segment containing intestinal metaplasia, a distinction needs to be made between 'long-segment' and 'short-segment' Barrett's in relation to the intensity of monitoring[1]. The aim must be to use differentiated monitoring strategies, following the recommendations of the American College of Gastroenterology – both for reasons of medical necessity and for reasons of cost[31]. Appropriate check-up intervals according to the grade of dysplasia are given in Figure 1.

PRIMARY TREATMENT OF BARRETT'S OESOPHAGUS

Since lifelong monitoring of patients with Barrett's oesophagus is very expensive, and issues of cost-effectiveness arise, an approach in which Barrett's mucosa is ablated using local endoscopic procedures, in addition to acid-suppression treatment, appears an attractive alternative.

In the pharmacological treatment of gastro-oesophageal reflux and Barrett's oesophagus, proton-pump inhibitors (PPI) have become established as the most important drugs for adequate acid suppression. Freedom from symptoms can be achieved far more often using PPI than with histamine H_2-receptor blockers (77.4% versus 47.6%)[32]. PPI have also proved to be much more potent in healing inflammation[33] and ulceration[34], and in preventing strictures[35,36]. Studies investigating the regression of Barrett's mucosa during PPI treatment have so far produced widely varying and sometimes contradictory results[37–42]. A total of 320 patients were treated for 672 months with a PPI (omeprazole 20–40 mg or lansoprazole 30–60 mg orally once or twice daily) in these studies. The reduction in the length of the Barrett's mucosa ranged from 0% to 54% (mean 13%), with reductions in the surface area ranging from 0% to 21%. The varying results are partly explained by bias and error in measuring the area and length of the Barrett's segment. In addition, the extent of acid suppression was not confirmed by pH-metry, and the individual studies used different PPI dosage protocols.

The influence of PPI therapy on the natural course of Barrett's oesophagus as it develops into dysplasia and carcinoma is not as yet clear. Maintenance of normal epithelial differentiation and proliferation is an important goal in cancer chemoprevention. *Ex-vivo* investigations have shown that continuous acid exposure induces differentiation in the mucosa in Barrett's oesophagus and reduces proliferation, whereas recurrent short-term exposure enhances proliferation[43]. It was shown in 42 patients that acid-suppression therapy with lansoprazole for 6 months increases cell differentiation and reduces proliferation[44]. The hypothesis that PPI treatment may reduce the likelihood of dysplasia–carcinoma development in Barrett's oesophagus has not yet been proved in any studies, and further long-term investigations are necessary.

In addition to thermocoagulation procedures for endoscopic ablation, such as argon plasma coagulation, potassium titanyl phosphate (KTP) laser and neodymium–yttrium aluminium garnet (Nd:YAG) laser, non-thermal procedures are also available, such as photodynamic therapy. However, even after complete removal of columnar epithelial metaplasia, regular monitoring is necessary to detect possible recurrences and administer repeat treatment. The high costs of ablation treatment are therefore incurred in addition to the costs of regular endoscopic check-up examinations, and the question arises as to whether ablation therapy for carcinoma prevention is useful and economically justifiable.

In summary, the data currently available show that routine ablation of Barrett's epithelium without dysplasia cannot be recommended – however, the issue needs to be investigated in controlled clinical studies.

Table 1 Thermal ablation therapy for Barrett's oesophagus

Reference	Therapy	No. of patients	Follow-up (months)	Outcome
Argon–plasma coagulation				
Berenson et al. 1993[45]	APC and PPI	10	1.5–9.5	CR 9/10, PR 1/10
Dumoulin et al. 1997[46]	APC and PPI	2	6	PR 2/2
Van Laethem et al. 1998[47]	APC and PPI	31	12	CR 19/31, PR 6/31, NR 3/31
Byrne et al. 1998[48]	APC and PPI	30	9	CR 16/30, PR 11/30
Grade et al. 1999[49]	APC and PPI	9	1.5	CR 7/9, PR 2/9
Mork et al. 1998[50]	APC and PPI		6–12	CR 13/ , PR 2/
Bohnacker et al. 1997[51]	APC and PPI	8	1	CR 8/8
Martin et al. 1998[52]	APC and PPI	18		
KTP laser				
Gossner et al. 1999[62]	KTP and PPI	10	6–15	CR 8/10, PR 2/10
Barham et al. 1997[61]	KTP and PPI	16	3–18	PR 16/16
Biddlestone et al. 1998[63]	KTP and PPI	10	–14	PR 9/10
Nd:YAG laser				
Sampliner et al. 1993[64]	Nd:YAG and PPI	1	11	CR 1/1
Ertan et al. 1995[68]	Nd:YAG and PPI	1	3	PR 1/1
Luman et al. 1996[69]	Nd:YAG and PPI	4	6	PR 4/4
Salo et al. 1998[65]	Nd:YAG	11	6–52	CR 11/11
Brandt and Kauvar 1992[66]	Nd:YAG	1		1992 TR,
Brandt et al. 1995[67]			Months	1995 CR
Multipolar electrocoagulation				
Sampliner et al. 1996[70]	MPEC and PPI	10	10–18	CR 10/10
Kovacs et al. 1999[71]	MPEC and PPI	27	4.5	CR 18/27, PR 9/27
Sharma et al. 1999[72]	MPEC and PPI	11	19–53	CR 11/11, recurrence 3/11
Montes et al. 1999[73]	MPEC and antirefl. surg.	14	18–30	CR 14/14

APC = argon plasma coagulation; MPEC = multipolar electrocoagulation; PR = partial regression ; CR = complete regression; TR = transient regression; PPI = proton-pump inhibitors; BM = Barrett's mucosa; HGD = high-grade dysplasia ; SC = superficial cancer.

Plasma coagulation

Argon plasma coagulation (APC) is a non-contact thermocoagulation procedure with the advantage of a limited depth of penetration – minimizing the risk of perforation. In comparison with the alternative of laser ablation, APC is substantially less expensive. In most cases partial or complete regression of Barrett's epithelium can be achieved[45–52].

The disadvantages of this procedure are the large number of sessions required to achieve complete ablation of Barrett's epithelium, and the relatively high risk of residual islands of metaplasia. In addition, it is possible for specialized tissue with a neoplastic potential to remain under the neo-epithelium. Despite the limited depth of mucosal destruction, massive haemorrhage or perforation resulting in mortality can occur[48,49].

Table 2 Photochemical ablation

Reference	Photosensitizer and wavelength (nm)	No. of patients	Follow-up (months)	Outcome
Laukka and Wang 1995[58]	HpD, 630	5 (1 HGD)	6	PR 5/5
Overholt et al. 1999[80]	DHE, 630	100 (13 SC)	4–84	BM: CR 43/100, HGD: CR 78, MC: CR 10/13
Barr et al. 1996[54]	ALA, 630	5 (HGD)	26–44	PR 5/5
Gossner et al. 1998[56]	ALA, 635	32 (10 HGD, 22 SC)	1–30	HGD: CR 10/10, SC: CR 12/22
Biddlestone et al. 1998[63]	ALA, 630	5	3–21	PR

HpD = haematoporphyrin derivative; DHE = dihaematoporphyrin ester/ether; ALA = 5-aminolavulinic acid; PR = partial regression; CR = complete regression, BM = Barrett's mucosa; HGD = high-grade dysplasia; SC = superficial cancer.

Photodynamic therapy

Photodynamic therapy (PDT), as a local endoscopically guided treatment approach, is based on selective sensitization of precancerous or malignant lesions and light-induced tissue destruction. The light sources now most often used are dye lasers in continuous-wave mode. Laser light with a defined wavelength is introduced into the gastrointestinal tract endoscopically via flexible optical fibres, and can be used for local irradiation of the sensitized dysplastic or malignant tissue. Photodynamic therapy exploits the phenomenon that light can activate photosensitized substances stored in the tissue, and can destroy the tissue by means of oxidation processes. In contrast to conventional high-energy lasers, the mode of action of PDT thus allows selective, non-thermal destruction of the target tissue while protecting the healthy surroundings as far as possible. To administer the light in tubular hollow organs such as the oesophagus, cylindrical diffusers are used for circumferential light application[53]. Using the appropriate irradiation applicators, an area of up to 8 cm can be ablated in a single treatment session, depending on the laser energy used. The light doses applied range from 20 J to 300 J, depending on the photosensitizer used, with a power density of 100–400 – a fraction of the power applied using the Nd:YAG laser.

PDT is an effective method of ablating Barrett's epithelium. Partial or complete regression of the columnar epithelial metaplasia, sometimes with biopsy-confirmed dysplasia, has been achieved in almost all of the studies published. In combination with long-term acid suppression using a proton-pump inhibitor, regeneration can be achieved, with ingrowth of normal squamous epithelium[54–59].

The advantage of PDT is that the ablation is homogeneous and extensive, allowing long Barrett's segments to be completely treated in a few sessions. In comparison with other techniques, PDT requires the lowest number of sessions to achieve ablation of Barrett's epithelium. Side-effects that have been observed involved phototoxic reactions in the skin, dysphagia and odynophagia, strictures and pleural effusion. However, these side-effects mainly occurred with first-generation and second-generation photosensitizers. PDT with 5-aminolaevulinic acid, a new endogenous photosensitizer, has a reduced depth of penetration and thus a lower rate of stenosis[56]. In addition, the agent has faster decay kinetics in comparison with other photosensitizers, so that the risk of phototoxic effects in the skin is present only for a period of 36–48 h[60]. This markedly improves the patients' quality of life, since they do not have to remain in darkened rooms for several weeks.

Other

In addition to the treatment procedures mentioned above, there are other methods of ablating Barrett's epithelium that are more rarely used, such as KTP and Nd:YAG laser ablation and monopolar or multipolar electrocoagulation.

The potassium titanyl phosphate (KTP) laser is a double-frequency neodymium–yttrium aluminium garnet (Nd:YAG) laser into which a KTP crystal is incorporated to reduce the wavelength from 1064 nm to 532 nm. This allows surface temperatures of more than 65°C in the oesophageal mucosa, with an external temperature on the serosa of only 21°C. KTP laser treatment allows complete ablation of Barrett's mucosa – but even with this procedure it is possible for residual specialized columnar epithelium to remain underneath the newly formed squamous epithelium[61–63].

Very few studies have been published on Nd:YAG laser ablation, and they have included only small numbers of patients. However, in most cases the reports have described good ablation results, although several sessions were required for complete ablation with this procedure. No severe complications were observed even when high power was used, but permanent high-dose acid-suppression therapy was needed to prevent recurrences[64–69].

Multipolar electrocoagulation has also been used successfully for ablation therapy, although the number of sessions required was higher than with any of the other methods. The success rate for complete removal of Barrett's epithelium correlated with the length of the Barrett's segment. Successful regression was achieved only in 25% of patients with segments longer than 4 cm. Another disadvantage of this procedure is the high rate of side-effects. Some 40–50% of the patients treated suffered complications, ranging from dysphagia and odynophagia to gastrointestinal haemorrhage[70–73].

TREATMENT OF DYSPLASIA AND EARLY CANCER

Surgical resection of the oesophagus is still regarded as the gold standard for treatment of high-grade dysplasia and early Barrett's carcinoma. Owing to the not-inconsiderable mortality rate and the high morbidity rate, further development of less invasive treatment procedures that can be offered to patients would be desirable. Published data are already available for endoscopic mucosal resection and photodynamic therapy. For the thermal procedures the published studies include only small numbers of patients, or consist of case reports.

An important consideration for adequate therapy is the interplay between the various treatment procedures – which should be regarded not as competitive, but as complementary.

Arguments in favour of local endoscopic therapy for mucosal carcinoma or dysplasia include the high morbidity (18–48%) and mortality (3–5% in high-volume departments) associated with surgical therapy and the fact that the risk of lymph-node metastases is virtually zero[74-76]. Endoscopic local treatment of early Barrett's carcinoma or dysplasia should at present be carried out only at experienced centres with appropriate expertise and in a research framework, since the data on local therapy are still uncertain. There is a complete lack of prospective data on the long-term survival rate – so that all local endoscopic treatment procedures for high-grade dysplasia or early carcinoma in Barrett's oesophagus must still be regarded as experimental.

Endoscopic mucosal resection

Based on experience with local endoscopic treatment in early gastric carcinoma[77,78], endoscopic mucosal resection (EMR) has been used by several research groups in the treatment of early malignancies in the oesophagus and at the oesophagogastric junction. The suck-and-cut technique, with or without prior ligation, allows large areas to be ablated with inclusion of the submucosa, even in the difficult conditions of the oesophagus. Several endoscopists also carry out conventional loop resections with or without injections into the target lesion.

The advantages of EMR in comparison with all other local endoscopic treatment procedures are obvious. The histological preparation of the resection specimen provides information on the depth of invasion of the individual wall layers, and allows complete resection within healthy margins. The patient is still able to undergo surgical treatment even if submucosal invasion (associated with positive lymph nodes in 20–25% of patients) is not initially recognized at EMR.

There are at present only a few publications on EMR in Barrett's oesophagus with severe dysplasia or early carcinoma. Our own published experience in 69 patients, 62 of whom had early Barrett's carcinoma while seven had high-grade dysplasia, showed that complete remission was obtained using EMR in 98% of cases. A mean of 2.2 sessions were required to achieve this. During a mean follow-up period of 13.5 months (4–38 months), recurrences or metachronous carcinomas were observed in 29% of the patients, but successful local therapy for these was also possible. The complication rate reported in the study was 9%; haemorrhage occurred in eight cases, but endoscopic haemostasis was possible, and transfusions were not required. The absence of method-specific mortality and the low morbidity in comparison with the surgical procedures underline the fact that this method is a minimally invasive one[79]. In spite of the initially good results, a definitive assessment of this technique will be possible only after a longer follow-up period.

Photodynamic therapy

Photodynamic therapy has become established in recent years as one of the most important local endoscopically guided treatment procedures for high-grade dysplasia in Barrett's oesophagus and early Barrett's carcinoma.

The largest study yet published, including 100 patients with Barrett's oesophagus and dysplasia or superficial carcinoma, was presented by Overholt's research group[80]. The photosensitizer used was haematoporphyrin, which up to now has been the agent most widely used for this purpose. The follow-up period was a mean of 19 months (4–84 months). Ten of 13 superficial carcinomas were successfully treated, and dysplasia was successfully eliminated in 78 patients. To optimize the treatment the investigators used Nd:YAG laser treatment for small residual lesions. These good results were purchased at the cost of a high rate of oesophageal strictures, but the incidence of this was reduced by using a longer balloon applicator.

The endogenous substance 5-aminolaevulinic acid, a second-generation photosensitizer, may offer advantages here. Its high specificity for the mucosa leads to ablation of the mucosa alone, without destruction of deeper layers of the oesophageal wall, and post-therapeutic stenoses and phototoxic side-effects in the skin have not been observed[55,56,81,82]. A study by Gossner et al. showed that severe dysplasia can be completely destroyed, although complete removal of carcinomas with a thickness of more than 2 mm was not possible[56]. Future studies will need to determine whether this implies a differential indication for the type of photosensitizer that needs to be used, in relation to the lesion being treated. Another alternative to the haematoporphyrins is provided by new photosensitizers from the chlorin group of substances, such as *meso*-tetrahydroxyphenylchlorin (mTHPC, temoporfin). The high photodynamic efficacy of mTHPC in comparison with 5-aminolaevulinic acid, and the shorter-term photosensitization of the skin it allows in comparison with the haematoporphyrins, appear to be very promising for clinical purposes[83,84].

The main disadvantages of PDT lie in the limited availability of the procedure, its high costs, and methodological problems that have not yet been fully solved. These affect dosimetry, the various photosensitizers that are undergoing testing, and also light application[83].

Argon plasma coagulation

Successful use of argon plasma coagulation in early Barrett's carcinoma is documented by only a single case report including a total of three patients[84]. The malignancies were completely ablated in all cases in one or two sessions, and complete re-epithelialization even occurred in two patients with additional omeprazole treatment. During a mean follow-up period of 24.3 months, a recurrence was observed in one case, which was in turn successfully treated using PDT.

Laser therapy

Again, almost no data are available regarding laser treatment of early carcinoma. In one study a total of 10 patients (four with low-grade dysplasia, four with high-grade dysplasia and two with early Barrett's carcinoma) underwent KTP laser therapy[62]. Complete remission and re-epithelialization during acid-suppression treatment were seen in all cases. Residual specialized columnar epithelium was also found under the neo-epithelium in biopsy samples in this group. The follow-up averaged 15 months, and no complications or recurrences were seen.

Conventional surgery

Oesophageal resection is still the gold standard for the treatment of early carcinoma and high-grade dysplasia in patients with Barrett's oesophagus. Only the surgical procedure allows dissection of involved lymph nodes and complete removal of the potentially malignant tissue that is left in the residual Barrett's segment when endoscopic local treatment is used. Another argument in favour of surgical treatment for high-grade dysplasia and early carcinoma in Barrett's oesophagus is the high rate of second carcinomas that are not detected during endoscopic examination. However, radicality in the surgical procedure, which is repeatedly required by surgeons, is purchased at the cost of high morbidity and mortality rates for the patients[75,76].

The results of surgical treatment mainly depend on the local tumour stage and on whether lymph-node metastases are present. In a retrospective study of 41 patients with early oesophageal adenocarcinomas who underwent transhiatal subtotal or right transthoracic *en-bloc* oesophageal resection, the 5-year survival rate for all patients was 83%. When the tumours were differentiated into mucosal carcinomas and tumours with submucosal invasion, it was found that all patients with a mucosal carcinoma survived 5 years, in contrast to 79% of the patients with submucosal involvement. In patients with an adenocarcinoma that was restricted to the mucosa, a lymph-node metastasis was observed in one case; in patients with submucosal involvement the rate of lymph-node metastasis was 16%. The mortality rate was 4.8%, and the complication rate was 44%[76].

The mortality and morbidity rates reported in this study are broadly in agreement with the data published by other research groups for patients with early Barrett's carcinoma[75]. However, these results were achieved at experienced centres in highly selected groups of patients, and certainly do not represent a widespread standard. Another aspect that needs to be taken into consideration is that patients require several months to recover a quality of life similar to that which they had before surgery.

SUMMARY

There has been a sudden increase in recent years in the incidence of Barrett's oesophagus, a form of specialized intestinal columnar epithelial metaplasia, and of the oesophageal adenocarcinoma that is associated with it.

Barrett's oesophagus is classified according to its length into micro-Barrett's, short-segment Barrett's oesophagus (<3 cm) and classic or long-segment Barrett's oesophagus. The risk of malignant transformation increases in proportion to the length of the metaplastic mucosal area.

Since Barrett's oesophagus is a precancerous condition, it requires a careful monitoring strategy corresponding to the grade of dysplasia grade (Figure 1). In addition to conventional endoscopic examinations using high-resolution video endoscopes and four-quadrant biopsies, a number of new diagnostic procedures are now available – such as chromoendoscopy, magnification endoscopy, high-resolution endoscopy and fluorescence detection. These methods allow easier detection of dysplastic areas or early carcinomas in Barrett's oesophagus.

Drug-induced regression of Barrett's epithelium has been only partly successful in studies conducted so far, and a number of endoscopic ablation procedures are therefore also now being used. These include thermal ablation procedures such as argon plasma coagulation, KTP or Nd:YAG laser treatment and multipolar electrocoagulation, as well as non-thermal procedures (PDT). The advantage of PDT lies in the homogeneous and circumferential irradiation it allows, with fewer treatment sessions being required.

On the basis of the data currently available, a general recommendation for ablation cannot yet be given, since it has not been shown that ablation is capable of reducing the incidence of Barrett's carcinoma. In addition, continued monitoring is still needed even after successful ablation of columnar epithelial metaplasia.

The treatment of choice in early carcinoma and high-grade dysplasia is oesophageal resection. Due to the high morbidity and mortality rates associated with surgery, local endoscopic treatment procedures are increasingly being used for these lesions. The best results have been obtained with endoscopic mucosal resection and photodynamic therapy. Both methods have low complication rates, and the mortality in studies carried out so far has been zero. However, long-term results are not yet available, and these must be awaited before a definitive assessment of the procedures can be made. Thermal ablation procedures have only a minor role here.

References

1. Sharma P, Morales TG, Sampliner RE. Short segment Barrett's esophagus – the need for standardization of the definition and of endoscopic criteria. Am J Gastroenterol. 1998;7: 103–6.
2. Spechler SJ, Zeroogian JM, Antoniolo DA et al. Prevalence of metaplasia at the gastroesophageal junction. Lancet. 1994;344:1533–6.
3. Pracht AT, MacDonald TA, Hopwood DA, Johnston DA. Increasing incidence of Barrett's esophagus: education enthusiasm or epidemiology? Lancet. 1997;350:933.

4. Winters CJ, Spurling T, Chobanian S, Curtis D, Espositos R, Hacker J. Barrett's esophagus: a prevalent occult complication of gastroesophageal reflux disease. Gastroenterology. 1987; 92:118–24.
5. Cameron A, Ott B, Payne W. The incidence of adenocarcinoma in columnar-lined (Barrett's) esophagus. N Engl J Med. 1985;313:857–9.
6. Spechler S, Robbins A, Rubins H. Adenocarcinoma and Barrett's esophagus: an overrated risk? Gastroenterology. 1984;87:927–33.
7. Drewitz DJ, Sampliner RE, Garewal HS. The incidence of adenocarcinoma in Barrett's esophagus: a prospective study of 170 patients followed 4.8 years. Am J Gastroenterol. 1997;92:212–15.
8. Lagergren J, Bergström R, Lindgren A, Nyren O. Symptomatic gastroesophageal reflux as a risk factor for esophageal adenocarcinoma. N Engl J Med. 1999;340:825–31.
9. Lagergren J, Bergström R, Nyrén O. Association between body mass and adenocarcinoma of the esophagus and gastric cardia. Ann Int Med. 1999;130:883–90.
10. Weston AP, Krmpotich PT, Cherian R, Dixon A, Topalosvki M. Prospective long-term endoscopic and histological follow-up of short segment Barrett's esophagus: comparison with traditional long segment Barrett's esophagus. Am J Gastroenterol. 1997;92:407–13.
11. Rudolph RE, Vaughan TL, Storer BE et al. Effect of segment length on risk for neoplastic progression in patients with Barrett esophagus. Ann Int Med. 2000;132:612–20.
12. Sampliner R, Garewal H, Fennerty M, Aickin M. Lack of impact of therapy on extent of Barrett's esophagus in 67 patients. Dig Dis Sci. 1990;35:93–6.
13. Sagar P, Achroyd R, Patterson J, Stoddard C, Kingsnorth A. Regression and progression of Barrett's esophagus after antireflux surgery. Br J Surg. 1995;82:806–10.
14. Canto MI, Setrakia S, Petras RE et al. Methylene blue selectively stains intestinal metaplasia in Barrett's esophagus. Gastrointest Endosc. 1996;44:1–7.
15. Canto MI. Methylene blue staining and Barrett's esophagus. Gastrointest Endosc. 1999; 49: S12–16.
16. Gossner L, Pech O, May A, Stolte M, Ell C. Methylene blue staining for the detection of dysplasia or mucosal cancer in Barrett's esophagus. Gastroenterology. 1999;116:G1812.
17. Pugliese V. The role of endoscopy in esophageal cancer. Summary of a videoendoscopy session. Endoscopy. 1993;25(Suppl.):645–7.
18. Stevens PD, Lightdale CJ, Green PHR, Siegel LM, Garcia-Carrasquillo RJG, Rotterdam H. Combined magnification endoscopy with chromoendoscopy for the evaluation of Barrett's esophagus. Gastrointest Endosc. 1994;40:747–9.
19. Tio TL, Cohen P, Coene PPLO, Udding J, den Hartog Jager FCA, Tytgat GNJ. Endosonography and computed tomography of esophageal carcinoma: preoperative classification compared to the new (1987) TNM system. Gastroenterology. 1989;96:1478–86.
20. Tio TL, Coene PPLO, den Hartog Jager FCA, Tytgat GNJ. Preoperative TNM classification of esophageal carcinoma by endosonography. Hepato-Gastroenterology. 1990;37:376–81.
21. Akahoshi K, Chijiwa Y, Hamada S et al. Pretreatment staging of endoscopically early gastric cancer with a 15 MHz ultrasound catheter probe. Gastointest Endosc. 1998;48:470–6.
22. Hünerbein M, Ghadimi BM, Haensch W et al. Transendoscopic ultrasound of esophageal and gastric cancer using miniaturized ultrasound catheder probes. Gastrointest Endosc. 1998;48:470–76.
23. Natsugoe S, Yoshinaka H, Morinage T et al. Ultrasonographic detection of lymph-node metastases in superficial carcinoma of the esophagus. Endoscopy. 1996;28:674–9.
24. Yanai H, Masahiro T, Karita M, Okita K. Diagnostic utility of 20-megahertz linear endoscopic ultrasonography in early gastric cancer. Gastrointest Endosc. 1996;44:29–33.
25. Gossner L, Sroka R, Stepp H, May A, Stolte M, Ell C. Photodynamic diagnosis versus random biopsies for dysplasia and invisible mucosal cancer in Barrett's esophagus – a prospective randomized trial. Gastroenterology. 1999;116:G0763.
26. Gossner L, Sroka R, Stepp H, May A, Stolte M, Ell C. Oral versus topical ALA for photodynamic diagnosis of dysplasia and invisible mucosal cancer in Barrett's esophagus. Gastrointest Endosc. 1999;49:AB576.

27. Messmann H, Knüchel R, Endlicher E et al. Photodynamische Diagnostik gastrointestinaler Präkanzerosen nach Sensibilisierung mit 5-Aminolävulinsäure. Dtsche Med Wochenschr. 1998;123:515–21.
28. Stepp H, Sroka R, Baumgartner R. Fluorescence endoscopy of gastrointestinal diseases: basic principles, techniques and clinical experience. Endoscopy. 1998;30:379–86.
29. Van Sandick JW, van Lanschot JJB, Kuiken BW et al. Impact of endoscopic biopsy surveillance of Barrett's esophagus on pathological stage and clinical outcome of Barrett's carcinoma. Gut. 1998;43:216–22.
30. Van den Burgh A, Dees J, Hop WCJ et al. Oesophageal cancer is an uncommon cause of death in patients with Barrett's esophagus. Gut. 1996;39:5–8.
31. Sampliner RE, and the Practice Parameters Committee of the American College of Gastroenterology. Practice guidelines on the diagnosis, surveillance, and therapy of Barrett's esophagus. Am J Gastroenterol. 1998;7:1028–32.
32. Chiba N, DeGara CJ, Wilkinson JM et al. Speed of healing and symptom relief in grade II to IV gastroesophageal reflux disease: a meta-analysis. Gastroenterology. 1997;112:1798–810.
33. Triadafilopoulos G, Sharma R. Features of symptomatic gastroesophageal reflux disease in elderly patients. Am J Gastroenterol. 1997;92:2007–11.
34. Ollyo JB, Monnier PH, Fontolliet CH et al. L'ulcer de Savary: une nouvelle complication du reflux gastro-oesophagienne. Schweiz Med Wochenschr. 1988;118:823–7.
35. Smith PM, Kerr GD, Cockel R et al. A comparison of omeprazole and ranitidine in prevention of recurrence of benign esophageal stricture. Gastroenterology. 1994;107:1312–18.
36. Swarbrick ET, Gough AL, Foster CS et al. Prevention of recurrence of oesophageal stricture, a comparison of lansoprazoile and high-dose ranitidine. Eur J Gastroenterol Hepatol. 1996;8:431–8.
37. Cooper BT, Neumann CS, Cox MA et al. Continous treatment with omeprazole 20 mg daily for up to 6 years in Barrett's oesophagus. Aliment Pharmacol Ther. 1998;12:893–7.
38. Malesci A, Savarino V, Zentilin P et al. Partial regression of Barrett's esophagus by long-term therapy with high-dose omeprazole. Gastrointest Endosc. 1996;44:700–5.
39. Gore S, Healey CJ, Sutton R et al. Regression of columnar-lined (Barrett's) esophagus with continous omeprazole therapy. Aliment Pharmacol Ther. 1993;7:623–8.
40. Neumann CS, Iqbal TH, Cooper BT. Long term continuous omeprazole treatment in patients with Barrett's esophagus. Aliment Pharmacol Ther. 1995;9:451–4
41. Sampliner RE. Effect of up to 3 years of high-dose lansoprazole on Barrett's esophagus. Am J Gastroenterol. 1994;89:1844–8.
42. Peters FTM, Ganesh S, Kuipers EJ et al. Endoscopic regression of Barrett's oesophagus during omeprazole treatment: a randomized double blind study. Gut. 1999;45:489–94.
43. Fitzgerald RC, Omary MB, Triadafilopoulos G. Dynamic effects of acid on Barrett's esophagus: an *ex-vivo* proliferation and differentiation model. J Clin Invest. 1996;98:2120–8.
44. Ouatu-Lascar R, Fitzgerald RC, Triadafilopoulos G. Differentiation and proliferation in Barrett's esophagus an the effects of acid suppression. Gastroenterology. 1999;117:327–35.
45. Berenson MM, Johnson TD, Markowitz NR et al. Restoration of squamous mucosa after ablation of Barrett's esophageal epithelium. Gastroenterology. 1993;104:1686–91.
46. Dumoulin FL, Terjung B, Neubrand M, Scheurlen C, Fischer HP, Sauerbruch T. Treatment of Barrett's esophagus by endoscopic argon plasma coagulation. Endoscopy. 1997;29:751–3.
47. Van Laethem JL, Cremer M, Peny MO, Delhaye M, Deviere J. Eradication of Barrett's mucosa with argon plasma coagulation and acid suppression: immediate and mid term results. Gut. 1999;43:747–51.
48. Byrne JP, Armstrong GR, Attwood SEA. Restoration of the normal squamous lining in Barrett's esophagus by argon plasma coagulation. Am J Gastroenterol. 1998;93:1810–15.
49. Grade AJ, Shah IA, Medlon SM, Ramirez FC. The efficacy and safety of argon plasma coagulation in Barrett's esophagus. Gastrointest Endosc. 1999;50:18–22.
50. Mork H, Barth T, Kreipe HH et al. Reconstituion of squamous epithelium in Barrett's oesophagus with endoscopic argon plasma coagulation: a prospective study. Scand J Gastroenterol. 1998;33:1130–4.

51. Bohnacker S, Brand B, Porthun M et al. Endoscopic therapy for Barrett's esophagus argon plasma coagulation (APC). Endoscopy. 1997;29:E10.
52. Martin WR, Benz C, Jakobs R et al. Argon plasma coagulation (APC) in patients with Barrett's esophagus. Gastroenterology. 1998;114:A217.
53. Gossner L, Sroka R, Ell C. A new long-range through-the-scope balloon applicator for photodynamic therapy in the esophagus and cardia. Endoscopy. 1999;31:370–6.
54. Barr H, Shepherd NA, Dix A et al. Eradication of high-grade dysplasia in columnar-lined (Barrett's) oesophagus by photodynamic therapy with endogenously generated protoporphyrin IX. Lancet. 1996;348:584–5.
55. Gossner L, Sroka R, Hahn EG, Ell C. Photodynamic therapy: successful destruction of gastrointestinal cancer after oral administration of aminolaevulinic acid. Gastrointest Endosc. 1995;41:55–8.
56. Gossner L, Stolte M, Sroka R et al. Photodynamic ablation of high-grade dysplasia and early cancer in Barrett's esophagus by means of 5-aminolevulinic acid. Gastroenterology. 1998;114:448–55.
57. Laukka MA, Wang KK, Cameron AJ, Alexander GL. The use of photodynamic therapy in the treatment of Barrett's esophagus. Gastrointest Endosc. 1993;39:A291.
58. Laukka MA, Wang KK. Initial results using low-dose photodynamic therapy in the treatment of Barrett's esophagus. Gastrointest Endosc. 1995;42:59–63.
59. Overholt BF, Panjehpour M. Photodynamic therapy for Barrett's esophagus: clinical update. Am J Gastroenterol. 1996;91:1719–23.
60. Kennedy JC, Pottier RH. Endogenous porphyrin IX, a clinically useful photosensitizer for photodynamic therapy. J Photochem Photobiol. 1992;14:275–92.
61. Barham OP, Jonas RL, Biddlestone LR et al. Photothermal laser ablation of Barrett's oesophagus: endoscopic and histological evidence of squamous re-epithelialization. Gut. 1997;41:281–4.
62. Gossner L, May A, Stolte M, Seitz G, Ell C. KTP-laser destruction of dysplasia and early cancer in columnar-lined Barrett's esophagus. Gastrointest Endosc. 1999;49:8–12.
63. Biddlestone LR, Barham CP, Wilkinson SP, Barr H, Shepherd NA. The histopathology of treated Barrett's esophagus. Squamous reepithelialization after acid suppression and laser and photodynamic therapy. Am J Surg Pathol. 1998;22:239–45.
64. Sampliner RE, Hixon LJ, Fennerty MB, Garewal HS. Regression of Barrett's esophagus by laser ablation in an anacid environment. Dig Dis Sci. 1993;38:365–8.
65. Salo JA, Salminen JT, Kiviluto TA et al. Treatment of Barrett's esophagus by endoscopic laser ablation and antireflux surgery. Ann Surg. 1998;227:40–4.
66. Brandt LJ, Kauvar CR. Laser-induced transient regression of Barrett's epithelium. Gastrointest Endosc. 1992;38:619–22.
67. Brandt LJ, Blansky RL, Kauvar DR. Repeat laser therapy of recurrent Barrett's epithelium: success with anacidity. Gastrointest Endosc. 1995;41:267 (letter).
68. Ertan A, Zimmerman M, Younes M. Esophageal adenocarcinoma associated with Barrett's esophagus: long-term management with laser ablation. Am J Gastroenterol. 1995;90:2201–3.
69. Luman W, Lessels AM, Palmer KR. Failure of Nd:YAG photocoagulation therapy as treatment of Barrett's esophagus: a pilot study. Ann Surg. 1998;227:40–4.
70. Sampliner RE, Fennerty MB, Garewal HS. Reversal of Barrett's esophagus with acid suppression and multipolar electrocoagulation: preliminary results. Gastrointest Endosc. 1996;44:523–5.
71. Kovacs BJ, Chen YK, Lewis TD, DeGuzman LJ, Thompson KS. Successful reversal of Barrett's esophagus with multipolar electrocoagulation despite inadequate acid suppression. Gastrointest Endosc. 1999;49:547–53.
72. Sharma P, Bhattacharyya A, Garewal HS, Sampliner RE. Durability of new squamous epithelium after endoscopic reversal of Barrett's esophagus. Gastrointest Endosc. 1999;50:159–64.
73. Montes CG, Brandalise NA, Deliza R, Novais de Magalhaes AF, Ferraz JG. Antireflux surgery followed by bipolar electrocoagulation in the treatment of Barrett's esophagus. Gastrointest Endosc. 1999;50:173–7.
74. Hölscher AH, Bollschweiler E, Schröder W, Gutschow C, Siewert JR. Prognostic differences between early squamous cell and adenocarcinoma of the esophagus. Dig Esophagus. 1997;10:179–84.

75. Heitmiller RF, Redmond M, Hamilton SR. Barrett's esophagus with high-grade dysplasia: an indication for prophylactic esophagectomy. Ann Surg. 1996;224:66–71.
76. Hölscher AH, Bollschweiler E, Schneider PM, Siewert JR. Early adenocarcinoma in Barrett's esophagus. Br J Surg. 1997;84:1470–3.
77. Soehendra N, Binmoeller KF, Bohnacker S et al. Endoscopic snare mucosectomy in the esophagus without any additional equipment: a simple technique for resection of flat early cancer. Endoscopy. 1997;29:380–3.
78. Takeshita K, Inoue H, Saeki I et al. Endoscopic treatment of early oesophageal or gastric cancer. Gut. 1997;40:123–7.
79. Ell C, May A, Gossner L et al. Endoscopic mucosal resection of early cancer and high-grade dysplasia in Barrett's esophagus. Gastroenterology. 2000;118:670–7.
80. Overholt BF, Panjehpour M, Haydek JM. Photodynamic therapy for Barrett's esophagus: follow-up in 100 patients. Gastrointest Endosc. 1999;49:1–7.
81. Loh CS, Mac Robert AJ, Bedwell J, Regula J, Krasner N, Bown SG. Oral versus intravenous administration of 5-aminolaevulinic acid for photodynamic therapy. Br J Cancer. 1993;68:41–51.
82. Loh CS, MacRobert AJ, Krasner N, Bown SG. Mucosal ablation using photodynamic therapy for the treatment of dysplasia: an experimental study in the normal rat stomach. Gut. 1996;38;71–8.
83. Ell C, Gossner L. Photodynamic therapy and its potential for the treatment of gastrointestinal malignancies and precancerous conditions. Endoscopy. 1994;26:262–3.
84. Ell C, Gossner L, May A et al. Photodynamic ablation of early cancers of the stomach by means of mTHPC and laser irradiation. Gut. 1998;43:345–9.
85. May A, Gossner L, Günter E, Stolte M, Ell C. Local treatment of early cancer in short Barrett's esophagus by means of argon plasma coagulation: initial experience. Endoscopy. 1999;31:497–500.

3
Selective COX-2 inhibitors – safety and side-effects

C. J. HAWKEY

INTRODUCTION

Aspirin was introduced over 100 years ago in an attempt to produce a better version of sodium salicylate that caused less dyspepsia[1]. This was achieved by acetylation of sodium salicylate, an approach that subsequently was shown to have rendered it capable of inhibiting prostaglandin synthesis[2]. Indications for aspirin developed rapidly, and its use in rheumatic fever led to concerns that it might cause the heart failure of rheumatic fever that in fact reflected the underlying disease. Consequently, early advertisements stressed that aspirin 'does not affect the heart1'! (Figure 1).

In 1938 Douthwaite and Lintot published the first report showing that aspirin could damage the stomach[3] (Figure 2). They used rigid endoscopy to study the acute affects of aspirin and painted water colours of the gastric erosions that they saw.

MODE OF ACTION OF ASPIRIN

It was not until 1971 that a successful unifying theory for the mode of action of aspirin was published[2]. John Vane produced evidence that aspirin was capable of inhibiting prostaglandin synthesis, and postulated that reduced prostaglandin production underlay both the efficacy in the joint and toxicity in the stomach of this drug[2]. It is now known that aspirin binds irreversibly to serine at the 516 position and thereby blocks entry of precursor arachidonic acid into the cyclooxygenase channel[3] (Figure 3). The duration of aspirin's actions varies from cell to cell and, because of its irreversible binding, is dependent upon the synthesis of new protein. In the case of platelets the duration of action is of the order of a week, because platelets do not synthesize new protein, and new platelets without cyclooxygenase inhibition arise only by the generation of new platelets. A neglected area is the question of how much other tissues vary in the turnover of cyclooxygenase.

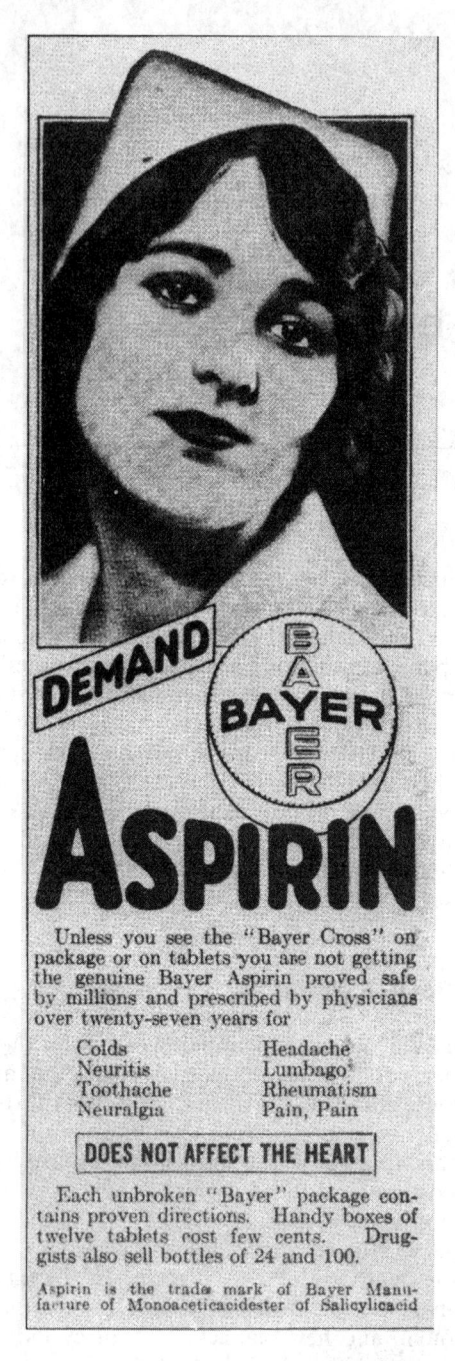

Figure 1 Early advertisement for aspirin. Today the claim 'Does not affect the heart' would not be made (Permission ref. 1)

SELECTIVE COX-2 INHIBITORS

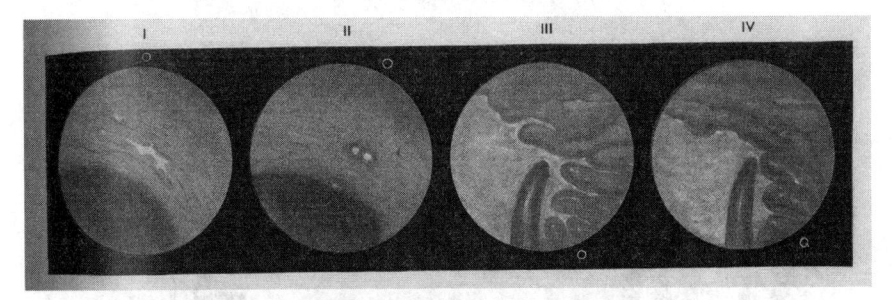

Figure 2 Effect of aspirin and other substances on the stomach (Permission ref. 3)

NON-ASPIRIN NSAIDs

Before the mode of action had been discovered the increasingly recognized gastrotoxicity of aspirin led to pressure for new non-aspirin drugs known as non-steroidal anti-inflammatory drugs (NSAIDs). Early examples included indomethacin, phenybutazone and ibuprofen, followed by diclofenac and naproxen, and into later azapropazone and piroxicam. These developments were largely driven pragmatically. Perhaps not surprisingly NSAIDs were found to have similar gastrotoxicity to aspirin, despite initial hopes to the contrary. The demonstration that they, like aspirin, inhibited prostaglandin synthesis, provided an explanation of their efficacy and this toxicity.

MODE OF ACTION OF NSAIDs

NSAIDs differ from aspirin in their mode of action in one critical way. Instead of binding to serine they bind to arginine at position 120 (Figure 3). Although the site of binding is the same the consequence is similar, with blockade of the entry of arachidonic acid into the cyclooxygenase channel. In contrast to aspirin, binding is reversible, so that the duration of action is much more closely related to drug pharmacokinetics.

IMPORTANCE OF NSAID ULCERS

Endoscopic studies have shown that an extraordinarily high proportion of patients taking NSAIDs (about 20%) have ulcers at any one time[4]. However, NSAIDs are associated with ulcer complications in about 1% or less of patients per annum, and in a causal way in perhaps 0.5%[5]. Based on odds ratio or relative risk, NSAIDs enhance the risk of ulcer complications by about 4-fold[5]. Others have suggested a larger proportion of ulcer complications are associated with NSAIDs, but these calculations are suspect[5]. Even on conservative estimates, if NSAID/aspirin is overall assumed to be fairly uniform throughout the world, it is plausible that they cause more than 100 000 ulcer deaths per annum worldwide.

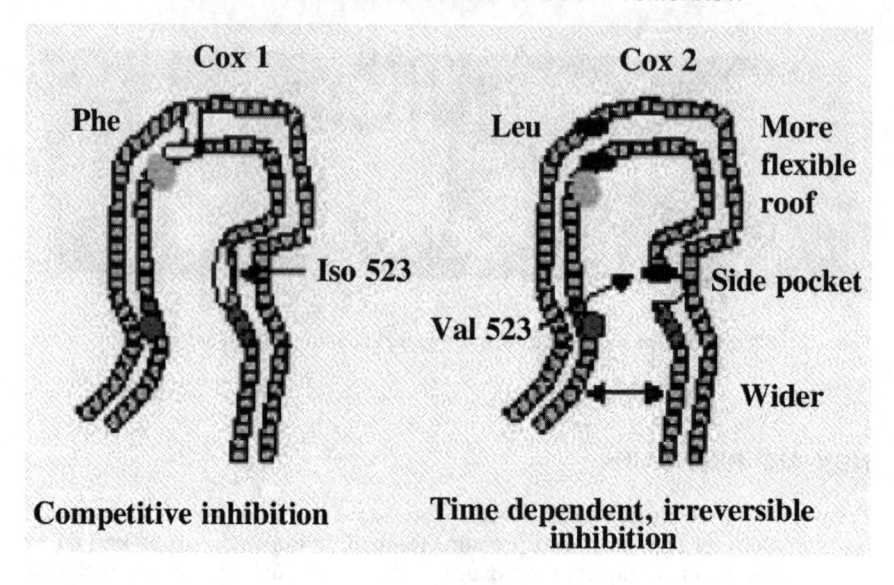

Figure 3 Important differences between COX-1 and COX-2

NSAIDs AND HYPERTENSION: THE NEGLECTED HAZARD

Such has been the concern regarding the gastric toxicity of NSAIDs that other, albeit recognized, side-effects have received less attention. In particular, NSAIDs have long been known to enhance hypertension, and meta-analyses in the 1990s suggest that, on average, NSAIDs may increase mean arterial blood pressure by 3–5 mm[6]. Data from the Framingham study can be used to calculate that, if untreated, this might over 10 years represent 6000 ischaemic/thrombotic cardiovascular events per annum[5]. In addition hypertension predisposed to heart failure, and two studies have shown directly that heart failure is more common in patients on NSAIDs than in controls who do not take the drugs[7]

DIRECT EVIDENCE ON NSAIDs AND MYOCARDIAL INFARCTION

The data on whether non-selective NSAIDs affect the risk of myocardial infarction are unclear. For reasons that are discussed below, naproxen may be a special case that, by different mechanisms, mimics the anti-platelet effects of aspirin. In general, epidemiological studies of the association between non-naproxen non-aspirin NSAIDs and myocardial infarction (or between all NSAIDs and myocardial infarction where naproxen use is uncommon) have suggested either no effect or a small but often non-significant increase in risk[8–16].

EFFECT OF NAPROXEN

Naproxen has a long half-life and in commonly used doses is very potent at inhibiting platelet thromboxane and platelet aggregation[17]. At normally used doses, even though naproxen is a reversible inhibitor, its potency on platelets and duration of action mean that its effect on platelets equals, or conceivably exceeds, those of aspirin. Since it is almost certainly true that the antithrombotic effects of aspirin are related to its ability to inhibit platelet thromboxane and aggregation, it would be surprising if this were not translated into an antithrombotic effect of naproxen. Several studies have shown this[9-11], whilst others have not[12-14]. Until recently (see below) there was no study suggesting enhanced risk of myocardial infarction with naproxen, and an overall assessment of the data would suggest a reduction in event rate of about 15-20% with naproxen[18], quite comparable to that seen with aspirin. Pharmacokinetic data suggest that NSAIDs might compete with aspirin for occupancy of the cyclooxygenase enzyme and thereby prevent its long-lasting effect on platelets[19]. Clinical studies have tended to suggest an increased incidence of myocardial infarction in aspirin users also taking an NSAID, but whether this is a direct effect of the NSAID, or interference with the effect of aspirin, is not known[20-22].

COX-2 INHIBITORS

The failure to produce a new super-aspirin with non-selective NSAIDs meant that the discovery that there were two cyclooxygenase enzymes was therapeutically very tempting[23]. It was convincingly demonstrated that COX-1 was a largely constitutive enzyme that is normally the dominant source of prostaglandins in the stomach[24,25], whilst COX-2 is expressed at sites of inflammation and in malignancy to become the dominant source of prostaglandins in these situations. Thus, COX-2 inhibitors should provide true mechanism-based anti-arthritis, analgesic and anti-inflammatory effects, whilst having little damaging potential for the normal stomach.

The mechanistic basis of currently available COX-2 inhibitors has been discovered[23]. Whilst COX-2 is extremely similar to COX-1 there are critical differences. It is similar in possessing arginine at position 120, which explains why non-selective drugs bind to and affect both COX-1 and COX-2. However, the COX-2 channel is wider than the COX-1 channel and, because of a valine for isoleucine substitution at position 523, there is a defect in the wall of COX-2 that provides a potential binding site. COX-2 inhibitors are bulkier drugs than COX-1 inhibitors and are able to access the COX-2 channel where they bind to this side-pocket. In contrast they are too large to enter the narrower COX-1 channel and hence biochemical cell activity is achieved.

In human studies COX-2 inhibitors have been shown to be highly selective in model systems and to spare prostaglandin synthesis in normal gastric mucosa[24,25]. An impressive set of acute studies has shown that there is no enhancement of acute injury compared to placebo, and a great reduction compared to non-selective NSAIDs[4,24,25]. Endoscopic studies over 3-6 months in patients have been reasonably consistent in suggesting a 4-fold reduction in the incidence of ulcers compared to non-selective NSAIDs[4,26,27]. In many, but not all, studies the ulcer incidence has been the same as on placebo. These data are therefore largely but not entirely compatible with the suggestion that the effects of COX-2 inhibitors on the stomach are comparable to those of non-use.

EFFECTS OF NSAIDs IN THE LOWER BOWEL

It has been known for a long time that NSAID use is associated with an increased risk of small bowel ulcers protected by entroscopy or at post-mortem[28,29], and one study suggested a 2–3-fold increase in the risk of small or large bowel perforation[20]. Studies with capsule endoscopy are starting to confirm that lesions are more common in small bowel on NSAIDs than on placebo[31], implying that NSAIDs could cause chronic ill-health by enhancing chronic blood loss and acute danger by predisposing to perforation and bleeding. Such studies have also suggested a lower rate of ulcers on selective COX-2 inhibitors compared, for example, to non-selective NSAIDs with proton pump inhibitor gastric protection[32].

OUTCOME STUDIES: VIGOR AND CLASS

Because COX-2 inhibitors were principally developed to reduce the risk of life-threatening ulcer complications it was important to study this directly. The VIGOR study of rofecoxib vs naproxen randomized approximately 8000 patients to naproxen 500 mg b.d. or rofecoxib 50 mg daily[33]. A supratherapeutic dose of rofecoxib was used to ensure the gastrointestinal findings were robust, and not just a consequence of using an ineffective dose. This study confirmed a reduction in clinically significant ulcers (primary endpoint) and serious events on rofecoxib compared to naproxen, although the reduction was in the 50–60% range rather than 4-fold (Figure 4a). Similar data on celecoxib are hard to interpret because only 6 months of data were originally published, although the study lasted over 1 year for some patients[34]. The 6-month data showed a trend towards reduction, whilst longer-term data did not; however, it is quite likely that this failure reflected trial design. Aspirin was taken by 20% of patients in this study and its effects may have masked the benefits of celecoxib compared to NSAIDs.

COX-2 INHIBITORS AND HYPERTENSION

Because sodium rejection is much more dependent on COX-2 than COX-1 it could be predicted that COX-2 inhibitors would replicate the effects of NSAIDs on sodium balance and blood pressure. Careful studies have shown there is a net sodium retention in the first 2 days of use with non-selective NSAIDs such as naproxen and selective COX-2 inhibitors such as rofecoxib

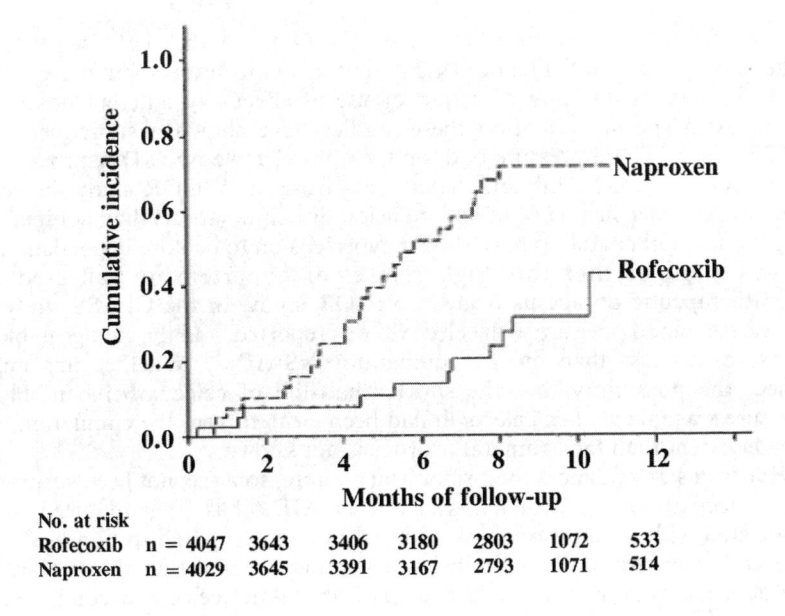

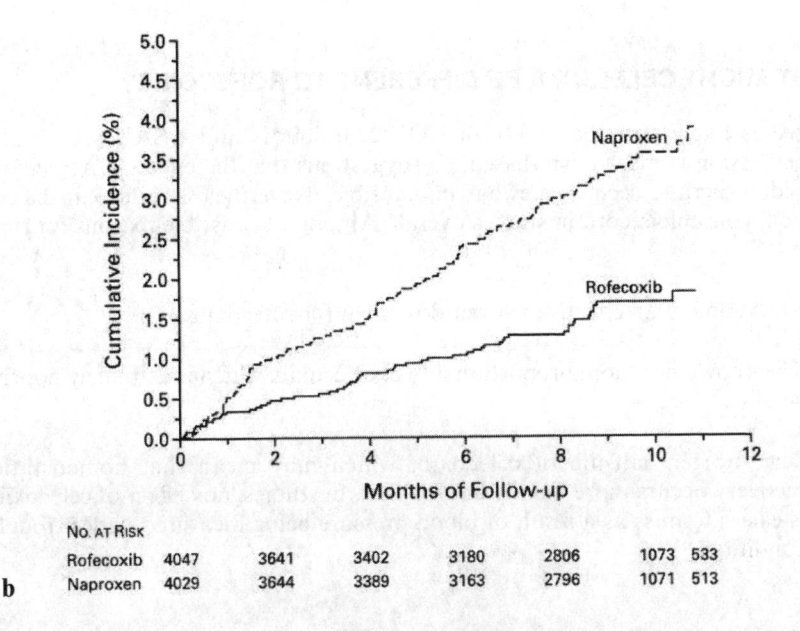

SELECTIVE COX-2 INHIBITORS

Figure 4 (a) Time to serious lower gastrointestinal clinical events in the naproxen and rofecoxib treatment group (incidence expressed as rate of events per 100 patient-years). (b) Cumulative incidence of the primary endpoint of a confirmed upper gastrointestinal event among all randomized patients (Permission ref. 37)

(25 mg daily) or celecoxib (200 mg b.d.)[35]. Other studies have suggested a difference between individual COX-2 inhibitors in this respect, but it is possible that this reflects duration of action or use of effectively different doses[36,37]. Along with sodium retention these studies have shown a subsequent 3–5 mmHg rise in blood pressure both on the non-selective NSAID naproxen and the selective COX-2 inhibitors. Safety data from the VIGOR study showed a somewhat higher incidence of hypertension discontinuations than comparator naproxen[33]. Other studies have shown hypertension to be dose-dependent, and it was thought that this higher level of hypertension reflected the supratherapeutic dosage used in the VIGOR study. In the CLASS study no increase in blood pressure with celecoxib was reported, and the change in blood pressure was less than on the comparator NSAIDs[34]. Whether this might reflect the possibility that the shorter half-life of celecoxib meant blood pressure was taken when celecoxib had been cleared from the circulation to a greater extent than the comparator drugs is not known.

Hypertension enhances the risk of heart failure, so it has not been surprising that rofecoxib, along with non-selective NSAIDs, has been reported to be associated with an increased risk of heart failure compared to non-use[8,9]. In one study there was a slight but insignificant increase in the unadjusted but not the adjusted risk of heart failure in patients taking celecoxib compared to reference[9].

WHY MIGHT CELECOXIB BE DIFFERENT TO ROFECOXIB?

It seems likely that the ability of COX-2 inhibitors and NSAIDs to cause hypertension is mechanism-based, so suggestions that the effects of rofecoxib are idiosyncratic seem somewhat implausible. Nevertheless, celecoxib has a more favourable record in studies overall. Among the possible reasons for this are:

1. Marketing of an effectively lower dose than for rofecoxib.

2. The known non-dose proportionality of celecoxib, which is extremely poorly soluble.

3. The shorter half-life of celecoxib, which may mean that homeostatic recovery occurs more readily and/or that, in studies, any effect of celecoxib is easier to miss as a result of blood pressure being measured under trough conditions.

NSAIDs, COX-2 INHIBITORS AND THE CARDIOVASCULAR SYSTEM

From the outset it was recognized that there were important questions to be asked about COX-2 inhibitors and vascular thrombosis[23]. Initially it was believed that most vascular prostacyclin derived from COX-1 in endothelial cells, making the effects of NSAIDs which would inhibit both this and platelet thromboxane difficult to predict. It seemed more likely that the direct effects of a COX-2 inhibitor would be neutral because both platelet thromboxane and COX-1-dependent endothelial prostacyclin would be unaffected. In addition, COX-2 overexpression in plaques was recognized, and thought possibly to play a role in plaque rupture, making it possible that COX-2 inhibitors might even be protective against cardiovascular disease. Thinking changed with the publication of data that suggested that whole-body production of prostacyclin, as measured by urinary metabolites, was more dependent on COX-2 than COX-1 (about 70% of the total)[20].

This shift in thinking about the biochemistry was paralleled by a shift in the evidence. Initial studies had been very encouraging[38–40], with a reduction in mortality from cardiovascular events on rofecoxib compared to ibuprofen in phase III studies that was large enough to have been 'statistically significant' if analysed[38]. However, in the VIGOR study there was a significant increase in cardiovascular events, and in particular in myocardial infarction (17 vs 5)[33] (Figure 4b). This provoked discussion about possible mechanisms, and the following were favoured.

1. A prothrombotic effect of rofecoxib (that may have reflected a supratherapeutic dose used).

2. The effect of the comparator naproxen.

3. The play of chance.

4. The consequences of hypertension.

5. Some combination of these.

The effect was too big to be due to chance, and was also greater than would be expected from what was known about the effect of naproxen on platelets[17]. The most widely held view was that the results of the VIGOR study represented a combination of an antithrombotic effect of naproxen and a prothrombotic effect of the supratherapeutic dose of rofecoxib. Epidemiological studies favoured this explanation by, on the whole, showing reduced myocardial infarction rates on naproxen and increased rates on rofecoxib only at supratherapeutic doses[12–14,16].

A belief that normal doses of rofecoxib posed no cardiovascular hazard contributed to a decision to compare the drug with placebo in the prevention of colorectal polyps, which are characterized by enhanced COX-2 expression. Such a study offered the opportunity to clarify once and for all the effect of rofecoxib by direct comparison with placebo (this is difficult to do in arthritis because of the need of patients for analgesia).

Data from the CLASS study are difficult to interpret because of small numbers, but there was not a significant decrease with celecoxib. Despite this, a number of authors who were convinced of the cardiotoxicity of COX-2 inhibitors published indirect data involving questionable comparisons between data from unrelated trials, suggesting possible differences.

RECENT DEVELOPMENTS

The initial concerns about cardiovascular safety of COX-2 inhibitors led the European Medicines Agency to review them. In 2003 the Agency declared itself broadly satisfied, and re-approved the use of COX-2 inhibitors. However, on 30 September 2004 Merck suddenly announced the withdrawal of rofecoxib because of unfavourable ongoing results from the APPROVe study that was terminated prematurely[41,42]. After a total of 2586 patients had been entered into the study, and accrued 6356 patients of exposure to rofecoxib 25 mg or placebo, there were 45 myocardial infarctions on rofecoxib compared to 25 on placebo. In absolute terms this was an increase in myocardial infarctions per 100 patient-years of approximately 0.75 to 1.5 events per 100 patient-years. No difference between the drugs appeared evident until after 18 months, leading some to conclude it was a consequence of long-term use. Pfizer took out major advertisements declaring celecoxib was different from rofecoxib, and safe and effective. An ongoing polyp study on celecoxib vs placebo, sponsored by industry, was immediately re-viewed by the Data Safety Monitoring Committee, who declared no reason to stop the trial, but the FDA terminated a similar agency-sponsored trial[43]. It was already known that paracoxib, the pro-drug for valdecoxib, had been associated with increased events when used after coronary artery bypass grafting, and Pfizer released the results of a second similar study that also showed a similar trend[44,45].

During the fallout from the withdrawal of rofecoxib several interesting but confusing results were reported; for example, a reported increase of myocardial infarction in patients who stopped NSAIDs[46], and a counterintuitive increase also in those taking naproxen[47].

LUMIRACOXIB AND THE TARGET STUDY

Lumiracoxib is a novel COX-2 inhibitor that has a different structure to existing COX-2 inhibitors. Potentially favourable characteristics of lumiracoxib are a short half-life, an acidic nature that might encourage accumulation at the sites of inflammation whilst allowing rapid clearance from the circulation, and the lack of a sulphur group. Lumiracoxib has been shown to be similar to other COX-2 inhibitors in having a clean safety profile in endoscopic studies[26,27]. Because of the concern over the cardiovascular safety of rofecoxib a large outcome study (the TARGET study with approximately 18 500 patients) was instituted and compared lumiracoxib both with naproxen and with ibuprofen[48–50]. Whilst the primary outcome of lumiracoxib was gastroduodenal, the choice of the two NSAIDs was based on the hope that this would help to distinguish a harmful effect of a COX-2 inhibitor and a beneficial effect of naproxen. The TARGET study was impressive in showing a 4–6-fold reduction in ulcer complication compared to naproxen or ibuprofen respectively (Figure 5a). Cardiovascular events were numerically lower on lumiracoxib compared to ibuprofen, and numerically higher on lumiracoxib compared to naproxen (Figure 5b); compatible with, but certainly not proof of, the hypothesis that benefits of naproxen were a major factor. Lumiracoxib also had significantly less effect on blood pressure than the comparators.

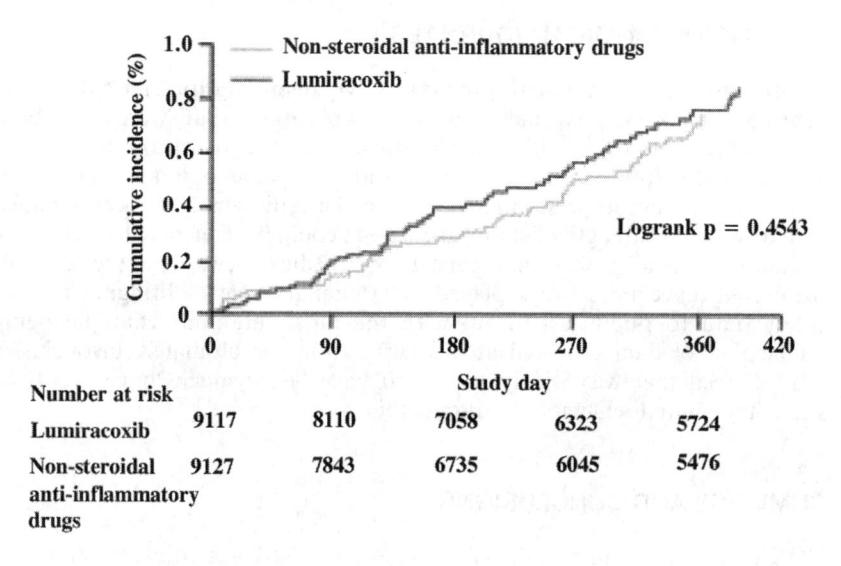

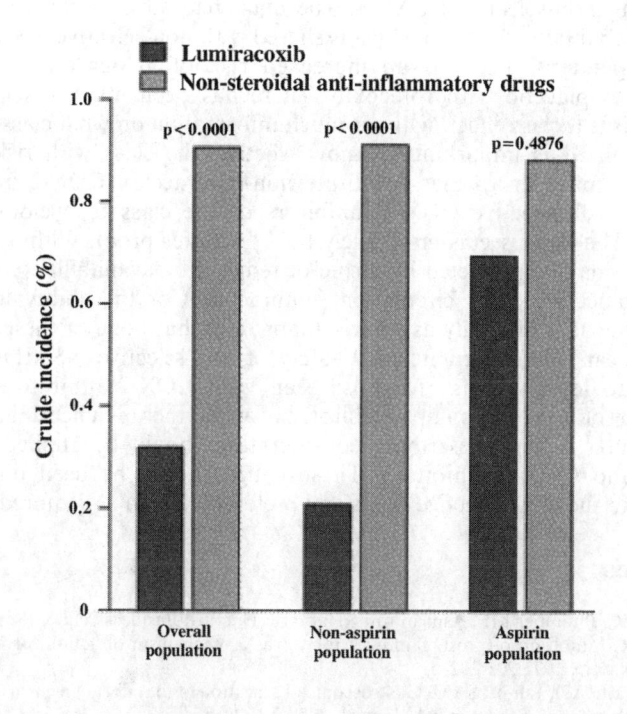

Figure 5 (a) Incidence of APTC composite endpoint for cardiovascular events. (b) Definite or probable upper gastrointestinal ulcer complications in all study populations (Permission ref. 50)

ROLE OF THE MEDICAL JOURNALS

Comments in the medical journals have been highly critical of the pharmaceutical industry, and there were implications that Merck had been concealing data[51,52]. This seems unlikely, since it would have been commercially unwise to conduct a study vs placebo if an increase in cardiovascular events was anticipated, and the criticisms have been rebuffed by industry. The strength of editorial criticism could be interpreted as reflecting a desire to make, rather than report, the medical news, and the journals themselves have not always played an exemplary role in bringing reliable safety data to public attention, with the most infamous example being publication of data censored at 6 months from the ultimately inconclusive CLASS trial that was widely known to have lasted much longer, and the subsequent initial reluctance to discuss this[34]

SUMMARY AND CONCLUSIONS

COX-2 inhibitors undoubtedly possess increased gastrointestinal safety compared to non-selective NSAIDs. The main real adverse effect is sodium retention (renal failure is rare) which is shared with non-selective NSAIDs and is dose-dependent. There is an increased risk of myocardial infarction compared to placebo with rofecoxib. There has been much discussion of whether this is a class effect, without much information on what class is under consideration. It is important to know whether the class with risks is the chemically similar drugs that constitute non-lumiracoxib COX-2 inhibitors, the class of all selective COX-2 inhibitors or the class of cyclooxygenase inhibitors. The latter seems most likely but it requires proof. Within the class some drugs may be protected by virtue of reduced bioavailability (celecoxib), rapid clearance from the circulation (lumiracoxib) or the ability to inhibit thromboxane as profoundly as aspirin (naproxen), but none of these issues is currently clear. The gastrointestinal safety of non-selective NSAIDs can be approved to levels similar to those seen with COX-2 inhibitors by co-prescription of a proton pump inhibitor, but while there is uncertainty about cardiovascular safety, prescribing consideration should be applied to both NSAIDs and COX-2 inhibitors. These drugs should be used only when necessary, in the most effective doses and preferably on an as-required basis.

References

1. Mann CC, Plummer ML. Aspirin wars. Harvard: Harvard Business School Press, 1991.
2. Vane JR. Inhibition of prostaglandin synthesis as a mechanism of action for aspirin-like drugs. Nature. 1971;231:232–5.
3. Douthwaite AH, Lintott SAM. Gastroscopic observation of the effect of aspirin and certain other substances on the stomach. Lancet. 1938;2:1222–5.
4. Hawkey CJ. Nonsteriodal anti-inflammatory drug gastropathy. Gastroenterology. 2000;119:521–35.
5. Hawkey CJ, Langman MJ. Non-steroidal anti-inflammatory drugs: overall risks and management – complementary roles for COX-2 inhibitors and proton pump inhibitors. Gut. 2003;52:600–8.

6. Johnson AG, Nguyen TV, Day RO. Do nonsteroidal anti-inflammatory drugs affect blood pressure? A meta-analysis [see comment]. Ann Intern Med. 1994;121:289–300
7. Mamdani M, Juurlink DN, Lee DS et al. Cyclo-oxygenase-2 inhibitors versus non-selective non-steroidal anti-inflammatory drugs and congestive heart failure outcomes in elderly patients: a population-based cohort study. Lancet. 2004;363:1751–6.
8. Garcia Rodriguez LA. Varas C. Patrono C. Differential effects of aspirin and non-aspirin nonsteroidal antiinflammatory drugs in the primary prevention of myocardial infarction in postmenopausal women [see comment]. Epidemiology. 2000;11:382–7.
9. Solomon DH, Glynn RJ, Levin R et al. Nonsteroidal anti-inflammatory drug use and acute myocardial infarction. Arch Intern Med. 2002;162:1099–104
10. Rahme E, Pilote L, LeLorier J. Association between naproxen use and protection against acute myocardial infarction. Arch Intern Med. 2002;162:1111—15.
11. Watson DJ, Rhodes T, Cai B, Guess HA. Lower risk of thromboembolic cardiovascular events with naproxen among patients with rheumatoid arthritis. Arch Intern Med. 2002;162:1105–10.
12. Ray WA, Stein CM, Hall K, Daugherty JR, Griffin MR. Non-steroidal anti-inflammatory drugs and risk of serious coronary heart disease: an observational cohort study [see comment]. Lancet. 359:118–23.
13. Mamdani M, Rochon P, Juurlink DN et al. Effect of selective cyclooxygenase 2 inhibitors and naproxen on short-term risk of acute myocardial infarction in the elderly. Arch Intern Med. 2003;163:481–6.
14. Solomon DH, Schneeweiss S, Glynn RJ et al. Relationship between selective cyclooxygenase-2 inhibitors and acute myocardial infarction in older adults [see comment]. Circulation. 2004;109:2068–73.
15. Garcia Rodriguez LA, Varas-Lorenzo C, Maguire A, Gonzalez-Perez A. Nonsteroidal antiinflammatory drugs and the risk of myocardial infarction in the general population. Circulation. 2004;109:3000–6.
16. Graham DJ, Campen D, Hui R et al. Risk of acute myocardial infarction and sudden cardiac death in patients treated with cyclo-oxygenase 2 selective and non-selective non-steroidal anti-inflammatory drugs: nested case–control study. Lancet. 2005;365:475–81.
17. Capone ML, Tacconelli S, Sciulli MG et al. Clinical pharmacology of platelet, monocyte, and vascular cyclooxygenase inhibition by naproxen and low-dose aspirin in healthy subjects. Circulation. 2004;109:1468–71.
18. Jüni P, Nartey L, Reichenback S, Sterchi R, Dieppe PA, Effer M. Risk of cardiovascular events and rofecoxib: cumulative meta-analysis. Lancet. 2004;364:2021–9.
19. Catella-Lawson F, Reilly MP, Kapoor SC et al. Cyclooxygenase inhibitors and the antiplatelet effects of aspirin. N Engl J Med. 2001;345:1809–17.
20. MacDonald TM, Wei L. Effect of ibuprofen on cardioprotective effect of aspirin. Lancet. 2003;361:573–4.
21. Kurth T, Glynn RJ, Walker AM et al. Inhibition of clinical benefits of aspirin on first myocardial infarction by nonsteroidal antiinflammatory drugs. Circulation. 2003;108:1191–5.
22. Patel TN, Goldberg KC. Use of aspirin and ibuprofen compared with aspirin alone and the risk of myocardial infarction. Arch Intern Med. 2004;164:852–6.
23. Hawkey CJ. COX-2 inhibitors. Lancet. 1999;353:307–14.
24. Wight NJ, Gottesdiener K, Garlick NM et al. Rofecoxib, a COX-2 inhibitor, does not inhibit human gastric mucosal prostaglandin production. Gastroenterology. 2001;120:867–73.
25. Atherton C, Jones J, McKaig B et al. Pharmacology and gastrointestinal satefysafety of lumiracoxib, a novel cyclooxygenase-2 selective inhibitor. An integrated study. Clin Gastroenterol Hepatol. 2004;2:113–20.
26. Hawkey CJ, Simon T, Beaulieu A et al. for the Rofecoxib Osteoarthritis Endoscopy Multinational Study Group. Comparison of the effect of rofecoxib (a cyclooxygenase 2 specific inhibitor), ibuprofen, and placebo on the gastroduodenal mucosa of patients with osteoarthritis. Arthritis Rheum. 2000;43:370–7.
27. Hawkey CJ. Gastrointestinal tolerability of lumiracoxib in patients with osteoarthritis and rheumatoid arthritis. Clin Gastrohepatol. 2005 (In press).

28. EnteroscopyBjarnason I, Hayllar J, MacPherson AJ, Russell AS. Side effects of non-steroidal anti-inflammatory drugs on the small and large intestine in humans. Gastroenterology. 1993;104:1832–47.
29. PMAllison MC, Howatson AG, Torrance CJ, Lee FD, Russell RI. Gastrointestinal damage associated with the use of non-steroidal anti-inflammatory drugs. N Engl J Med. 1992;327: 749–54.
30. WorralLangman MJ, Morgan L, Worrall A. Use of anti-inflammatory drugs by patients admitted with small or large bowel perforations and hemorrhage. Br Med J Clin Res. 1985;290:347–9.
31. Chutkan R, Toubia N. Effect of nonsteroidal anti-inflammatory drugs on the gastrointestinal tract: diagnosis by wireless capsule endoscopy. Gastrointest Endosc Clin N Am. 2004; 14:67–85.
32. Goldstein JL, Eisen G, Lewis B, Gralned I, Fort JG, lotnick S. Celecoxib is associated with fewer small bowel lesions than naproxen + omeprazole in healthy subjects as determined by capsule endoscopy. Gut. 2003;6(Suppl. A16).
33. Bombardier C, Laine L, Reicin A et al. VIGOR Study Group. Comparison of upper gastrointestinal toxicity of rofecoxib and naproxen in patients with rheumatoid arthritis. VIGOR Study Group. N Engl J Med. 2000;343:1520–8.
34. Silverstien FE, Faich G, Goldstein JL et al. Gastrointestinal toxicity with celecoxib vs non-steroidal anti-inflammatory drugs for osteoarthritis and rheumatoid arthritis: the CLASS study: a randomised controlled trial. J Am Med Assoc. 2000;284:1247–55.
35. Brune K, Hinz B. Selective cyclooxygenase-2 inhibitors: similarities and differences. Scand J Rheumatol. 2004;33:1–6.
36. Whelton A, Fort JG, Puma JA, Normandin D, Bello AE, Verburg KM. Cyclooxygenase-2-specific inhibitors and cardiorenal function: a randomised, controlled trial of celecoxib and rofecoxib in older hypertensive osteoarthritis patients. Am J Ther. 2001;8:85–95.
37. Whelton A, White WB, Bellow AE, Puma JA, Fort JG. Effects of celecoxib and rofecoxib on blood pressure and edema in patients $\geqslant 65$ years of age with systemic hypertension and osteoarthritis. Am J Cardiol 2002;90:959–63.
38. Daniels B, Seidenberg B. Cardiovascular safety profile of rofecoxib in controlled clinical trials. Arthritis Rheum. 1999:42Suppl. S143).
39. Weir MR, Sperling RS, Reicin A, Gertz BJ. Selective COX-2 inhibition and cardiovascular effects: a review of the rofecoxib development program. Am Heart J. 2003;146:591–604.
40. Reicin A, Shapiro D, Sperling RS, Barr E, Yu Q. Comparison of cardiovascular thrombotic events in patients with osteoarthritis treated with rofecoxib versus nonselective nonsteroidal anti-inflammatory drugs (ibuprofen, diclofenac, and nabumetone). Am J Cardiol. 2002;89:204–9.
41. http://www.vioxx.com/rofecoxib/vioxx/consumer/index.jsp. APPROVe.
42. Bresalier RS, Sandler RS, Quan H et al. Cardiovascular events associated with rofecoxib in a colorectal adenoma chemoprevention trial. N Engl J Med. 2005;352:1092–102.
43. Solomon SD, McMurray JJ, Pfeffer MA et al. Cardiovascular risk associated with celecoxib in a clinical trial for colorectal adenoma prevention. N Engl J Med. 2005;352:1071–80.
44. Ott E, Nussmeier NA, Duke PC et al., Multicenter Study of Perioperative Ischemia (McSPI) Research Group; Ischemia Research and Education Foundation (IREF) Investigators. Efficacy and safety of the cyclooxygenase 2 inhibitors parecoxib and valdecoxib in patients undergoing coronary artery bypass surgery. J Thorac Cardiovasc Surg. 2003;125:1481–92.
45. Nussmeier NA, Whelton AA, Brown MT et al. Complications of the COX-2 inhibitors parecoxib and valdecoxib after cardiac surgery. N Engl J Med. 2005;352:1081–91.
46. Fischer LM, Schlienger RG, Matter CM, Jick H, Meier CR. Discontinuation of nonsteroidal anti-inflammatory drug therapy and risk of acute myocardial infarction. Arch Intern Med. 2004;164:2472–6.
47. FDA statement on naproxen. (http://www.fda.gov/bbs/topics/news/2004/NEW01148.html.
48. Hawkey CJ, Farkouh M, Gitton X, Ehrsam E, Huels J, Richardson P. Therapeutic arthritis research and gastrointestinal event trial of lumiracoxib – study design and patient demographics. Aliment Pharmacol Ther. 2004;20:51–63.
49. Farkouh ME, Kirshner H, Harrington RA et al., TARGET Study Group. Comparison of lumiracoxib with naproxen and ibuprofen in the Therapeutic Arthritis Research and

Gastrointestinal Event Trial (TARGET), cardiovascular outcomes: randomised controlled trial. Lancet. 2004;364:675–84.
50. Schnitzer TJ, Burmester GR, Mysler E et al., TARGET Study Group. Comparison of lumiracoxib with naproxen and ibuprofen in the Therapeutic Arthritis Research and Gastrointestinal Event Trial (TARGET), reduction in ulcer complications: randomised controlled trial. Lancet. 2004;364:665–74.
51. Topol EJ. Failing the public health – rofecoxib, Merck, and the FDA. N Engl J Med. 2004;351:1707–9.
52. Dieppe PA, Ebrahim S, Martin RM, Juni P. Lessons from the withdrawal of rofecoxib [Editorial]. Br Med J. 2004;329:867–8.

Section II
Stomach

Chair: J. MÖSSNER and E.O. RIECKEN

4
Pathogenesis of peptic ulcer and distal gastric cancer

A. AXON

INTRODUCTION

Spiral organisms were recognized in the mammalian stomach at the end of the nineteenth century[1]. Towards the beginning of the twentieth century they were shown to have a pathogenic potential and to respond to chemotherapy[2]. Similar organisms were observed in the human stomach in the beginning of the 20th century and were rediscovered on a number of occasions; however, they were considered to be commensals. The first suggestion that they might be responsible for peptic ulcer was in 1975[3] when Steer and Colin-Jones drew attention to the gastritis that accompanied the infection and its association with peptic ulcer. This observation, however, was not followed up because the authors mistakenly believed the infecting organism to be *Pseudomonas* sp. In 1983[4] Marshall and Warren successfully cultured the organism known as *Helicobacter pylori*. They recognized the pathogenic potential of the bacterium and postulated a role for it in the development of gastritis, peptic ulcer and gastric cancer. Marshall subsequently went on to infect himself, causing a gastritis, and by confirming Koch's postulate that it is an infectious pathogen[5]. Work by others identified a bismuth and antibiotic combination that successfully eradicated the infection. This led to a number of prospective randomized studies proving conclusively that *H. pylori* was the underlying cause of both duodenal and gastric ulcer.

The hypothesis that *H. pylori* is the single critical factor necessary for the development of distal gastric cancer has been more difficult to prove because prospective randomized studies cannot be done in a condition with such a long evolution; however, a large amount of circumstantial evidence has accumulated, leaving no doubt that this organism is responsible for all but a small proportion of non-cardia gastric cancer.

HELICOBACTER-ASSOCIATED GASTRITIS

H. pylori is a Gram-negative, curved, flagellate organism that is able to colonize the gastric mucosa. The infection usually occurs during childhood, but the mode of transmission is unknown. A number of iatrogenic epidemics have arisen as a result of gastric intubation using inadequately disinfected gastric tubes, and this has enabled the natural history of the infection to be documented. Initial infection causes an acute dyspeptic illness comprising epigastric pain, nausea and mucusy vomit. During the initial illness there is an acute gastritis with polymorphonuclear infiltration and total achlorhydria. This gradually progresses to an acute on chronic infection with a gradual recovery of gastric acid secretion such that, in the majority of individuals, normal acid secretion is resumed within a year. In spite of the marked host inflammatory reaction the organism thrives within the mucus layer overlying the gastric epithelium, and this has led some workers to postulate that the inflammatory reaction is probably beneficial rather than harmful for the organism because it increases gastric permeability, thus providing more nutrition for the parasite. *H. pylori* is relatively acid-resistant because it produces a urease which breaks down gastric luminal urea to produce bicarbonate, thus creating a microenvironment of relative neutrality in spite of the presence of gastric acid. In spite of this, however, *H. pylori* is unable to proliferate at a low pH and this may account for why a more widespread gastritis is seen when host acid secretion is reduced. Its ability to colonize the acidic mammalian stomach gives it a survival advantage over other organisms less well adapted.

Over 50% of the world's population is chronically infected by *H. pylori*. The organism is closely applied to the apical membrane of the gastric mucus-secreting cell. Its presence stimulates the epithelial cell to produce cytokines[6] that attract inflammatory cells which initiate the inflammatory cascade. The epithelial cells themselves are disorganized and cuboidal. Treatment with a suitable antibiotic regimen eliminates the infection and returns the gastric mucosa to normal. Within a month the acute inflammation has disappeared, but the chronic inflammatory cell infiltration can take a year to dissipate. Long-continued *H. pylori* infection leads to destruction of the gastric epithelium, with atrophy and the development of intestinal metaplasia[7].

GASTRIC ULCER

Gastric acid is strongly conserved throughout the mammalian species. The internal lumen of the human stomach is maintained at an acidic pH throughout the 24 h. Some buffering occurs when food is ingested, but the thought of a meal, and the presence of nutrition within the stomach, stimulates a complex series of reflexes that cause rapid and maximal acid secretion by the gastric parietal cells that quickly returns the lumen to a strongly acid pH. The reason for this widespread acidity in different animal species is unclear, but it has probably evolved in order to protect the gastrointestinal tract from infection by ingested pathogens. The gastric epithelium has evolved to contain this acidic environment and with an ability to resist the destructive effects of the acid. A series of mechanisms described as 'cytoprotection' are present within the epithelium lining the luminal surface.

Superficial gastric epithelial cells secrete mucus which forms a thick layer separating the cell from the acid within the lumen of the stomach[8]; in addition they secrete a small amount of alkali that diffuses into the mucus layer. The effect of acid diffusing from the lumen into the mucus layer from one side is balanced by the alkali coming from the opposite direction, and this leads to a pH gradient of around 2 at the outer point of the gel mucus layer to 7.5 at the epithelial surface. In the event that this protection fails, causing the cells to be eroded, they have a remarkable ability to migrate from the gastric pits, and by changing shape to rapidly cover the eroded area. These mechanisms are dependent upon the anatomical integrity of the mucosal cell and the secretion of prostaglandins that enhance the cytoprotective properties of the cell.

A further protection intrinsic to the mucosal cell comprises the phospholipid membrane of the cell that provides a non-wettable or hydrophobic surface such that hydrophilic molecules have difficulty in achieving penetration. In the presence of *H. pylori* infection these mechanisms of cytoprotection fail[9]. Hydrophobicity is lost, mucus and alkaline secretion is reduced and cell migration impaired.

This collapse of the protective mechanism allows acid to erode and destroy the epithelial continuity, penetrating to the lamina propria submucosa and eventually to the muscularis propria itself. The mechanism can be reversed either by pharmacological suppression of gastric acid or treatment of the underlying infection that has undermined the cytoprotective mechanism.

Gastric ulcer may arise in individuals who are not infected by *H. pylori* but have some other inflammatory condition of the mucosa such as Crohn's disease. However, an increasing number of gastric ulcers are now caused by the prescription of non-selective, non-steroidal anti-inflammatory drugs which antagonize the action of cyclo-oxygenase I. The effect of this is to limit the secretion of prostaglandins, thereby impairing the cytoprotective mechanism.

DUODENAL ULCER

The epithelial lining of the duodenum is totally different from that of the stomach. The mucosa comprises an intestinal absorptive epithelium interspersed with goblet cells. Mucus is secreted by the Brunner's glands and goblet cells but, as with the stomach, the cells lining the surface of the duodenum secrete alkali. The pancreas produces bicarbonate which is secreted rapidly when the duodenum becomes acidified. The risk of acid attack is therefore less in the duodenum than in the stomach, where the pH is constantly acidic. Furthermore, *H. pylori* is not capable of colonizing intestinal epithelium; it can infect only gastric epithelial tissue. At first sight therefore it is surprising that duodenal ulceration became the predominant peptic ulcer of the mid-twentieth century.

To understand why duodenal ulcers occur it is necessary to understand something of the ecology of *H. pylori*. Although it is beautifully adapted to survive within an acidic environment, its preferred niche is the neutral slightly acid environment on the apical surface of the gastric epithelial cell. It is here that it is able to reproduce, and where it can gain sustenance from the nutrition that exudes from the underlying mucosa on which it stations itself. There is a wide range of acid secretion between different human subjects. Both basal acid secretion and maximal acid output vary substantially from one individual to another, and it appears that in those persons who have a high acid secretion *H. pylori* gastritis is limited to the antrum of the stomach (antral-predominant gastritis). In other persons who have a lower acid secretion the whole of the gastric mucosa may be inflamed. Once the pattern of gastritis has been established in the host it will tend to persist either as antral-predominant or corpus-predominant, and the reason for this is that an antral gastritis, for reasons that are unclear, affects the antral G and D cells which are responsible for the secretion of somatostatin and gastrin, and have the effect of causing increased acid secretion[10]. This has the effect of limiting the inflammation even more to the antrum and protecting the corpus. On the other hand if the corpus of the stomach becomes significantly inflamed the inflammatory reaction inhibits parietal cell secretion, thereby inducing further hypochlorhydria, and thus enhancing the corpus-predominant pattern. Long-continued inflammation of the corpus eventually leads to atrophy of the specialized acid-secreting epithelium in the corpus, giving rise to permanent hypochlorhydria and eventual achlorhydria in some cases.

It has been well recognized for many years that duodenal ulcer is associated with a high acid secretion. Those who develop it have a constitutional tendency to secrete more acid, and the antral-predominant gastritis affects gastrin secretion causing an even higher acid output. A high acid output itself affects the nature of the duodenal epithelium; it causes the epithelial lining to change from an intestinal type histology to a gastric morphology[11]; so-called 'gastric metaplasia'. This happens in patches and is often found in Zollinger Ellison syndrome, a well-recognized cause of a continuously high acid state; however, patients who have naturally high acid secretion also develop gastric metaplasia within the duodenal epithelium. Under these circumstances *H. pylori* is able to migrate to the duodenum and infect the patches of metaplastic gastric epithelium. Having done so an inflammatory reaction is induced, i.e. a 'gastritis' of the duodenum. This leads to failure of the cytoprotection mechanism, acid attack and ulceration.

GASTRIC CANCER

It was relatively simple to prove that peptic ulcer was a complication of *H. pylori* gastritis. Prospective, randomized studies clearly demonstrated that ulcers healed by eradication of *H. pylori* do not recur, while those treated by acid suppression alone usually returned within a year. No similar study is possible with gastric cancer. Nevertheless it was observed at an early stage that there was an association between *H. pylori* gastritis and gastric cancer, and convincing data have been obtained from nested studies.

Over the years serum has been saved (nested) from normal subjects and patients as a result of prospective research studies unrelated to *H. pylori*. More recently the sera have been unthawed and tested for *H. pylori* serology and the results compared with the outcome of the population studied. A meta-analysis[12] demonstrates that infection with *H. pylori* gives an odds ratio of 3.5 for developing cancer compared with control groups. These findings suggest that *H. pylori* may be responsible for a good deal of non-cardia gastric cancer. However, the odds ratio is insufficiently high to confirm that *H. pylori* is a necessary as opposed to a contributory factor for its development. An interesting subanalysis of this data, however, showed that serum taken more than 15 years before the analysis, as opposed to a shorter period, gave a higher odds ratio of 8, suggesting that *H. pylori* might have disappeared in a substantial proportion of those whose serum had been taken closer to the time when a cancer developed.

Gastric cancer usually arises on the background of gastric atrophy with extensive intestinal metaplasia; however, *H. pylori* does not thrive in this environment. Achlorhydria enables faecal-type intestinal bacteria to proliferate, thus creating an environment in which *Helicobacter* is less able to compete. Furthermore, the organism is capable of colonizing only gastric mucosal cells, not those that have undergone intestinal metaplasia. By the time the cancer has developed, therefore, *H. pylori* may have disappeared from the stomach, and the antibodies stimulated by its presence may also have declined.

It is now apparent that this is what had happened. A paper from Kikuchi et al. in 1995[13] described Japanese patients who had developed cancer under the age of 40; serology in these patients gave an odds ratio of 13, and when early gastric cancer was assessed the odds ratio rose to 21. A further important breakthrough was the discovery that, whereas standard ELISA serology declines rapidly after the disappearance of *H. pylori*, the antibody to CagA, a protein found in the more virulent *H. pylori* strains, remains in the blood for a longer period. Ekstrom et al.[14], in a serological study, showed that 96% of patients with cancer had at some time been infected with *H. pylori* compared with 57% of controls. This provided an odds ratio of 21, thus confirming the concept that infection with the organism confers roughly 20 times the risk of developing cancer compared with someone who is uninfected.

Further evidence to support the hypothesis that *H. pylori* is responsible for gastric cancer is the observation that Mongolian gerbils experimentally infected with this organism develop gastric cancer[15,16] and that early treatment of the infection will protect them[17].

It should be emphasized that these data relate only to patients with non-cardia gastric cancer. Cancer that arises within the cardia region of the stomach (the 5 mm or so of mucosa just below the gastro-oesophageal junction) is not associated with *H. pylori*.

It is not, however, the presence of *H. pylori* within the stomach that appears to be the immediate cause of cancer. As indicated earlier, cancer tends to develop only in those with extensive atrophy, achlorhydria and intestinal metaplasia. Indeed the disease often arises after the organism has disappeared. It seems that it is the destruction of the corpus mucosa that predisposes to the development of neoplasia. A prospective study of 1526 patients[18] has shown that those with antral-predominant gastritis do not have an increased risk of cancer compared with a 16 times increased risk for those with pan-gastritis and a 35 times increase for those with corpus-predominant gastritis. These data also confirm an observation recognized for many years, which is that patients with duodenal ulcer (a condition associated with a high gastric acid secretion and an antral-predominant gastritis) are relatively protected from developing gastric cancer, while those who have the predilection for gastric ulcer (relative hypochlorhydria and a pan-gastritis) are the ones who are more likely to develop cancer.

The implication is that it is not *H. pylori* that directly causes cancer. If that was so one would expect individuals with antral-predominant gastritis to develop antral cancer. This does not happen. It is not that the antrum itself is resistant to cancer: on the contrary, cancer of the gastric antrum is common in patients who have a pan-gastritis, achlorhydria and intestinal metaplasia.

In spite of these observations a great deal of data has accumulated to suggest that *H. pylori* infection itself might be an initiating factor for the carcinogenic process. The infection is known to stimulate the production of reactive oxygen metabolites[19] to increase gastric cell turnover[20] and to impair the secretion of ascorbic acid into the stomach[21]. Each of these mechanisms in theory increases the likelihood of a mutagenic change. Nevertheless, when exfoliated cells from patients infected with *H. pylori* are assessed for single-strand breaks using the Comet technique, the cells obtained from infected individuals have fewer strand breaks than controls[22]. It is interesting that patients with duodenal ulcer, a condition with a high cell turnover, the presence of metaplastic gastric epithelium and severe duodenitis never develop cancer in the duodenum. It appears therefore that the development of gastric cancer arises in individuals with a low gastric secretion, a pan-gastritis, and in whom there has been long-standing gastric atrophy, achlorhydria and intestinal metaplasia. It may be, as suggested many years ago by Correa et al.[23], that the faecal-type organisms colonizing the achlorhydric stomach are ultimately responsible for the production of the carcinogens that cause gastric cancer.

The above analysis relates mainly to patients who develop intestinal-type cancer. This is the commonest type of non-cardia cancer; however, there is a second histological type classified as 'diffuse' gastric cancer. This lesion is also strongly associated with *H. pylori*, but tends to occur in younger individuals. It arises in mucosa which is closer to the actively inflamed mucosa[24] and is less strongly associated with intestinal metaplasia. It is possible that this form of cancer is more directly associated with active *Helicobacter* infection; however, this cannot be the whole truth because it is not associated with antral-predominant gastritis; the principle that gastric cancer is associated with extensive inflammation in the stomach remains the most important observation.

Gastric cancer does occur in a small minority of patients who are not, and have never been, infected by *H. pylori*, it includes those with a genetic susceptibility to the disease and those with pernicious anaemia.

The third type of gastric cancer unassociated with *H. pylori* is that which occurs at the gastro-oesophageal junction in the cardia mucosa. The cause of this lesion is still debated, but may be a result of a highly acidic micro-environment possibly linked to nitrogen metabolism[25].

It seems, however, that not all people have the same predilection for gastric cancer. Host polymorphisms that control the inflammatory cytokines secreted in response to *H. pylori* infection influence the severity and pattern of the gastritis, thus influencing susceptibility to cancer[26]. The virulence of the infecting organism is also of considerable importance[27].

If gastric cancer does result from a pan-gastritis with atrophy and intestinal metaplasia, and is not associated with an antral-predominant gastritis, one would predict that those countries with a high incidence of the disease will have a different pattern of gastritis compared to a low cancer area. In order to test this hypothesis we have recently undertaken a prospective, comparative study of patients in the UK and in Japan[28] (where there is a four times higher incidence of gastric cancer), and have compared 20 individuals in each decennial and in each centre from the ages of 20 to 70. We have shown that the prevalence of *H. pylori* in the two populations is similar, but that English patients have an antral-predominant gastritis while in Japan it is corpus-predominant. In the English patients atrophy and intestinal metaplasia were uncommon, but in the Japanese they were much more frequently found.

GASTRIC ULCER, DUODENAL ULCER, GASTRIC CANCER – WHY THE DIFFERENCES IN EPIDEMIOLOGY?

It is interesting that, although gastric cancer has been recognized for many years, gastric ulcer came to prominence only during the nineteenth century, and duodenal ulcer was almost unknown until the end of that century. At the beginning of the twentieth century gastric ulcer in Western societies began to decline, while duodenal ulcer increased to reach a peak in the 1950s. The end of the century saw a decline in both gastric and duodenal ulcer, accompanied by a rise in gastro-oesophageal reflux disease[29]. Today we are seeing a change in the developing countries in the Far East, where the incidence of gastric cancer and gastric ulcer was high, but is now beginning to decline with a concomitant increase in duodenal ulcer and more recently gastro-oesophageal reflux disease.

It is possible that these geographical differences and temporal changes reflect alterations in acid secretion. Acid secretion is rarely measured today; however, a study from Japan has shown a remarkable increase in acid secretion since the 1970s[30]. Looking at three birth cohorts comprising elderly people in the 1970s, young people in the 1970s and young people in the 1990s, the study demonstrated a considerable increase in both basal and maximal acid secretion over time when comparing the three birth cohorts. Interestingly, although *H. pylori* causes a slight diminution in acid secretion, similar changes also occurred in these. According to these data there has been a significant rise in acid secretion over a period of about 40 years in Japan. If this increase is a genuine one, and can be applied to history as well as geography, it may be that in the eighteenth century there was a very low acid secretion in the Western population with a concomitantly severe and corpus-predominant *Helicobacter* infection that caused gastric cancer. An increase in acid secretion in nineteenth and early twentieth centuries could have caused gastric ulcer to come into prominence, and with the further increase in acid secretion in the twentieth century a change from pan-gastritis to an antral-predominant pattern causing duodenal ulcer to come to the fore. An increased acid secretion could be responsible for the rise in gastro-oesophageal reflux disease. It is possible that the decline in *H. pylori* infection throughout the developed world might have resulted from a high acid secretion that could have protected people from becoming infected in the first place. There is no direct evidence that a high acid level protects from *H. pylori* infection, but it is interesting that those who have tried to infect themselves or others experimentally have used an acid-suppressant during the infection phase, on the presumption that it will make it easier for *H. pylori* to colonize them. Furthermore, gastro-oesophageal reflux disease which is associated with a higher acid secretion is negatively associated with *H. pylori* infection[31]. This concept would also tie in with the observation that a high acid secretion restricts *H. pylori* gastritis to the antrum.

If gastric acid secretion has risen over the past 200 years what is the likely explanation for it?

One of the most obvious changes that has occurred in our population in the last century has been the increase in the physical stature of the population. In Western Europe the linear height in men has risen by roughly 1 cm per decade[32]. More recently there has also been an increase in body mass. The reason for this consistent trend is unclear, but it has been attributed to better (or more abundant) nutrition. While this may explain the increasing obesity in the Western world it may not be the explanation for the increase in linear height, because it is possible to accurately predict the adult height of a child at the age of 2. This suggests that the cause may operate *in utero*, infancy or early childhood. There is clear evidence from work done in the 1960s[33] and 1970s[34] that maximal acid secretion correlates with lean body mass (a measurement that includes height and weight). It is possible therefore that the increase in body size during the twentieth century might be responsible for the rise in acid secretion. It is also possible that the varying geographical differences relating to the complications of *H. pylori* infection (duodenal ulcer, gastric ulcer and gastric cancer) might also be a result of differences in gastric acid secretion, and they may possibly also be related to the height and weight of the indigenous population. There is, however, little published data available to support this hypothesis.

CONCLUSION

The rediscovery of *H. pylori* in 1983 has provided a convincing explanation for the development of peptic ulcer. The organism causes an acute on chronic gastritis that inhibits the cytoprotective mechanisms within the stomach, allowing for gastric erosion and ulceration. In individuals with a high gastric acid output and antral-predominant gastritis, gastric acid secretion is enhanced by the effect of inflammation on the endocrine cells of the antrum, causing hypergastrinaemia. The increased acid secretion causes gastric metaplasia to develop in the duodenum, which in turn becomes infected by *H. pylori*, leading to a duodenitis and the same sequence of ulceration as occurs within the stomach.

Non-cardia gastric cancer arises in an individual with a naturally low acid secretion in whom long-standing, widespread inflammation has given rise to gastric atrophy, intestinal metaplasia, achlorhydria and an overgrowth of faecal organisms within the stomach. The specific mechanism that induces the carcinogenic change is as yet unknown, but in the case of the intestinal-type cancer, which is the commonest gastric cancer, it is unlikely to be a direct effect of the *H. pylori* infection on the gastric mucosa. The infection may however contribute directly to the development of the diffuse type of gastric cancer in those with widespread inflammation. Cancer of the cardia of the stomach is not associated with gastric cancer. Cancer may also arise in the absence of *H. pylori* in patients with pernicious anaemia or those with a genetic susceptibility to the disease.

References

1. Bizzozero G. Ueber die Schlauchformigen Drusen des Magendarmkanals unde die Beziehungen ihres Epithels zu dem Obertflachenepithel der Schleimhaut. Arch Mikr Anat. 1893;42:82–152.
2. Kasai K, Kobayashi R. The stomach spirochete occurring in mammals. J Parasitol. 1919; 6:1–10.
3. Steer H, Colin-Jones DG. Mucosal changes in gastric ulceration and their response to carbenoxolone sodium. Gut. 1975;16:590–7.
4. Marshall BJ, Warren JR. Unidentified curved bacilli in the stomach of patients with gastritis and peptic ulceration. Lancet. 1984;1:1311–14.
5. Marshall BJ, Armstrong JA, McGechie DB, Glancy RJ. Attempt to fulfil Koch's postulates for pyloric campylobacter. Med J Aust. 1985;142:436–9.
6. Crabtree JE, Covacci A, Farmery SM et al. *Helicobacter pylori*induced interleukin-8 expression in gastric epithelial cells is associated with CagA positive phenotype. J Clin Pathol. 1995;48:41–5.
7. Asaka M, Kato M, Kudo M et al. Atrophic changes of gastrtic mucosa are caused by *Helicobacter pylori* infection rather than ageing: studies in asymptomatic Japanese adults. Helicobacter. 1996;1:52–6.
8. Quigley EM, Turnberg LA. pH of the microclimate lining human gastric and duodenal mucosa *in vivo*. Studies in control subjects and in duodenal ulcer patients. Gastroenterology. 1987;92:1876–84.
9. Goggin PM, Marrero JM, Spychal RI, Jackson PA, Corbishley CM, Northfield TC. Surface hydrophobicity of gastric mucosa in *Helicobacter pylori* infection: effect of clearance and eradication. Gastroenterology. 1992;103:1486–90.
10. Calam J, Beales ILP, Gibbons A, Ghatei M, Del Valle J. Effects of abnormalities of gastrin and somatostatin in *Helicobacter pylori* infection on acid secretion. In: Hunt RH, Tytgat GNJ, editors. *Helicobacter pylori*: Basic Mechanisms to Clinical Cure. Dordrecht: Kluwer Academic Publishers, 1996:108–21.
11. Wyatt JI, Rathbone BJ, Dixon MF, Heatley RV. *Campylobacter pyloridis* and acid induced gastric metaplasia in the pathogenesis of duodenitis. J Clin Pathol. 1987;40:841–8.
12. Helicobacter and Cancer Collaborative Group. Gastric cancer and *Helicobacter pylori*: a combined analysis of 12 case control studies nested within prospective cohorts. Gut. 2001; 49:347–53.
13. Kikuchi S, Wada O, Nakajima Tet al. Serum anti-*Helicobacter pylori* antibody and gastric carcinoma among young adults. Cancer. 1995;75:2789–93.
14. Ekstrom AM, Held M, Hansson LE, Engstrand, L, Nyren O. *Helicobacter pylori* in gastric cancer established by CagA immunoblot as a marker of past infection. Gastroenterology. 2001;121:784–91.
15. Honda S, Fujioka T, Tokieda M, Satoh R, Nishizono A, Nasu M. Development of *Helicobacter pylori*-induced gastric carcinoma in Mongolian gerbils. Cancer Res. 1998;58: 4255–9.

16. Watanabe T, Tada M, Nagai H, Sasaki S, Nakao M. *Helicobacter pylori* infection induces gastric cancer in Mongolian gerbils. Gastroenterology. 1998;115:642-648.
17. Keto Y, Ebata M, Okabe S. Gastric mucosal changes induced by long term infection with *Helicobacter pylori* in Mongolian gerbils: effects of bacteria eradication. J Physiol Paris. 2001;95:429–36.
18. Uemura N, Okamoto S, Yamamoto S et al. *Helicobacter pylori* infection and the development of gastric cancer. N Engl J Med. 2001;345:784–9.
19. Drake IM, Mapstone NP, Schorah CJ et al. Reactive oxygen species activity and lipid peroxidation in *Helicobacter pylori* associated gastritis: relation to gastric mucosal ascorbic acid concentrations and effect of *H. pylori* eradication. Gut. 1998;42:768–71.
20. Lynch DAF, Mapstone NP, Clarke AMT et al. Cell proliferation in *Helicobacter pylori* associated gastritis and the effect of eradication therapy. Gut. 1995;36:346–50.
21. Sobala GM, Schorah CJ, Sanderson M et al. Ascorbic acid in the human stomach. Gastroenterology. 1989;97:357–63.
22. Everett SM, White KL, Drake IM et al. The effect of *Helicobacter pylori* infection on levels of DNA damage in gastric epithelial cells. Helicobacter. 2002;7:271–80.
23. Correa P, Haenszel W, Cuello C, Tannenbaum S, Archer M. A model for gastric cancer epidemiology. Lancet. 1975;2:58–60.
24. Yoshimura T, Shimoyama T, Fukuda S, Tanaka M, Axon ATR, Munakata A. Most gastric cancer occurs on the distal side of the endoscopic atrophic border. Scand J Gastroenterol. 1999;34:1077–81.
25. Iijima K, Fyfe V, McColl KEL. Studies of nitric oxide generation from salivary nitrite in human gastric juice. Scand J Gastroenterol. 2003;38:246–52.
26. El Omar EM, Carrington M, Chow WH et al. Interleukin-1 polymorphisms associated with increased risk of gastric cancer. Nature. 2000;404:398–402.
27. Figueiredo C, Machado JC, Pharoah P et al. *Helicobacter pylori* and interleukin-1 genotyping: an opportunity to identify high-risk individuals for gastric carcinoma. J Natl Cancer Inst. 2002;94:1680–7.
28. Naylor G, Gotoda T, Gatta L et al. A comparison of gastritis in a UK and Japanese population. Gut. 2004;53(Suppl. 3):O84 (abstract).
29. El-Serag HB, Sonnenberg A. Opposing time trends of peptic ulcer and reflux disease. Gut. 1998;43:327–33.
30. Kinoshita Y, Kawanami C, Kishi K et al. *Helicobacter pylori* independent chronological change in gastric acid secretion in the Japanese. Gut. 1997;41:452–8.
31. Raghunath A, Hungin AP, Wooff D, Childs S. Prevalence of *Helicobacter pylori* in patients with gastro-oesophageal reflux disease: systematic review. Br Med J. 2003;326:737.
32. Cole TJ. Secular trends in growth. Proc Nutr Soc. 2000;59:317–24.
33. Baron JH. Lean body mass, gastric acid and peptic ulcer. Gut. 1969:10:637–42.
34. Elder JB, Smith IS. Gastric acid output, pepsin output and lean body mass in normal and duodenal ulcer subjects. Lancet. 1975;1:100–3.

5
Vaccination against *Helicobacter pylori* revisited

P. MICHETTI

INTRODUCTION

Helicobacter pylori is a Gram-negative human gastric bacterium that infects approximately 50% of adults in the developed world and over 90% of inhabitants in the developing world. The geographic strains distribution suggests coevolution of mankind and *H. pylori* for thousands of years[1,2]. Transmission has been reported by faecal–oral, oral–oral, and iatrogenic spread. *H. pylori* acquisition seems to occur mainly during the first years of life in high-risk groups of children and correlates well with low socioeconomic status[3,4]. Although spontaneous elimination of *H. pylori* infection occurs in young children and the elderly[5], *H. pylori* normally causes a lifelong chronic gastritis. The infection plays an important role in peptic ulcer disease and gastric B-cell mucosa-associated lymphoid tissue (MALT) lymphoma, and is associated with gastric adenocarcinoma[6–8]. The International Agency for Research and Cancer (IARC, USA) classified *H. pylori* as a group I carcinogen, a definite cause of human gastric cancers[9]. More recently it has been shown in Japan that *H. pylori*-positive men have a higher risk of developing gastric adenocarcinoma than do *H. pylori*-negative men[10]. Eradication of *H. pylori* is now accepted as the primary therapy of peptic ulcer disease associated with this infection, and indications to *H. pylori* eradication therapy have been progressively expanded[11]. Interventional studies in high-risk groups even suggest that eradication may contribute to the prevention of gastric adenocarcinoma development[12]. Treatment regimens to eliminate gastric *H. pylori* infection are based on the association of two antibiotics and an antisecretory agent, most often a proton pump inhibitor. Success rates of various antibiotic combinations ranged between 70% and 85%[13]. However, antibiotic resistance and poor compliance significantly affect the effectiveness of these strategies. Furthermore antibiotic-based therapies are not suited for large-scale eradication in populations with high cancer risk, e.g. some large groups of subjects in emergent societies.

The mechanisms underlying the persistence of *H. pylori* in the human stomach remain largely unclear. *H. pylori* antigens are recognized and presented by professional antigen-presenting cells such as dendritic cells, and innate and adaptive immune responses are generated[14,15]. Despite this seemingly vigorous and comprehensive immune response, *H. pylori* infection becomes persistent in the majority of infected subjects. Observational and experimental data accumulated in the past decade have shown that the degree of gastric inflammation in response to *H. pylori* is down-regulated both by bacterial and host mechanisms. These mechanisms are not uniformly expressed by all strains and hosts, and this may explain, according to large epidemiological studies, why only 15–20% of subjects infected with *H. pylori* will develop peptic ulcer or gastric malignancies in their lifetime.

SUPPRESSIVE EFFECT OF *H. PYLORI* ON IMMUNE RESPONSES

Pathogens that cause chronic infections, such as *H. pylori*, have to develop strategies allowing them to survive the environmental and immunological factors that would limit their survival. Some of these strategies may be specifically addressed at limiting the effectiveness of the induction, of the effector function, and/or of the memory function of the immune responses. It has been shown in humans that *H. pylori* infection impairs *H. pylori*-specific memory $CD4^+$ T cell responses through antigen-specific $CD4^+CD25^{high}$ regulatory T cells, and this could be involved in the persistence of the infection[16]. In mice $CD4^+CD25^+$ regulatory cells have been associated with the control of severe gastric pathology following infection with *H. pylori*[17].

Specific virulence factors also contribute to the persistence of *H. pylori*. The vacuolating cytotoxin VacA has been shown to be able to interfere with Ii-mediated antigen presentation[18] and to inhibit T cell activation through mechanisms depending on the formation of anion-specific channels, blocking the translocation of the transcription factor NFAT to the nucleus, thus interfering with the cytokine signalling pathway[19,20] in $CD4^+$ and $CD8^+$ cells. In addition, VacA inhibits the activation of intracellular signalling through protein kinases MKK3/6 and p38 and the Rac-specific nucleotide exchange factor, Vav[20]. Taken together, these data suggest that VacA can hamper an effective response against *H. pylori*, allowing the persistence of colonization and the establishment of a chronic gastric inflammation. It remains to be demonstrated how these *in-vitro* findings apply to the *in-vivo* situation.

VACCINATION AGAINST GASTRIC *HELICOBACTER* INFECTIONS

Multiple studies have shown that effective protective immunity against *H. pylori* can be induced in experimental animal models after immunization, using various routes of delivery, e.g. mucosal (oral, intranasal, rectal) and parenteral, co-administering the soluble antigen(s) with appropriate antigens, such as bacterial toxins and their mutants for the mucosal immunization, with aluminium hydroxide or Freund's adjuvant for parenteral immunization (for review, see ref. 21).

Initial studies tested the safety and immunogenicity of oral immunization with urease and were performed in volunteers infected with *H. pylori*. These studies showed that urease was safe, but unable by this route to elicit an immune response above the one naturally present in infected subjects[22]. If urease was administered with the heat-labile enterotoxin of *Escherichia coli* as a mucosal adjuvant, however, a B cell response could be seen, that included mainly IgA-secreting cells[23]. This response was even associated with decreased *H. pylori* density at the surface of the gastric mucosa. Later, and with the exception of a very recent trial still in progress, all the other human vaccine studies have been performed in *H. pylori*-negative volunteers, precluding any evaluation of a potential efficacy of the antigen–adjuvant combination tested. Several trials, conducted by two independent groups of investigators, tested the safety and immunogenicity of various transformed *Salmonella* strains expressing urease. Di Petrillo et al. administered a PhoP/PhoQ-deleted *S. enterica typhimurium* vaccine strain and could see no seroconversion to *H. pylori* urease, constitutively expressed by this strain[24]. The same group of investigators later tested the same antigen in a PhoP/PhoQ-deleted *S. enterica typhimurium* strain and obtained a seroconversion in three out of six of the volunteers[25]. Using a novel *in-vivo* conditional expression system to express urease in the commercially available *S. typhi* Ty21a human vaccine strain, Bumann et al. obtained a 50% seroconversion rate in 12 volunteers[26]. This group recently embarked on testing the efficacy of their vaccine construct by challenging the volunteers with a *H. pylori* strain isolated specifically for this purpose[27], a model that is not without questions regarding its value for vaccine development[28]. In these conditions, four out of nine volunteers were protected (or with minimal residual infection) against *H. pylori* compared with none of the four controls[29]. In this small series, only four out of 16 volunteers showed any immune response to the vaccine antigen before challenge. This work is still in progress and is likely, if the preliminary results are confirmed, to boost the search for the human vaccine against *H. pylori*.

Parenteral vaccination is also currently being tested in humans, as this strategy was shown as effective in animal models as oral vaccination[30]. The vaccine preparation tested in this setting included three antigens, VacA, the protein GagA, and HP-NAP, the neutrophil-activating protein of *H. pylori*. The adjuvant added to the antigen preparation was aluminium hydroxide, the only vaccine adjuvant approved for human use. Again this strategy was tested in non-infected volunteers, precluding any efficacy assessment, but the preparation elicited vigorous B and T cell responses with an IgG response in 85% of 57 subjects. T cell responses to GagA and VacA, dominated by interferon gamma production, were also observed[31]. Further work with this vaccine is ongoing.

Recent data have shown that the best way to induce strong immune responses both at local and systemic levels was to prime animals mucosally (e. g. orally or intranasally) using LT mutants as adjuvants, and then to boost them systemically. This was demonstrated using purified *H. pylori* antigens, such as CagA and HP-NAP[32]. In humans infected with *H. pylori* the best route to induce vaccine-specific immune responses at the local level (as judged by the ability to induce antigen-specific IgA in the stomach and duodenum) was the oral or the intrajejunal route, but not the rectal or the nasal route[33]. In non-infected human volunteers, similar response patterns were observed, suggesting that infection with *H. pylori* does not alter recruitment of T and B lymphocytes at the gastric level. In non-infected volunteers, increased numbers of activated CD69[+] and of CD4[+] circulating lymphocytes were measured following oral and intestinal immunization with *H. pylori* urease administered with the heat-labile toxin of *E. coli*. In a trial of vaccination with a whole-cell *H. pylori* vaccine formulation given orally, antigen-specific B cells were also induced in *H. pylori* non-infected individuals[34]. The exact mechanisms of priming and recruitment of antigen-specific B and T cells to the gastric mucosa still remain to be elucidated.

Infection with *H. pylori* is primarily acquired at paediatric age, and in developing countries infection can take place very early in life[35]. Prophylactic vaccination given during the very first months of life would then be desirable to prevent the long-term effect of chronic colonization and to reduce transmission among the population. Recent work in mice has shown that passive transfer of *H. felis*-specific antibodies through breast feeding protects pups against colonization, although infection reappears at weaning[36]. Interestingly, parenteral immunization of mice within the first day of life with *H. pylori* whole-cell lysate prepared with Freund's adjuvant has been shown to confer protection against a challenge with *H. pylori*, at levels comparable to those observed in adult mice[37].

BALANCE OF Th1/Th2 LYMPHOCYTE PHENOTYPES AND IMMUNITY

A great deal of work in recent years, mainly in animals experimentally infected with *H. pylori* or *H. felis*, has strongly supported the concept that infection induces a prominent Th1-type (inflammatory) immune response, whereas Th2-type immune responses are more frequently associated with protection, for example induced by active immunization, either because of a direct effect of antigen-specific antibodies, or because of the inhibitory effect of Th2-type cytokines (e.g. IL-10) on Th1-type responses and on the colonization itself.

New *in-vitro* data shed light on possible mechanisms responsible for this Th1 bias. *H. pylori* appears able to preferentially trigger IL-12 secretion by human dendritic cells[38]. This IL-12 response, however, may be important in controlling the infection as higher colonization levels were observed in IL-12 knockout mice with wild-type and colonization-impaired mutants of *H. pylori*[39]. In human gastric tissue, however, both IFN-γ and IL-10 are increased, as measured by immunohistochemistry with monoclonal antibodies[40]. This observation suggests that *H. pylori* has a dual effect; on the one hand driving a Th1 response dominated by IFN-γ, and on the other hand inducing IL-10, which may dampen the inflammatory and cytotoxic effects of Th1 cells.

The key role of IL-4 in limiting the degree of gastritis caused by infection with *H. pylori* has been further stressed in recent work. Treatment of mice with IFN-γ induced gastritis, enhanced levels of gastrin and reduced levels of somatostatin, whereas IL-4 suppressed expression and secretion of gastrin and reduced colonization with *H. pylori* in chronically infected mice[41]. As *H. pylori* suppresses IL-4-induced Stat6 tyrosine phosphorylation, the bacterium suppresses polarization towards an anti-inflammatory Th2-type immune response, thus favouring the establishment of a chronic infection[42].

Another Th2-type cytokine known to limit the degree of gastritis following *Helicobacter* infection is IL-10. Indeed, infection of IL-10 knockout mice with *H. felis* induces a more severe chronic gastric pathology and a Th1-type immune response much more prominent than in wild-type animals[43]. Depleting complement during *H. pylori* infection in IL-10 knockout mice led to decreased gastritis, reduced gastric mucosa neutrophil counts, and delayed bacterial clearance[43]. These recent data, taken together with prior evidence, strongly suggest that Th2-type immune responses are crucial in mediating protective immunity and these Th2-type immune responses should be induced by active immunization in order to prevent or to treat *H. pylori* infection.

Studies in strains of mice knocked out at the levels of genes coding for cytokines suggest that the fine mechanisms underlying the balance of the quality of the immune responses required for protection against *H. pylori* are most likely multifactorial, depending on various host-related and pathogen-related factors. Double knocked-out mice lacking antibodies and IL-4 were still protected against a challenge with *H. pylori* after intranasal immunization with a whole-cell lysate. Immunization-induced protection was also achieved in mice deficient for IL-5, suggesting that these cytokines may not be essential for protection[44]. These data appear to be in agreement with others from the same and other groups showing that protection after intranasal or intragastric immunization can be associated with a Th1 response, as shown by increased expression of IL-12 p40 subunit, but not of IFN-γ nor of inducible nitric oxide synthase. In addition, protection was not achieved in mice knocked-out for the gene encoding the p40 subunit of Il-12[44]. However, these results require some caution in their analysis as the genetic background of the host affects the outcome of *H. pylori* infection. This has been exemplified in a study looking at the impact of gene deletion for IL-12 or IL-4 in various mouse strains. While gene-targeted C57BL/6 mice showed reduced susceptibility to gastric colonization, the same deletion in BALB/c mice strongly enhanced the level of gastric colonization. With the exception of IL-10 and IL-12 knockout mice (which exhibited the highest levels of colonization), all other knocked-out strains of mice were successfully protected by prophylactic oral immunization at a level similar to that achieved in wild-type animals[45].

IDENTIFYING CORRELATES OF PROTECTION

Despite all efforts made so far, no correlates of protection have been clearly defined in the experimental animal models of infection with *H. pylori* and of immunization. An intriguing finding has been reported recently, suggesting that mechanisms of protection against *Helicobacter* may involve not only lymphocyte-mediated effector functions, but also paracrine functions of adipocytes surrounding resident lymphocytes. Indeed, mice immunized and protected against challenge with the bacterium exhibited a peculiar gene expression, absent in non-protected and in control mice, with up-regulation of adipocyte-specific factors such as adipsin, resistin, adiponectin, and CD36, and increased presence of T and B cells in the fat tissue surrounding the stomachs of protected mice[46]. This finding suggests the existence of crosstalk between adipose tissue and lymphoid cells.

Another aspect of protection is the cooperation between mucosally homing $\alpha 4\beta 7$ integrin$^+$ CD4$^+$ T cells, shown to be required for protection, and mast cells, also expressing this integrin complex. Using monoclonal antibodies blocking $\alpha 4\beta 7$ integrin function, we showed that this function is required for protection in mice[47]. More recently we sought to discover whether mast cells also participate in vaccination-mediated protection against *Helicobacter* infection. We first showed that mast cell numbers increase in the gastric mucosa as early as CD4$^+$ T cells and that mast cells are activated, as indicated by increased mRNA expression of their granule proteases in the gastric mucosa and increased levels of mast cell protease 1 in serum. These changes occur only in mice immunized with *H. pylori* urease and cholera toxin (CT) and challenged with *Helicobacter*, in contrast to mice challenged only following CT immunization. To prove that mast cells are required for protection, deficient mice (strain WBB6F1-Kit^W/Kit^{W-v}) were vaccinated with urease and CT, using as controls wild-type WBB6F1-Kit$^{+/+}$ littermates. Urease-vaccinated mast cell-deficient Kit^W/Kit^{W-v} mice were unable to eliminate *H. felis* and *H. pylori* after challenge, while controls cleared these infections. If Kit^W/Kit^{W-v} mice were reconstituted with bone marrow-derived mast cells from wild-type WBB6F1-Kit$^{+/+}$ mice, protection was restored, confirming that mast cells are crucial for gastric protection. The precise mechanism by which mast cells contribute to gastric mucosa protection is currently under study. Mast cells have been shown to have a direct bacteria clearance capacity in a murine model of bacterial peritonitis[48,49], and in our preliminary experiments seem able to kill *H. pylori in vitro*. In remains to be demonstrated whether this direct effect of mast cells occurs in the gastric mucosa, or whether mast cells act indirectly via the induction of immune and/or non-immune changes in the mucosa.

CONCLUSION

Studies in recent years have provided important new insights and research avenues into the mechanisms by which *H. pylori* ensures its persistence in the human stomach. These host–pathogen interactions that participate in the development of the clinically relevant complications of the infection are probably also central in the transmission of the infection. A better understanding of these regulatory mechanisms may also lead to the development of novel treatment strategies and to effective prophylactic and therapeutic vaccines against *H. pylori*. These research goals are relevant to a global control of this infection that remains, despite the decreasing incidence of the infection in fully industrialized countries, an important public health issue in most areas of the world.

References

1. Covacci A, Telford JL, Del Giudice G, Parsonnet J, Rappuoli R. *Helicobacter pylori* virulence and genetic geography. Science. 1999;284:1328–33.
2. Falush D, Wirth T, Linz B et al. Traces of human migrations in *Helicobacter pylori* populations. Science. 2003;299:1582–5.
3. Malaty HM, Graham DY. Importance of childhood socioeconomic status on the current prevalence of *Helicobacter pylori* infection. Gut. 1994;35:742–5.
4. Rowland M, Kumar D, Daly L, O'Connor P, Vaughan D, Drumm B. Low rates of *Helicobacter pylori* reinfection in children. Gastroenterology. 1999;117:336–41.
5. Rothenbacher D, Bode G, Berg G et al. Prevalence and determinants of *Helicobacter pylori* infection in preschool children: a population-based study from Germany. Int J Epidemiol. 1998;27:135–41.
6. Marshall BJ, Goodwin CS, Warren JR et al. Prospective double-blind trial of duodenal ulcer relapse after eradication of *Campylobacter pylori*. Lancet. 1988;2:1437–42.
7. Forman D, Newell DG, Fullerton F et al. Association between infection with *Helicobacter pylori* and risk of gastric cancer: evidence from a prospective investigation [see comments]. Br Med J. 1991;302:1302–5.
8. Wotherspoon AC, Doglioni C, Diss TC et al. Regression of primary low-grade B-cell gastric lymphoma of mucosa-associated lymphoid tissue type after eradication of *Helicobacter pylori*. Lancet. 1993;342:575–7.
9. IARC Working Group on the Evaluation of Carcinogenic Risks to Humans. Schistosomes, liver flukes and *Helicobacter pylori*, Lyon, 7–14 June 1994. IARC Monogr Eval Carcinog Risks Hum. 1994;61:1–241.
10. Uemura N, Okamoto S, Yamamoto S et al. *Helicobacter pylori* infection and the development of gastric cancer. N Engl J Med. 2001;345:784–9.
11. Bazzoli F. Key points from the revised Maastricht Consensus Report: the impact on general practice. Eur J Gastroenterol Hepatol. 2001;13(Suppl. 2):S30-7.
12. Uemura N, Mukai T, Okamoto S et al. Effect of *Helicobacter pylori* eradication on subsequent development of cancer after endoscopic resection of early gastric cancer. Cancer Epidemiol Biomarkers Prev. 1997;6:639–42.
13. Suerbaum S, Michetti P. *Helicobacter pylori* infection. N Engl J Med. 2002;347:1175–86.
14. Hafsi N, Voland P, Schwendy S et al. Human dendritic cells respond to *Helicobacter pylori*, promoting NK cell and Th1-effector responses *in vitro*. J Immunol. 2004;173:1249–57.
15. Voland P, Hafsi N, Zeitner M, Laforsch S, Wagner H, Prinz C. Antigenic properties of HpaA and Omp18, two outer membrane proteins of *Helicobacter pylori*. Infect Immun. 2003;71:3837–43.
16. Lundgren A, Suri-Payer E, Enarsson K, Svennerholm AM, Lundin BS. *Helicobacter pylori*-specific CD4$^+$ CD25^{high} regulatory T cells suppress memory T-cell responses to *H. pylori* in infected individuals. Infect Immun. 2003;71:1755–62.
17. Raghavan S, Fredriksson M, Svennerholm AM, Holmgren J, Suri-Payer E. Absence of CD4$^+$CD25$^+$ regulatory T cells is associated with a loss of regulation leading to increased pathology in *Helicobacter pylori*-infected mice. Clin Exp Immunol. 2003;132:393–400.
18. Montecucco C, de Bernard M. Immunosuppressive and proinflammatory activities of the VacA toxin of *Helicobacter pylori*. J Exp Med. 2003;198:1767–71.
19. Gebert B, Fischer W, Weiss E, Hoffmann R, Haas R. *Helicobacter pylori* vacuolating cytotoxin inhibits T lymphocyte activation. Science. 2003;301:1099–102.
20. Boncristiano M, Paccani SR, Barone S et al. The *Helicobacter pylori* vacuolating toxin inhibits T cell activation by two independent mechanisms. J Exp Med. 2003;198:1887–97.
21. Ruggiero P, Peppoloni S, Rappuoli R, Del Giudice G. The quest for a vaccine against *Helicobacter pylori*: how to move from mouse to man? Microbes Infect 2003;5:749–56.
22. Kreiss C, Buclin T, Cosma M, Corthesy-Theulaz I, Michetti P. Safety of oral immunization with recombinant urease in patients with *Helicobacter pylori* infection. Lancet. 1996;347:1630–1.
23. Michetti P, Kreiss C, Kotloff KL et al. Oral immunization with urease and *Escherichia coli* heat-labile enterotoxin is safe and immunogenic in *Helicobacter pylori*-infected adults [see comments]. Gastroenterology. 1999;116:804–12.

24. DiPetrillo MD, Tibbetts T, Kleanthous H, Killeen KP, Hohmann EL. Safety and immunogenicity of phoP/phoQ-deleted *Salmonella typhi* expressing *Helicobacter pylori* urease in adult volunteers. Vaccine. 1999;18:449–59.
25. Angelakopoulos H, Hohmann EL. Pilot study of phoP/phoQ-deleted *Salmonella enterica* serovar *typhimurium* expressing *Helicobacter pylori* urease in adult volunteers. Infect Immun. 2000;68:2135–41.
26. Bumann D, Metzger WG, Mansouri E et al. Safety and immunogenicity of live recombinant *Salmonella enterica* serovar *Typhi* Ty21a expressing urease A and B from *Helicobacter pylori* in human volunteers. Vaccine. 2001;20:845–52.
27. Graham DY, Opekun AR, Osato MS et al. Challenge model for *Helicobacter pylori* infection in human volunteers. Gut. 2004;53:1235–43.
28. Michetti P. Experimental *Helicobacter pylori* infection in humans: a multifaceted challenge. Gut. 2004;53:1220–1.
29. Aebischer T, Bumann D, Epple HJ et al. Development of a human vaccination cum challenge model with live recombinant *Salmonella* against *H. pylori*. Helicobacter. 2004;9:589.
30. Guy B, Hessler C, Fourage S et al. Systemic immunization with urease protects mice against *Helicobacter pylori* infection. Vaccine. 1998;16:850–6.
31. Malfertheiner P, Schultze V, Del Giudice G et al. Phase I safety and immunogenicity of a three-component *H. pylori* vaccine. Gastroenterology. 2002;122:A585.
32. Vajdy M, Singh M, Ugozzoli M et al. Enhanced mucosal and systemic immune responses to Helicobacter pylori antigens through mucosal priming followed by systemic boosting immunizations. Immunology. 2003;110:86–94.
33. Johansson EL, Bergquist C, Edebo A, Johansson C, Svennerholm AM. Comparison of different routes of vaccination for eliciting antibody responses in the human stomach. Vaccine. 2004;22:984–90.
34. Losonsky GA, Kotloff KL, Walker RI. B cell responses in gastric antrum and duodenum following oral inactivated *Helicobacter pylori* whole cell (HWC) vaccine and LT(R192G) in *H. pylori* seronegative individuals. Vaccine. 2003;21:562–5.
35. Frenck RW Jr, Clemens J. *Helicobacter* in the developing world. Microbes Infect. 2003;5:705–13.
36. Corthesy-Theulaz I, Corthesy B, Bachmann D, Velin D, Kraehenbuhl JP. Passive immunity in *Helicobacter*-challenged neonatal mice conferred by immunized dams lasts until weaning. Infect Immun. 2003;71:2226–9.
37. Eisenberg JC, Czinn SJ, Garhart CA et al. Protective efficacy of anti-*Helicobacter pylori* immunity following systemic immunization of neonatal mice. Infect Immun. 2003;71:1820–7.
38. Guiney DG, Hasegawa P, Cole SP. *Helicobacter pylori* preferentially induces interleukin 12 (IL-12) rather than IL-6 or IL-10 in human dendritic cells. Infect Immun. 2003;71:4163–6.
39. Hoffman PS, Vats N, Hutchison D et al. Development of an interleukin-12-deficient mouse model that is permissive for colonization by a motile KE26695 strain of *Helicobacter pylori*. Infect Immun. 2003;71:2534–41.
40. Holck S, Norgaard A, Bennedsen M, Permin H, Norn S, Andersen LP. Gastric mucosal cytokine responses in *Helicobacter pylori*-infected patients with gastritis and peptic ulcers. Association with inflammatory parameters and bacteria load. FEMS Immunol Med Microbiol. 2003;36:175–80.
41. Zavros Y, Rathinavelu S, Kao JY et al. Treatment of *Helicobacter* gastritis with IL-4 requires somatostatin. Proc Natl Acad Sci USA. 2003;100:12944–9.
42. Ceponis PJ, McKay DM, Menaker RJ, Galindo-Mata E, Jones NL. *Helicobacter pylori* infection interferes with epithelial Stat6-mediated interleukin-4 signal transduction independent of cagA, cagE, or VacA. J Immunol. 2003;171:2035–41.
43. Ismail HF, Fick P, Zhang J, Lynch RG, Berg DJ. Depletion of neutrophils in IL-10(-/-) mice delays clearance of gastric *Helicobacter* infection and decreases the Th1 immune response to *Helicobacter*. J Immunol. 2003;170:3782–9.
44. Garhart CA, Nedrud JG, Heinzel FP, Sigmund NE, Czinn SJ. Vaccine-induced protection against *Helicobacter pylori* in mice lacking both antibodies and interleukin-4. Infect Immun. 2003;71:3628–33.

45. Panthel K, Faller G, Haas R. Colonization of C57BL/6J and BALB/c wild-type and knockout mice with *Helicobacter pylori*: effect of vaccination and implications for innate and acquired immunity. Infect Immun. 2003;71:794–800.
46. Mueller A, O'Rourke J, Chu P et al. Protective immunity against *Helicobacter* is characterized by a unique transcriptional signature. Proc Natl Acad Sci USA. 2003;100:12289–94.
47. Michetti M, Kelly CP, Kraehenbuhl JP, Bouzourene H, Michetti P. Gastric mucosal alpha (4)beta(7)-integrin-positive CD4 T lymphocytes and immune protection against *Helicobacter* infection in mice. Gastroenterology. 2000;119:109–18.
48. Echtenacher B, Mannel DN, Hultner L. Critical protective role of mast cells in a model of acute septic peritonitis. Nature. 1996;381:75–7.
49. Malaviya R, Ikeda T, Ross E, Abraham SN. Mast cell modulation of neutrophil influx and bacterial clearance at sites of infection through TNF-alpha. Nature. 1996;381:77–80.

6
Mucosa-associated lymphoid tissue lymphoma: lessons from Germany

W. FISCHBACH

INTRODUCTION

Based on new insights into the aetiology and pathogenesis of gastrointestinal lymphomas and their histomorphological and molecular characteristics, important progress in diagnostic and therapy has been made during recent years. The lessons we learnt become particularly evident when we remember our knowledge in the early 1990s:

1. The MALT (mucosa-associated lymphoid tissue) concept had just been introduced in clinical routine diagnostics.

2. The relevance of *Helicobacter pylori* (Hp) infection in the pathogenesis of gastric MALT lymphoma had just became evident. The therapeutic potential of *H. pylori* eradication was unknown.

3. The contribution of endoscopic ultrasound (EUS) to the local staging of gastric lymphoma was not yet defined.

4. No prospective studies based on the MALT classification were available.

This was the starting-point when we designed our first German–Austrian multicentre study which was initiated in 1993. This study simultaneously focused on the histopathological, immunohistochemical and molecular biological characterization of gastric lymphoma, as well as on the accuracy of endoscopic biopsy diagnosis and EUS compared to the gold standard of evaluation of the resected specimen and pathohistological staging[1]. Based on surgery as the standard therapeutic procedure at that time grade of malignancy and stage, having proved to be the decisive prognostic factors[2,3], served as treatment stratifiers. In parallel to the activities of the 'Würzburg study group' two other groups from Germany performed large multicentre trials. Their results essentially contributed to our current understanding of the disease[4–7].

The lessons from Germany arising from these studies are summarized in this chapter and discussed in the light of findings from abroad.

DEFINITION, AETIOLOGY, PATHOGENESIS AND CLASSIFICATION

Based on the outstanding work of Isaacson and Spencer, and the establishment of the concept of MALT, primary gastrointestinal lymphomas are nowadays considered to be a distinct entity. This is reflected by the new WHO classification of 2002[8] (Table 1). The vast majority of gastric lymphomas are extranodal marginal zone-B cell-lymphomas of MALT, which can be identified by means of histopathological, immuno-histochemical and molecular biological characteristics[9]. The WHO classification no more considers a differentiation of low- and high-grade lymphoma, although such a classification would be helpful from the clinical point of view considering the grade of malignancy (low-grade, secondary high-grade, high-grade) as a decisive prognostic factor and therapeutic determinant. It takes into account the fact that no conclusive data are available suggesting a sequential development of high-grade lymphoma from low-grade precursors.

Table 1 WHO classification of gastrointestinal Non-Hodgkin's lymphoma[8]

B cell lymphoma	T cell lymphoma
Marginal zone B cell lymphoma of MALT type	Enteropathy-associated T cell lymphoma (EATCL)
Follicular lymphoma (grade I–III)	Peripheral T cell lymphoma (non-EATCL)
Mantle cell lymphoma (lymphomatous polyposis)	
Diffuse large B cell lymphoma with/without MALT type components	
Burkitt lymphoma	
Immundeficiency-associated lymphoma	

Intensive basic scientific and clinical studies during the past 10–15 years have dealt with the origin of acquired MALT. In the late 1980s Stolte and others identified *H. pylori*, still named *Campylobacter pylori* at that time, as the cause of chronic gastritis with consequent acquisition of intramucosal lymph follicles and accumulation of immunoglobulin A-producing cells showing morphological characteristics of MALT[10,11]. This acquired lymphatic tissue proved to regress after successful eradication of the bacterium[12]. In 1991 Wotherspoon et al. demonstrated for the first time that patients with primary gastric MALT lymphoma are regularly infected by *H. pylori*[13]. With a positivity rate of 90% to almost 100% this finding has been confirmed by our group also, demonstrating a distinct association with CagA-positive *H. pylori* strains[14]. In addition to these histomorphological and serological studies, recent epidemiological, molecular biological and experimental data clearly indicate that *H. pylori* plays a decisive role both in the development and progression of gastric MALT lymphoma[15]. Figure 1 summarizes our current understanding of the pathogenesis of gastric MALT lymphoma. The initial antigen-dependent proliferation is of major importance for an antibiotic treatment approach, as discussed later. As long as antigen-driven tumour proliferation is evident, successful elimination of this stimulus may be followed by regression of the lymphoma. There is a need, however, to identify the parameters for the progression from *H. pylori*-dependent lymphoma to autonomous tumour growth. Genetic alterations are obviously involved in this process. There is some evidence that high-grade lymphomas do not always follow this sequence, but develop to a substantial part *de novo*. The pathogenetic concept as demonstrated in Figure 1 does not explain the few cases of *H. pylori*-negative (including serological status) gastric MALT lymphoma. It seems conceivable that other microorganisms may also be of potential pathogenetic importance. Stolte and co-workers reported an association of *H. heilmannii* with gastric MALT lymphoma[16]. These considerations are also supported by our findings of lymphoma regression in some serologically and histologically *H. pylori*-negative individuals following usual eradication therapy[17].

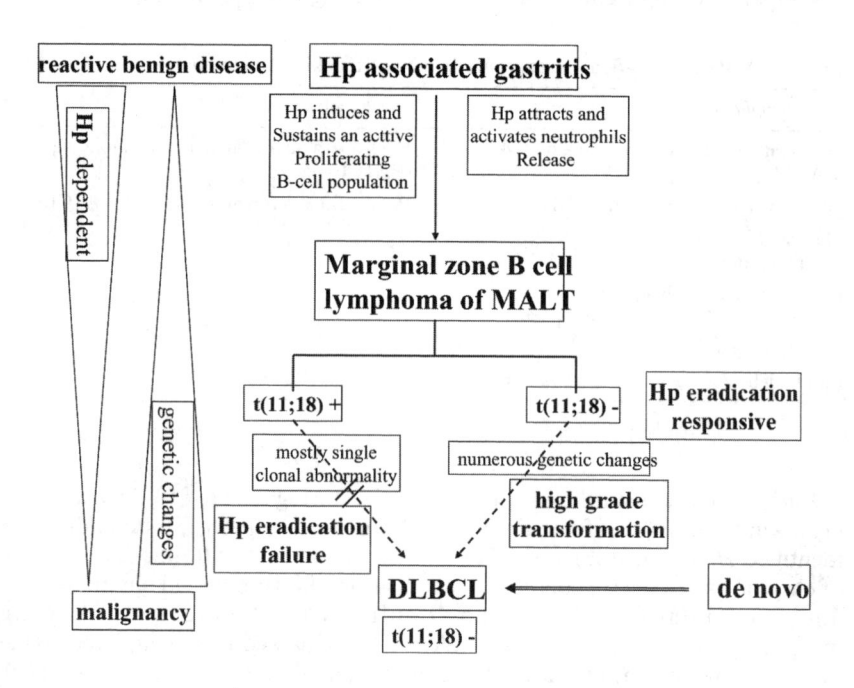

Figure 1 Summary of current understanding of the pathogenesis of gastric MALT lymphoma

DIAGNOSIS AND CLINICAL STAGING

As already mentioned above, grade of malignancy and stage are the two major prognostic factors and therapeutic determinants[2,3]. Against this background, *endoscopic biopsy diagnosis* and clinical staging are particularly important. Although in our first prospective multicentre study it was possible to diagnose the overwhelming majority of lymphomas (95%) by endoscopic biopsies, pathological work-up of the gastrectomy specimens showed that exact typing and grading were missed in 26%[1]. These discrepancies were caused mainly by overlooking low- or high-grade components in the biopsies reflecting the multifocality and focal high-grade transformation in some lymphomas. Considering these findings subtle endoscopic bioptic techniques are needed, including a minimum of 10–12 biopsies from visible lesions and macroscopically normal-appearing areas ('gastric mapping'), as well as repeated examinations and the use of large forceps in the individual case.

The *stage* of gastric lymphoma is usually described by the Musshoff classification for extranodal lymphoma and its modification of stage EI by Radaszkiewicz et al.[3] (Table 2). Another classification system – the Lugano classification – is not widely used as it offers no significant advantages and has considerable problems in practical use. Against the background of several limitations of both staging systems the EGILS (European Gastrointestinal Lymphoma Study Group) developed the Paris staging system, which is based on the TNM classification and which better reflects the specifics of gastrointestinal lymphoma[18]. Independent of which staging system is used a differentiation of stages I1, I2, and II1, and of stages T1-4/N0-1, respectively

Table 2 Staging classification systems of gastrointestinal lymphoma

Ann Arbor system	Lugano system	TNM classification	Spread of lymphoma
EI 1*	I1	T1 N0 M0	Mucosa, submucosa
E I 2	I2	T2 N0 M0	Muscularis propria, subserosa
E I 2	I2	T3 N0 M0	Serosal penetration
E I 2	IIE**	T4 N0 M0	Infiltration of adjacent organs or tissues
E II 1	II1E	T1-4 N1 M0	Infiltration of regional lymph nodes (compartments I+II)
E II 2	II2E	T1-4 N2 M0	Infiltration of lymph nodes beyond the regional stations (compartment III), including retroperitoneal, mesenteral and para-aortal lymph nodes
III	–	T1-4 N3 M0	Infiltration of infradiaphragmatic and supradiaphragmatic lymph nodes
IV	IV	T1-4 N0-3 M1	Dissemination of the lymphoma

*E = primary extranodal localization; **E = infiltration of adjacent organs per continuitatem.

Table 3 Stage stratified treatment of low grade and high grade gastric lymphoma

Stage	Low grade	High grade
I1/2	H. pylori eradication	Chemotherapy ± radiation (surgery + chemotherapy)
	If H. pylori is negative, no complete remission or relapse: radiation (surgery)	
	Minimal residual disease – watch-and-wait	
II1/2	Radiation (surgery)	Chemotherapy ± radiation (surgery ± chemotherapy)
III, IV	Chemotherapy	Chemotherapy ± radiation

(Table 2), is clinically important due to its prognostic and therapeutic impact. *Endoscopic ultrasound (EUS)* is the only morphological procedure able to visualize the different layers of the gastric wall and the perigastric lymph nodes. It is therefore suitable for the local staging of gastric lymphoma. The treatment strategy of our first prospective study was based on surgery[1]. With respect to the increasingly favoured stomach-conserving treatment approach it was probably the last chance to compare the diagnostic accuracy of EUS with the gold standard of the pathohistological stage. Given an overall diagnostic accuracy of 53% the results were rather disappointing[19]. The main source of error was endosonographically 'positive' lymph nodes that were found at histology to represent inflammatory reactions rather than lymphoma infiltration. It has to be kept in mind that the study was performed in the mid-1990s when the technique of EUS was still new for most gastroenterologists. It can be assumed that, with increasing familiarity with EUS, the potential of endosonographically guided puncture of lymph nodes, and the use of miniechoendoscopes, the diagnostic accuracy of EUS has been substantially improved recently. The value of EUS in estimating the response of gastric lymphoma to radiation or chemotherapy is still not well documented; yet there is evidence from a small German series that success or failure of *H. pylori* eradication therapy can be predicted by EUS[20]. In another series published recently by our group we could confirm the prognostic validity of EUS with respect to the rate of lymphoma regression following eradication therapy[21]. The results on staging procedures have to be discussed against the fact that 90% of both low-grade and high-grade gastric lymphoma present as stage I or II based on the surgical and pathohistological staging in our first multicentre study[1].

THERAPY

The convincing evidence for a pathogenetic role of *H. pylori* infection, as pointed out above, inevitably involved a therapeutic effort. In 1993, Wotherspoon et al. reported a complete regression of low-grade gastric MALT lymphoma following successful eradication of the bacterium in five of six cases[22]. Since then, several prospective trials have confirmed this observation. Bayerdörffer and co-workers found lymphoma regression in 23 of 33 patients[6], and the same group later reported on a successful treatment in 100 out of 125 cases[23]. The results of our study, with complete lymphoma regression in 89% of cases[1], are in good agreement with these findings and the literature suggesting an overall success rate of *H. pylori* eradication therapy of about 80% in low-grade gastric MALT lymphoma of stage I[15]. However, the ultimate value of this fascinating therapeutic option was under debate until very recently with respect to lacking long-term data. In 2004, we presented our follow-up of 44.6 (12–89) months in 95 patients suffering from gastric low-grade MALT lymphoma and being exclusively treated by eradication therapy[21]. A long-lasting complete remission was documented in 62%, offering a real chance of cure to these patients. 18% revealed *minimal residual disease*, which is defined as histologically persisting lymphoma infiltrates at 1 year after successful eradication therapy and normalization of the macroscopic findings. Up to now these patients were classified as non-responders to *H. pylori* eradication and transferred to radiation or surgery. We believe that such a treatment procedure is not necessary. In a first series of seven patients with minimal residual disease we did not find a single case revealing lymphoma progression, dissemination or high-grade transformation[24]. The favourable natural course of minimal residual disease was confirmed in a larger clinical series recently[25]. We therefore clearly favour a watch-and-wait strategy in this situation.

In our first multicentre study we have convincingly shown that a *surgical approach* followed by radiation and/or chemotherapy, depending on grade of malignancy, stage and residual tumour status, represents a successful concept for localized gastric lymphoma of stages I and II[1]. In good agreement with a French study[26] we identified R0 resection as an independent prognostic factor. However, simultaneously it became increasingly evident that combined radio-/chemotherapy offers a comparable therapeutic efficiency. In a non-randomized prospective trial the 'Münster Study Group' found no difference with respect to overall survival and lymphoma-free survival between surgically and conservatively treated patients[5]. In our eyes the main clinical challenge was therefore to clarify whether the surgical or conservative approach is preferable with respect to both cure of disease and quality of life. To give a satisfying answer to this question we performed a second prospective study comparing, in a randomized trial, surgery and radiation in low-grade and surgery plus chemotherapy and chemotherapy alone in high-grade gastric lymphoma, respectively. According to our first results we could not find any differences with respect to treatment failure, relapse or survival[27]. The advantage of an organ-preserving treatment contributing to a better quality of life seems not to be related to a negative outcome.

CURRENT RECOMMENDATIONS AND FUTURE ASPECTS

Lessons from Germany include new insights into aetiology and pathogenesis of gastric MALT lymphoma and their histomorphological and molecular biological characteristics offering a much more precise differential diagnosis and prognostic estimation. We have learnt that, due to the unspecific macroscopic appearance of gastric lymphoma and the uncertainty of random endoscopic biopsies, a gastric mapping procedure is essential to establish a correct diagnosis and typing of the lymphoma. Endoscopic ultrasound has become an obligatory part of the initial staging procedure. *H. pylori* eradication therapy has proven to be highly efficacious in gastric low-grade MALT lymphoma of stage I, offering a real chance of cure to a considerable number of patients. A watch-and-wait strategy seems to be a good choice in the individual case of minimal residual disease after successful *H. pylori* eradication. A conservative approach based on radiation in low-grade and chemotherapy in high-grade lymphoma, respectively, is preferred to surgery. The current treatment recommendations are summarized in Table 3. The three German study groups have considerably contributed to these statements. To concentrate and harmonize their future activities the German study group on gastrointestinal lymphoma (DSGL: Deutsche Studiengruppe Gastrointestinale Lymphome) has been established recently. The DSGL has activated new study protocols in 2004 and invites everybody to include patients into the ongoing trials (detailed information from the author).

References

1. Fischbach W, Dragosics B, Koelve-Goebeler ME et al. Primary gastric B-cell lymphoma: results of a prospective multicenter study. Gastroenterology. 2000;119:1191–202.
2. Cogliatti SB, Schmid U, Schumacher U et al. Primary B-cell gastric lymphoma: a clinicopathological study of 145 patients. Gastroenterology. 1991;101:1159–70.
3. Radaszkiewicz Th, Dragosics B, Bauer P. Gastrointestinal malignant lymphomas of the mucosa-associated lymphoid tissue. Factors relevant to prognosis. Gastroenterology. 1992; 102:1628–38.
4. Koch P, delValle F, Berdel WE et al. Primary gastrointestinal non-Hodgkin's lymphoma: I. Anatomic and histologic distribution, clinical features, and survival data of 371 patients registered in the German multicenter study GIT NHL 01/92. J Clin Oncol. 2001;19:3861–73.
5. Koch P, Del Valle F, Berdel W et al. Primary gastrointestinal non-Hodgkin's lymphoma: II. Combined surgical and conservative or conservative management only in localized gastric lymphoma. Results of the prospective German multicenter study GIT NHL 01/92. J Clin Oncol. 2001;19:3874–83.
6. Bayerdörffer E, Neubauer A, Rudolph B et al. Regression of primary gastric lymphoma of mucosa-associated lymphoid tissue type after cure of *Helicobacter pylori* infection. Lancet. 1995;345:1591–4.
7. Neubauer A, Thiede Ch, Morgner A et al. Cure of *Helicobacter pylori* infection and duration of remission of low-grade gastric mucosa-associated lymphoid tissue lymphoma. J Natl Cancer Inst. 1997;89:1350–5.
8. Jaffe ES, Harris NL, Stein H, Vardiman JW. World Health Organization Classification of Tumours: Pathology and Genetics: Tumours of Haematopoetic and Lymphoid Tissues. Lyon: IARC Press, 2002.
9. Fischbach W. Gastrointestinale Lymphome. Ätiologie, Pathogenese und Therapie. Internist. 2000;41:831–40.

10. Stolte M, Eidt S. Lymphoid follicles in antral mucosa: immune response to *Campylobacter pylori*? J Clin Pathol. 1989;42:1269–71.
11. Greiner A, Marx A, Heesemann J, Leebmann J, Schmausser B, Müller-Hermelink HK. Idiotype identity in a MALT-type lymphoma and B-cells in *Helicobacter pylori* associated chronic gastritis. Lab Invest. 1994;70:572–8.
12. Stolte M. *Helicobacter pylori* gastritis and gastric MALT-lymphoma. Lancet. 1992;339:745
13. Wotherspoon A, Ortiz-Hidalgo C, Falzon MR, Isaacson PG. *Helicobacter pylori*-associated gastritis and primary B-cell gastric lymphoma. Lancet. 1991;338:1175–6.
14. Eck M, Schmausser W, Haas R et al. MALT-type lymphoma of the stomach is associated with *Helicobacter pylori* strains expressing the CagA protein. Gastroenterology. 1997;112:1482–6.
15. Fischbach W. MALT-Lymphome des Magens. Dtsch Med Wochenschr. 1999;124:1142–7.
16. Stolte M, Kroher G, Meining A et al. A comparison of *Helicobacter pylori* and H. heilmannii gastritis. A matched control study involving 404 patients. Scand J Gastroenterol. 1997;32:28–33.
17. Kolve ME, Greiner A, Müller-Hermelink HK, Wilms K, Fischbach W. Eradication of *Helicobacter pylori* (*Hp*) in gastric MALT-type lymphoma is still an experimental therapy. Gastroenterology. 1997;112:A594
18. Ruskone-Fourmestraux A, Dragosics B, Morgner A. Paris staging system for primary gastrointestinal lymphomas. Gut. 2003;52:912–16.
19. Fischbach W, Goebeler-Kolve ME, Greiner A. Diagnostic accuracy of EUS in the local staging of primary gastric lymphoma: results of a prospective, multicenter study comparing EUS with histopathologic stage. Gastrointest Endosc. 2002;56:696–700.
20. Sackmann M, Morgner A, Rudolph B, et al. Regression of gastric MALT lymphoma after eradication of *Helicobacter pylori* is predicted by endosonographic staging. MALT Lymphoma Study Group. Gastroenterology. 1997;113:1087–90.
21. Fischbach Goebeler-Kolve ME, Dragosics B, Greiner A, Stolte M. Long-term outcome of patients with gastric marginal zone B-cell lymphoma of MALT following exclusive *Helicobacter pylori* eradication therapy. Experience from a large prospective series. Gut. 2004;53:34–7.
22. Wotherspoon AC, Doglioni C, Diss TC et al. Regression of primary low-grade B-cell gastric lymphoma of mucosa-associated lymphoid tissue type after eradication of *Helicobacter pylori*. Lancet. 1993;342:575–7.
23. Morgner A, Bayerdörffer E, Neubauer A et al. Cure of *Helicobacter pylori* infection in 125 patients with primary gastric low-grade MALT lymphoma. Gastroenterology. 1998;114:A814.
24. Fischbach W, Goebeler-Kolve M, Starostik P et al. Minimal residual low-grade gastric MALT-type lymphoma after eradication of *Helicobacter pylori*. Lancet. 2002;360:547–8.
25. Goebeler-Kolve ME, Savio A, Greiner A, Fischbach W. Management of patients with minimal residual gastric low-grade lymphoma of MALT-type after eradication of *Helicobacter pylori*: increased experience from a clinical series. Gastroenterology. 2003;124 (Suppl. 1):A242.
26. Ruskone-Fourmestraux A, Aegerter P, Delmer A, Lavergne A, et al. Primary digestive tract lymphoma: a prospective multicentric study of 91 patients. Gastroenterology. 1993;105:1662–71.
27. Goebeler ME, Greiner A, Stolte M et al. Results of the German Randomized Prospective Multicenter Study in 42 patients with localized primary gastric B-cell lymphoma. Gastroenterology. 2004;126:A1362.

7
Who gets gastric cancer – predisposition or bad luck?

K. E. L. McCOLL

INTRODUCTION

Cancers arise from interactions between environmental influences and human genes. The relative and precise contribution of these two factors varies widely from cancer to cancer and from case to case. In addition, the nature of the interaction between the environmental factors and the human genome is to a certain extent random and the outcome therefore unpredictable. As a consequence the risks of a particular individual developing cancer can be predicted with only a limited degree of accuracy.

This chapter does not address cancer at the gastro-oesophageal junction or proximal cardia region of the stomach, but only gastric cancers occurring more distally. Such cancers can be subdivided into 'familial' and 'sporadic' in type.

FAMILIAL GASTRIC CANCER

This term is used to describe cancers arising in a person with a strong family history of the same tumour and usually presenting at a relatively young age. Such subjects are thought to have a strong genetic predisposition to the cancer. In some families there is a clear autosomal dominant pattern of inheritance and the cancers usually present before 50 years of age. Such cancers are usually of the diffuse histological subtype and develop against a background of a histologically and functionally normal gastric mucosa. A number of germline mutations have been identified to explain hereditary diffuse gastric cancer. The best documented is that involving the E-cadherin gene where there is deletion of one of the alleles[1–4]. Sixty-seven per cent of men and 83% of women who inherit the genetic abnormality will develop gastric cancer by the age of 80 years[5]. This cancer represents one extreme end of the spectrum where genetic predisposition is the paramount factor explaining the development of the lesion. Hereditary diffuse cancers are relatively rare, accounting for less than 3% of gastric cancers[6]. Germline mutations of the E-cadherin gene account for approximately 25% of hereditary diffuse gastric cancers[1].

SPORADIC GASTRIC CANCER

The vast majority of gastric cancers are of the 'sporadic' type, occurring in subjects with little if any family history of the lesion and usually presenting in later life. This chapter will focus on these 'sporadic' gastric cancers and on the role of predisposing factors, and bad luck, in the development of these tumours.

Role of *Helicobacter pylori*

A number of environmental factors are associated with an increased risk of sporadic gastric cancer. The most important of these is colonization of the gastric mucosa by *H. pylori*. This is a Gram-negative helical flagellated bacterium present in the stomach of approximately 50% of the world's human population. The organism was first reported by Warren and Marshall in 1983[7]. The infection is usually acquired in childhood and, unless treated, persists indefinitely. It is more common in populations of low socioeconomic status[8]. The bacterium adheres to the luminal surface of the gastric epithelial cells protected from the gastric acid by the overlying mucus layer. The organism does not invade the underlying mucosa but induces an infiltrate of both chronic and acute inflammatory cells. Half of the world's population thus have a histological gastritis induced by this chronic infection. Epidemiological studies have shown a strong association between *H. pylori* and gastric cancer. Subjects with the infection have a six-fold higher risk of developing gastric cancer than uninfected subjects[9]. It is estimated that 75% of cases of gastric cancer can be attributed to *H. pylori* infection[9].

Role of other environmental factors

Other environmental risk factors for gastric cancer had been identified before the discovery of *H. pylori* infection. These include smoking, a diet high in salt and a diet low in fruit and antioxidants[10–12]. It has been important to re-examine the associations between these various risk factors and gastric cancer, to ensure that they are not due to confounding by each other. The potential problem relates to the fact that *H. pylori* and a low antioxidant intake and high salt intake are all associated with low socioeconomic status. Consequently, one risk factor might merely be a surrogate marker for the other. Studies from South America suggest that *H. pylori* and low fruit intake are independent risk factors[12] and studies from Norway confirm the same with respect to *H. pylori* and smoking[10].

Multistage progression to sporadic gastric cancer

Over the past 20 years there has been considerable progress in our understanding of the mechanism by which *H. pylori* infection increases the risk of gastric cancer. The infection produces a superficial gastritis in all infected subjects, and this is usually most severe in the distal antral region of the stomach. However, in infected subjects who go on to develop gastric cancer, the pattern of gastritis changes over the years[13]. The inflammation extends to involve the proximal body region of the stomach and this becomes the predominant site of the gastritis. In addition, the inflammation produces atrophy of the gastric mucosa. This process leads to areas of gastric mucosa being replaced by mucosa whose phenotype resembles that of the small or large intestine, a process referred to as intestinal metaplasia. This progressive histological change in the appearance of the gastric mucosa is accompanied by changes in gastric function, with a progressive decrease and eventual complete loss of acid secretory capacity[14]. The loss of acid secretion allows a variety of bacterial species to colonize the stomach, including those able to generate potentially carcinogenic N-nitroso compounds[15]. When achlorhydria develops the *H. pylori* infection which initiated the progressive process disappears[14]. Subjects who develop this body-predominant atrophic gastritis and achlorhydria have a much higher risk of developing gastric cancer than those who have only a persisting superficial gastritis[16]. Most sporadic gastric cancers have an intestinal phenotype and are thought to arise from the areas of histological intestinal metaplasia. Progression from intestinal metaplasia to cancer proceeds through an intermediate stage of dysplasia.

There is therefore a clear multistage histological pathway for the development of most cases of sporadic gastric cancer. The process starts with superficial gastritis induced by *H. pylori* infection. This progresses to atrophic gastritis with loss of acid secretion, then to intestinal metaplasia, dysplasia and finally cancer. Subjects with the more virulent CagA-positive strains of *H. pylori* are more likely to progress along this pathway[17,18]; however, a number of other factors influence the likelihood of progression along this pathway leading to cancer.

It seems likely that the other environmental risk factors for sporadic gastric cancer may exert their effect by influencing the rate of progression from superficial gastritis to atrophic gastric and to gastric cancer. The progressive damage to the gastric epithelium by the inflammatory gastritis is likely to be a consequence, at least in part, of the damaging effects of free radicals produced by the inflammatory cells. The protective effect of a diet high in fruit and antioxidants may provide protection from these radicals and thus reduce the chance and rate of progression from superficial gastritis to atrophic gastritis. Likewise, antioxidants may prevent the free radicals from inducing DNA damage, leading eventually to metaplasia, dysplasia and cancer. The increased risk of gastric cancer associated with a high salt intake may be explained by the ability of salt to erode the surface mucus layer which protects the gastric epithelium from various chemicals within the gastric lumen[19,20]. This may include ingested carcinogens or mutagenic chemicals generated by the nitrosating bacterial species which colonize the achlorhydric stomach[21]. Cigarette smoke contains a wide range of carcinogens which will contribute to the progression of the mutagenic process.

Role of host genetic factors in progression to sporadic gastric cancer

Recent studies indicate that host genetic factors play an important role in determining the risk of sporadic as well as familial gastric cancer. Functionally relevant genetic polymorphisms of the interleukin (IL)-1B gene affect the nature of the gastric mucosal response to *H. pylori* infection at both a histological and physiological level. El-Omar et al. demonstrated that polymorphisms of the IL-1B gene encoding IL-1B and of the IL-1RN gene encoding the naturally occurring receptor antagonist markedly increase the risk of developing atrophic gastritis and achlorhydria in response to *H. pylori* infection[22]. IL-1B is a powerful inhibitor of acid secretion as well as a stimulus of the inflammatory cascade. These proinflammatory polymorphisms have also been shown to increase the risk of gastric cancer[22]. More recent studies have shown a similar but weaker role for polymorphisms of the TNF-α gene that correlates with high tumour necrosis factor (TNF)-α levels[23]. Toll-like receptor 4 is an important host pattern recognition receptor that is key to initiating an inflammatory response against bacterial lipopolysaccharide. Recent studies by El-Omar et al. have shown that polymorphisms that cause aberrant lipopolysaccharide handling increase the risk of *H. pylori*-infected subjects developing atrophy, hypochlorhydria and gastric cancer[24]. It can therefore be seen that a variety of host genetic factors influence the inflammatory response to *H. pylori* infection, and consequently the probability of progressing to gastric cancer. It is likely that many other functional genetic polymorphisms will be found to exert a similar influence.

Role of gender

Another important host genetic factor which influences the risk of gastric cancer is male gender[25]. *H. pylori* infection, atrophic gastritis and achlorhydria are equally common in males and females. However, the risk of gastric cancer is higher in males. This suggests that something related to male sex increases the risk of progressing from atrophic gastritis to cancer. Alternatively, something related to female sex may be protective. The reduced risk of gastric cancer in females is in fact a delay in the age at which the risk of sporadic cancer increases[25]. This is consistent with something related to the female reproductive years being protective. It is possible that female sex hormones exert a protective effect. In addition, the lower tissue iron levels associated with the female reproductive years may protect against the generation of free radicals and DNA damage. In laboratory animals tissue iron levels are known to be associated with increased risk of certain cancers, including those of the upper gastrointestinal tract[26].

Multistage multifactorial multicombination

Three points are therefore apparent with respect to sporadic gastric cancer: (1) it is usually a multistage process with progression from superficial gastritis to atrophic gastritis, dysplasia and cancer; (2) it is a multifactorial process as the progression is a consequence of the complex interaction of a substantial number of host genetic and environmental factors, many of which are probably still unrecognized; (3) in addition, many different combinations of these genetic host and environmental factors are likely to enable progression to cancer.

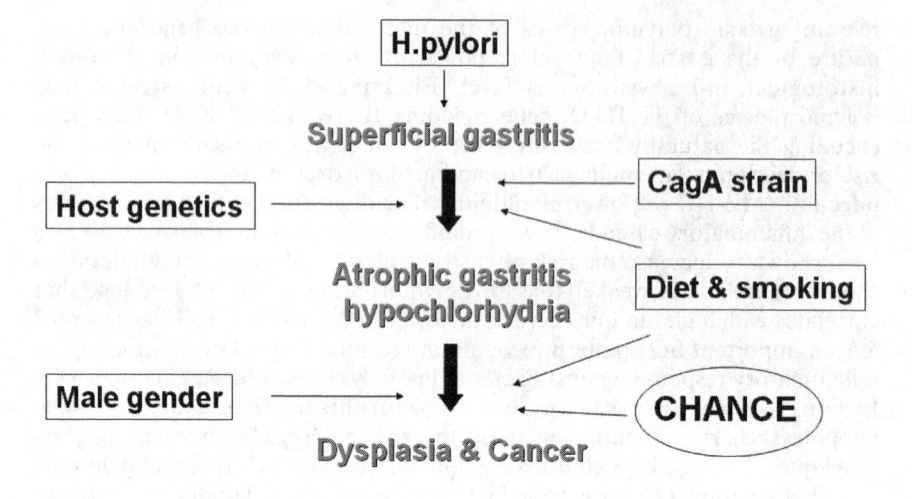

Figure 1 The development of sporadic gastric cancer is a multistage process progressing from *H. pylori* superficial gastritis to atrophic gastritis and intestinal metaplasia to dysplasia and cancer. Multiple factors influence advancement from one stage to the next. There is also an element of chance in the final development of cancer due to the random nature of DNA dosage

Molecular events introduce chance into risk of sporadic cancer

We can therefore see that predisposition as a consequence of host genetic and environmental factors plays an important role in sporadic gastric cancer. Is there a place for bad luck? To appreciate the role of luck it is important to understand what is happening at a molecular level, and the changes which are taking place within the genome of the epithelial stem cells which eventually manifest themselves as cancer.

Gastric cancer cells are characterized by having alterations of genes controlling cell growth and proliferation, apoptosis, ageing and angiogenesis. The pattern of genetic alteration varies markedly between individual gastric cancers[27]. Thus, a variety of different genetic aberrations can result in a similar cancer phenotype. The genetic alterations causing sporadic gastric cancer are the result of individual mutations of DNA base, and again these seem to arise at random sites and thus result in the variety of genetic aberrations.

What is the association between the alterations in DNA and the well-recognized progression from *H. pylori* superficial gastritis to atrophic gastritis with achlorhydria and on to cancer? It seems likely that the inflammation induced by *H. pylori* infection results in progressive DNA damage. This damage is likely to be induced by free radicals produced by the inflammatory cells. In addition, *H. pylori* increases epithelial cell proliferation, which makes the cells more susceptible to DNA damage. It is also possible that chemical mutagens generated by nitrosating bacteria colonizing the achlorhydric stomach may add to the DNA damage. This damage to DNA by free radicals or chemical carcinogens is random, and will therefore produce a variety of genetic aberrations, only some of which may lead to cancer. Consequently, there is an element of good and bad luck determining the outcome and the development of this cancer (Figure 1).

CONCLUSIONS

In summary, it can be seen that both predisposition and bad luck play a role in the development of gastric cancer. In the familial gastric cancers genetic predisposition is the dominant factor, with only a minor role for environmental influences and luck. However, in the more common sporadic cancers there is an important role for each of those three factors.

CLINICAL IMPLICATIONS

Our understanding of the mechanisms by which sporadic gastric cancer arises does indicate ways of potentially reducing its incidence. *H. pylori* infection appears to be an essential though inadequate factor in most cases of sporadic cancer. Consequently, preventing patients from developing *H. pylori* infection in the first place is likely to be the single most effective means of reducing the incidence of sporadic gastric cancer. Alterations in other environmental risk factors, such as reducing salt intake, increasing fruit intake and reducing smoking, is likely to be helpful even in those harbouring the infection. Evidence that such measures are effective is provided by the marked fall in incidence of gastric cancer over the past 50 years, which has coincided with a fall in *H. pylori* prevalence, a fall in salt intake and a rise in fruit consumption. Though we can never eliminate bad luck, we can reduce our chances of developing sporadic gastric cancer by appropriate modification to important environmental co-factors.

References

1. Fitzgerald RC, Caldas C. Clinical implications of E-cadherin associated hereditary diffuse gastric cancer. Gut. 2004;53:775–8.
2. Hunjtsman DG, Carneiro F, Lewis FR et al. Early gastric cancer in young, asymptomatic carriers of germ-line E-cadherin mutations. N Engl J Med. 2001;344:1904–9.
3. Handschuh G, Candidus S, Luber B et al. Tumour-associated E-cadherin mutations alter cellular morphology, decrease cellular adhesion and increase cellular motility. Oncogene. 1999;18:4301–12.
4. Kim HC, Wheeler JMD, Kim JC et al. The E-cadherin gene (*CDH1*) variants T340A and L599V in gastric and colorectal cancer patients in Korea. Gut. 2000;47:262–7.
5. Pharoah PDP, Guilford P, Caldas C and the international gastric cancer linkage consortium. Incidence of gastric cancer and breast cancer in CDH1 (E-cadherin) mutation carriers from hereditary diffuse gastric cancer families. Gastroenterology. 2001;121:1348–53.
6. Huntsman DG, Carneiro F, Lewis FR et al. Hereditary diffuse gastric cancer: more answers or more questions? Gastroenterology. 2002;122:830–2.
7. Warren JR, Marshall BJ. Unidentified carved bacilli on gastric epithelium in active chronic gastritis. Lancet. 1983;1:1273–5.

8. Woodward M, Morrison C, McColl K. An investigation into factors associated with *Helicobacter pylori* infection. J Clin Epidemiol. 2000;53:175–81.
9. *Helicobacter* and Cancer Collaborative Group. Gastric cancer and *Helicobacter pylori*: a combined analysis of 12 case control studies nested within prospective cohorts. Gut. 2001; 49:347–53.
10. Hansen S, Melby K, Aase S, Jellum E, McColl KEL, Vollset SE. *H. pylori* infection and smoking have strong joint effects as risk factors of non-cardia gastric cancer but have opposing effects on cardia cancer. Gut. 2000;46(Suppl. No: 2):A40 (abstract).
11. Joossens JV, Hill MJ, Elliott P et al. Dietary salt, nitrate and stomach cancer mortality in 24 countries. Int J Epidemiol. 1996;25:494–504.
12. Bluck LJ, Izzard AP, Bates CJ. Measurement of ascorbic acid and kinetics in man using stable isotopes and gas chromatography/mass spectrometry. J Mass Spectr. 1996;31:741–8.
13. Kuipers EJ. Review article: Relationship between *Helicobacter pylori*, atrophic gastritis and gastric cancer. Aliment Pharmacol Ther. 1998;12(Suppl. 1):25–36.
14. El-Omar E, Penman ID, Ardill JES, Chittajallu RS, Howie C, McColl KEL. *Helicobacter pylori* infection and abnormalities of acid secretion in patients with duodenal ulcer disease. Gastroenterology. 1995;109:681–91.
15. Reilly JP. Safety profile of the proton pump inhibitors. Am J Health-System Pharm. 1999; 56(Suppl. 4):S11–17.
16. Uemura N, Okamoto S, Yamamoto S et al. *Helicobacter pylori* infection and the development of gastric cancer. N Engl J Med. 2001;345:784–9.
17. Blaser MJ, Perez-Perez GI, Kleanthous H et al. Infection with *Helicobacter pylori* strains possessing CagA is associated with an increased risk of developing adenocarcinoma of the stomach. Cancer Res. 1995;55:2111–15.
18. Parsonnet J, Friedman GD, Orentreich N, Vogelman H. Risk for gastric cancer in people with CagA positive or CagA negative *Helicobacter pylori* infection. Gut. 1997;40:297–301.
19. Kodama M, Kodama T, Suzuki H, Kondo K. Effect of rice and salty rice diets on the structure of mouse stomach. Nutr Cancer. 1984;6:135–47.
20. Bergin IL, Sheppard BJ, Fox JG. *Helicobacter pylori* infection and high dietary salt independently induce atrophic gastritis and intestinal metaplasia in commercially available outbred Mongolian gerbils. Dig Dis Sci. 2003;48:475–85.
21. Tatematsu M, Takahashi M, Fukushima S, Hananouchi M, Shirai T. Effects in rats of sodium chloride on experimental gastric ancers induced by N-methyl-N'-nitrosoguanidine or 4′Nitroquinoline-1-oxide. J Natl Cancer Inst. 1975;55:101–6.
22. El-Omar EM, Carrington M, Wong-Ho C et al. Interleukin-1 polymorphisms associated with increased risk of gastric cancer. Nature. 2000;404:398–99.
23. Machado JC, Figueiredo C, Canedo P et al. A proinflammatory genetic profile increases the risk for chronic atrophic gastritis and gastric carcinoma. Gastroenterology. 2003;125:364–71.
24. Hold GL, Smith MG, Chow WH, Rabkin CS, El-Omar EM. A functional toll-like receptor 4 polymorphism increases risk of gastric cancer. Gut. 2004;53(Suppl. 3):A23.
25. Sipponen P, Hyvarinen H, Seppala K, Blaser MJ. Review article: Pathogenesis of the transformation from gastritis to malignancy. Aliment Pharmacol Ther. 1998;12(Suppl. 1): 61–71.
26. Goldstein SR, Yang GY, Curtis SK et al. Development of esophageal metaplasia and adenocarcinoma in a rat surgical model without the use of a carcinogen. Carcinogenesis. 1997;18:2265–70.
27. Moss SF. Review article: Cellular markers in the gastric precancerous process. Aliment Pharmacol Ther. 1998;12(Suppl. 1):91–109.

8
Future of endoscopic imaging

G. N. J. TYTGAT

INTRODUCTION

Several novel endoscopy methods have been developed over the past few years[1-13]. The most exciting is bioendoscopy, the molecular characterization of tissue by endoscopic means. All methods have common aims: (a) to enhance the resolution (the optical distinction between two points) and by doing so producing a detailed analysis of tissue microarchitecture; and (b) to characterize the biochemical characteristics of the various tissues. A further ultimate objective of all novel developments, in addition to more precise tissue characterization, is to eliminate the need for conventional biopsy. Yet a more realistic goal at this stage is still largely the identification of suspicious areas likely to harbour neoplastic change for targeted biopsy.

This overview will summarize some of those novel developments. Methods for spectroscopic analysis of tissue will not be discussed, except fluorescence spectroscopy.

HIGH-RESOLUTION–HIGH-MAGNIFICATION ENDOSCOPY

High-resolution endoscopes provide detailed images of the intestinal surface lining. Image resolution is further enhanced by optical/electronic magnification at the expense of reducing the surface area that is visualized[14-16].

With further development of endoscopic and digital image technologies, incorporating optical zooming and digital image enhancement, new options may become available to detect and characterize minute mucosal abnormalities which may have the potential to be disease-specific. Digital processing, for example, of videoendoscopic images of reflux oesophagitis may offer promise for interpreting mucosal colour changes with a potential to provide earlier diagnosis, improved reproducibility and comparison. Novel chip design may further increase the resolution. The realization of super-CCD chip technology has the potential to advance the detection of minute structural detail through increase of the light-sensitive photodiode area[17].

High-resolution–high-magnification endoscopy is often combined with chromoscopy to further enhance the visibility of the surface microarchitecture which allows detailed inspection of villous and especially pit patterns in the intestinal tract. The latter application is rapidly expanding worldwide to facilitate the detection of flat (adenomatous) neoplastic change[18].

NARROW-BAND IMAGING (NBI)

NBI was recently developed to improve the overall quality and detail of endoscopic images and to accentuate the microvasculature and villous or pit patterns of the mucosal surface. The sequential illumination method in videoendoscopes has a rotation disc with RGB (red, green, blue) filters in front of a white-light source (xenon lamp). NBI is a novel technique that changes these optical filters to narrow-band spectral filters. The NBI system narrows the bandwith of the spectral transmittance of the optical filters used in the light source. The penetration depth of light is dependent on its wavelength. Visible blue light penetrates only the very superficial layer. The narrow-band blue image is therefore somewhat enhanced compared to the narrow-band red and green signal. NBI accentuates the relief pattern of the mucosa without the need for chromoscopy. In addition, the identification of the size and distribution of superficial capillaries is accentuated[19–21].

LASER-SCANNING CONFOCAL MICROSCOPY (LCM)

LCM images are obtained by measuring the reflective light of a 405 nm wavelength diode laser. Virtual histological images can be obtained successfully from fresh unstained tissue[22–24]. The special resolution of LCM is around 1 µm. The light penetration depth is limited to about 200 µm. Staining with 2% cresyl violet facilitates identification of nuclei and cell membranes[25]. *In-vivo* detection of morphological and microvascular changes of the colon in association with colitis using fibreoptic confocal imaging has been desscribed[26–27].

ENDOCYTOSCOPY

Inoue and colleagues developed a catheter-type contact endomicroscope which has a 1100 times magnifying power at maximum. After 1% methylene blue vital staining of the mucosa, living normal cells and cancer cells can be successfully observed in high-quality images, comparable to conventional cytology. The cellular architecture and composition can be analysed at micron-scale resolution. Mobility of erythrocytes in capillaries is readily identified. Neoplastic cells have blurred and irregularly enlarged nuclei. This technology approaches virtual biopsy and virtual histology[9].

FLUORESCENCE SPECTROSCOPY

Fluorescence spectroscopy allows the determination of biochemical properties from tissue. Photons of fluorescent light are scattered and absorbed during their path to the tissue surface where they are collected via an optical fibre. Fluorescence occurs when tissue emits light of slightly longer wavelengths following excitation by light of a shorter wavelength. One can exploit either fluorescence generated by excitation of naturally occurring tissue fluorophores such as collagen, porphyrins, NADH, etc. (autofluorescence) or fluorescence emitted after excitation of exogenously administered drugs (5-aminolaevulinic acid or haematoporphyrin derivative). In autofluorescence the detection of dysplastic lesions depends on changes in tissue microarchitecture and in the concentration, spatial distribution and metabolic activity of endogenous fluorophores. Using excitation wavelength in the violet blue, Barrett's epithelium generally emits a fluorescence spectrum characterized by a relative increase in the red-to-green fluorescence intensity ratio. This ratio rises as the mucosa evolves from grades of dysplasia (neoplasia) to carcinoma. Thus neoplastic tissue exhibits slightly weaker red fluorescence but markedly weaker green fluorescence than normal tissues when illuminated by blue light[28-32].

The latest videoautofluorescence imaging endoscope has one CCD chip for white light endoscopy and another chip for integration of total autofluorescence after blue light excitation (395–475 nm) plus green (550 nm) and red (610 nm) reflectance components to create pseudocolour image of neoplastic areas.

BIOENDOSCOPY

The use of optically detectable affinity ligands to target molecules of interest allows further more precise characterization of tissue. The identification of targets that are highly specific for a the disease process, together with high-affinity attachment of the labelling substance to the target, is obviously critical for more refined tissue characterization. Such fluorophores typically emit light in the near-infrared zone, and the fluorescent signal is often rather strong. An example of this technique is the use of fluorescently labelled antibodies against carcinoembryonic antigen, which may facilitate the detection of gastric tumour cells[33]. Whole-body imaging with green fluorescent protein may be useful to test the efficiency of gene carriers for *in-vivo* transduction experiments[34]. Reporter molecules or molecular beacons such as fluorescent indocyanine fluorochromes, linked to a peptide backbone carried by a pegylated polymer, accumulate in neoplastic tissue and strongly fluoresce after proteolysis by cathepsin B and stimulation with excitation light[35]. Such beacons may perhaps also be sprayed on suspected targets instead of being infused systemically. Topical administration of antibodies carrying a fluorescent tag to various luminally exposed epitopes would be another possibility for *in-situ* chemical tissue characterization. Another example of bioendoscopy is the use of the FISH technique to analyse chromosomal changes and mutations at the cellular level. So far cells need to be harvested by brush cytology, but perhaps future technology might eliminate the need for cell harvesting.

DISCUSSION

Random tissue sampling remains a 'hit-or-miss' process when searching for (neoplastic) lesions without suspicious morphological change. If histological confirmation of a lesion is required before deciding on topical treatment, the time lag associated with tissue processing necessitates a second procedure, which is a major and costly disadvantage. In addition there is a pressing need to improve the accuracy for targetting surveillance biopsies to genuine dysplastic areas such as in patients with long-standing ulcerative colitis or Barrett's oesophagus. This can be achieved only through more precise endoscopic tissue analysis.

Several novel imaging modalities have been developed to improve the detailed endoscopic inspection and analysis of the mucosal surface of the gastrointestinal tract. The main purpose of these novel developments is to facilitate the detection of microarchitectural changes suspicious of neoplastic aberration, allowing targeted biopsy or local ablation, preferably with mucosal resection to allow adequate ultimate histopathological analysis.

High-resolution–high-magnification endoscopy, usually combined with chromoscopy (lugol, indigocarmine, methylene blue) allows high-resolution analysis of the mucosal microarchitecture (pit patterns, villous growth). The applications of such technology are increasing for the detection of villous areas in Barrett's oesophagus or abnormal pit patterns in flat adenoma/neoplasia of the colon.

Narrow-band imaging is an emerging method for highlighting features of the mucosal surface that are invisible with standard white light videoendoscopy. NBI accurately depicts a villous relief and various pit patterns, and accentuates the vascular microcirculation.

In fluorescence endoscopy, tissue fluorophores are activated with bluish light to emit minute quantities of fluorescent light (autofluorescence). Fluorescent spectra from normal and neoplastic mucosa, differ sufficiently to allow computer-generated false colouring of abnormal areas for targeted biopsy or targeted destruction.

Probe-based laser-scanning confocal microscopic imaging may characterize suspicious areas as frankly malignant because malignant tissue architecture is readily identifiable and distinguishable from normal.

Bioendoscopy is defined as any endoscopic technique that either provides biological information about the target tissue or exploits unique biological features of the target tissue. The potential of bioendoscopy is dazzling. The possibility to monitor the function of a variety of proteins *in vivo* by designing appropriate beacons is on the horizon.

New optical techniques will continue to emerge, such as multiphoton, second harmonic and magnetic resonance microscopy, which can look deeper and in a less destructive way into living tissue. Green fluorescence protein, a reporter of gene expression and protein localization in living cells, unifies digitized fluorescence microscopy/endoscopy to molecular biology. By using blue, cyan, yellow and red fluorescent protein tags, confocal fluorescence microscopy and related imaging technologies will allow tracking of multiple proteins within living tissue.

It is readily obvious from the bewildering array of novel developments that the role of imaging in future biomedical research will only continue to accelerate at an unprecedented rate.

References

1. Bruno MJ. Magnification endoscopy, high resolution endoscopy, and chromoscopy; towards a better optical diagnosis. Gut. 2003;52(Suppl. 4):iv7-11.
2. Tajiri H, Matsuda K, Fukisaki J. What can we see with the endoscope? Present status and future perspectives. Dig Endsc. 2002;14:131-7.
3. Dacosta RS, Wilson BC, Marcon NE. New optical technologies for earlier endoscopic diagnosis of premalignant gastrointestinal lesions. J Gastroenterol Hepatol. 2002;17 (Suppl.):S85-104.
4. Dacosta RS, Wilson BC, Marcon NE. Photodiagnostic techniques for the endoscopic detection of premignant gastrointestinal lesions. Dig Endosc. 2003;15:153-73.
5. Yao K, Yoa T, Matsui T et al. Hemoglobin content in intramucosal gastric carcinoma as marker of histologic differentiation: a clinical application of quantitative electronic endoscopy; Gastrointest Endosc. 2000;52:241-9
6. Nakamura K. The future of new diagnostic techniques in gastroenterology. Development of real-time endoscopic image processing technology: adaptive index of haemoglobin color enhancement processing. Dig Endosc. 2002;14:S40-7.
7. Pasricha PJ, Motamedi M. Optical biopsies, 'bioendoscopy' and why the sky is blue: the coming revolution in gastrointestinal imaging. Gastroenterology. 2002;122:571-4.
8. Aabakken L. Endoscopic tumor diagnosis and treatment. Endoscopy. 2003;35:887-90.
9. Kumagai Y, Monma K, Kawada K. Magnifying chromoendoscopy of the esophagus: in-vivo pathological diagnosis using an endocytoscopy system. Endoscopy. 2004;36:590-4.
10. Ohkawa A, Miwa H, Namihisa A et al. Diagnostic performance of light-induced fluorescence endoscopy for gastric neoplasms. Endoscopy. 20004;36:515-21.
11. Lambert R. Diagnosis of esophagogastric tumors. Endoscopy. 2004;36:110-19.
12. Pasricha PJ. The future of therapeutic endoscopy. Clin Gastroenterol Hepatol. 2004;2:286-9.
13. Riemann JF. Wo liegt die zukunft der gastroenterologischen endoskopie? Z Gastroenterologie. 2004;42:495-6.
14. Otsuka Y, Niwa Y, Ohmiya N et al. Usefulness of magnifying endoscopy in the diagnosis of early gastric cancer. Endoscopy. 2004;36:165-9.
15. Hurlstone DP, Cross SS, Adam I et al. Efficacy of high magnification chromoscopic colonoscopy for the diagnosis of neoplasia in flat and depressed lesions of the colorectum: a prospective analysis. Gut. 2004;53:284-90.
16. Kiesslich R, Jung M. Magnification endoscopy: does it improve mucosal surface analysis for the diagnosis of gastrointestinal neoplasias? Endoscopy. 2002;34:819-22.
17. Udagawa T, Amano M, Okada F. Development of magnifying video endoscopes with high resolution. Dig Endosc. 2001;13:163-9.
18. Participants in the Paris Workshop. The Paris endoscopic classification of superficial neoplastic lesions: esophagus, stomach, and colon. Gastrointest Endosc. 2003;58:S3-50.
19. Sharma P, McGregor D, Cherian R, Weston A. Use of narrow band imaging, a novel imaging technique, to detect intestinal metaplasia and high-grade dysplasia in patient with Barrett's esophagus. Gastrointest Endosc. 2003;57:AB77
20. Kara MA, Bergman JJ, Fockens P et al. Narrow band imaging for improved mucosal pattern recognition in Barrett's esophagus. Gastrointest Endosc. 2003;57:AB176
21. Fujisaki J, Saito N, Matsuda K et al. Clinicopathological analysis of superficial type Barrett's esophageal cancer and efficacy of magnifying endoscopy with narrow band image system for specialized columnar epithelium. Gastrointest Endosc. 2003;57:AB179.

22. Inoue H, Igari T, Nishikage T, Ami K, Yoshida T, Iwai T. A novel method of virtual histopathology using laser-scanning confocal microscopy *in-vitro* with untreated fresh specimens from the gastrointestinal mucosa. Endoscopy. 2000;32:439-43.
23. Inoue H, Cho JY, Satodate H et al. Development of virtual histology and virtual biopsy using laser-scanning confocal microscopy. Scand J Gastroenterol. 2003;(Suppl. 237):37-9.
24. Sakashita M, Inoue H, Kashida H et al. Virtual histology of colorectal lesions using laser-scanning confocal microscopy. Endoscopy. 2003;35:1033-8.
25. George M, Meining A. Cresyl violet as a fluorophore in confocal laser scanning microscopy for future *in-vivo* histopathology. Endoscopy. 2003;35:585-9.
26. McLaren W, Anikijenko P, Barkla D. *In vivo* detection of experimental ulcerative colitis in rats using fiberoptic confocal imaging (FOCI). Dig Dis Sci. 2001;46:2263-76.
27. McLaren W, Anikjenko P, Thomas S. *In vivo* detection of morphological and microvascular changes of the colon in association with colitis using fiberoptic confocal imaging. Dig Dis Sci. 2002;47:2424-33.
28. Haringsma J, Tytgat GN, Yano H et al. Autofluorescence endoscopy: feasibility of detection of GI neoplasms unapparent to white light endoscopy with an evolving technology. Gastrointest Endosc. 2001;53:642-50.
29. Tajiri H, Kobayashi M, Izuishi K, Yoshida S. Fluorescence endoscopy in the gastrointestinal tract. Dig Endosc. 2000;12: S28-31.
30. Prosst RL, Gahlen J. Fluorescence diagnosis of colorectal neoplasms: a review of clinical applications. Int J Colorectal Dis. 2002;17:1-10.
31. Bhunchet E, Hatakawa H, Sakai Y, Shibata T. Fluorescein electronic endoscopy: a novel method for detection of early stage gastric cancer not evident to routine endoscopy. Gastrointest Endosc. 2002;55:562-71.
32. Mayinger B, Jordan M, Horbach T et al. Evaluation of in vivo endoscopic autofluorescence spectroscopy in gastric cancer. Gastrointest Endosc. 2004;59:191-8.
33. Keller R, Winde G, Terpe HJ, Foerster EC, Domschke W. Fluorescence endoscopy using a fluorescein-labeled monoclonal antibody against carcinoembryonic antigen in patients with colorectal carcinoma and adenoma. Endoscopy. 2002;34:801-7.
34. Wack S, Hajri A, Heisel F et al. Feasibility, sensitivity, and reliability of laser-induced fluorescence imaging of green fluorescent protein-expressing tumors *in vivo*. Mol Ther. 2003;7:765-73.
35. Marten K, Bremer C, Khazaie K et al. Detection of dysplastic intestinal adenomas using enzyme-sensing molecular beacons in mice. Gastroenterology. 2002;122:406-14.

Section III
Liver I

Chair: R. SCHMID and R. WILLIAMS

9
Portal hypertension: diagnosis and treatment

D. LEBREC

INTRODUCTION

Portal hypertension signifies an elevation of pressure in the portal vein and its venous territory. In the normal person portal pressure is around 12 mmHg with a pressure gradient between the portal and systemic vascular system lower than 5 mmHg. In patients with portal hypertension, portal pressure ranges from 17 to 40 mmHg with a portacaval pressure gradient ranging from 6 to 30 mmHg. Portal hypertension is present in approximately 20% of patients with cirrhosis but in decompensated cirrhosis, portal hypertension is present in all. The syndrome may be complicated by the development of portosystemic shunts that are responsible in part for variceal bleeding, hepatopulmonary syndrome and pulmonary arterial hypertension. When liver failure is associated with portal hypertension, ascites, spontaneous bacterial peritonitis and hepatic encephalopathy may occur. Portal hypertension depends on an increase in both portal tributary blood flow and hepatic vascular resistance. It is well known that a decrease in the degree of portal hypertension is associated with a decrease in certain complications. In this chapter the diagnosis and treatment of portal hypertension are discussed.

DIAGNOSIS OF PORTAL HYPERTENSION

The diagnosis of portal hypertension may be difficult in patients with chronic liver disease. Portal hypertension may be moderate and asymptomatic or severe. Non-invasive and invasive evaluations have been tested.

Physical signs

Splenomegaly

Splenomegaly is frequent but not always present in portal hypertension. There is no clear relationship between portal pressure and splenic size[1]. The only consequence of splenomegaly is hypersplenism (most frequently a low platelet count) with a normal bone-marrow function. Hypersplenism is not only associated with portal hypertension but can be present in any condition associated with splenomegaly and peripheral cytopenia.

Abdominal collateral circulation

The abdominal collateral circulation can be visualized if the obstacle is distal from or at the level of the left branch of the portal vein corresponding to a recanalization of the umbilical or paraumbilical veins. In Cruveilhier–Baumgarten syndrome an association with umbilical varicosities (caput medusa) and a collateral ascending circulation between the umbilicus and the xyphoid process may be observed. The collateral circulation in portal hypertension must be distinguished from cavocaval circulation, which is not ascending and is located in the flanks.

Ascites

The presence of ascites in patients with chronic liver disease suggests the presence of severe portal hypertension. All patients need investigation of the causes of ascites even when cirrhosis is suspected. Ascitic fluid should be sent for determination of albumin or protein concentration. The use of ascitic fluid protein in the differential diagnosis of the causes of ascites is overrated and misinterpreted.

Blood tests

In patients with cirrhosis the degree of portal hypertension is correlated with the severity of liver failure[2]. Thus, low levels of albumin and prolongation of prothrombin time – two markers of the severity of liver failure – have been tested in patients with chronic liver disease to evaluate the presence of portal hypertension. However, these values do not estimate the degree of portal hypertension.

Since hepatic fibrosis is responsible in part for the development of portal hypertension, different markers of fibrosis have been evaluated to correlate with portal pressure. For example, serum levels of laminin and aminoterminal propeptide of type III procollagen have been suggested to correlate with the hepatic venous pressure gradient[3,4]. The results showed an association between these markers of fibrosis and the degree of portal hypertension, i.e. elevated in patients with portal hypertension, but no significant correlation was found. Moreover, these findings were observed in alcoholics but not in other forms of liver disease.

Preliminary results showed that fibrotest, a component of different tests, are correlated with portal hypertension in patients with cirrhosis[5]. In this study it has been shown that, under a certain level of the fibrotest score, portal hypertension is always moderate, i.e. the hepatic venous pressure gradient is lower than 12 mmHg. Further studies are needed to confirm these results.

Endoscopic evaluation

Esophagogastroendoscopy

Endoscopy investigation is essential for evaluating portal hypertension. This procedure may detect the three main lesions responsible for gastro-oesophageal bleeding in portal hypertension: gastro-oesophageal varices, hypertensive gastropathy and antral vascular ectasia. The presence of oesophageal varices is considered to be pathognomonic of portal hypertension. Variceal size and wall abnormalities seem to be the most accurate predictive factors for the risk of bleeding, but are not correlated with the degree of portal hypertension.

Endoscopic sonography

The portal venous system is studied by exploring the oesophagus and stomach[6]. Oesophageal and gastric varices are seen at endoscopic sonography as anechoic structures beneath the mucosal and submucosal layers. Detection of oesophageal or gastric varices depends on the grade of the varices. In patients with oesophageal varices the sensitivity of endoscopic sonography is inferior to endoscopy in patients with small varices[6]. In patients with gastric varices endoscopic sonography is more sensitive than endoscopy, especially for fundal varices. Peri-oesophageal and perigastric veins are seen as anechoic structures outside the esophageal or gastric walls. The azygos vein is observed in all subjects and in patients with portal hypertension. The diameter of the azygos vein is significantly larger in patients with portal hypertension.

HAEMODYNAMIC EVALUATION

Portal and hepatic venous pressures

Many methods have been described to measure portal pressure. Direct methods of inserting a needle or a catheter in the portal vein have been used, but these are invasive and must be performed under general anaesthesia, which modifies haemodynamic values. Indirect methods by direct puncture of the splenic pulp or the liver are also invasive and unreliable.

At present the procedure of choice is measurement of the hepatic venous pressure gradient by inserting a catheter in the internal jugular, femoral or humeral vein, under local anaesthesia. The catheter is guided under fluoroscopic control into a hepatic vein. Wedged hepatic venous pressure, which is similar to the occluded pressure obtained with balloon catheters, is recorded when the tip of the catheter is wedged in a small hepatic venule. Free hepatic venous pressure is measured with the tip of the catheter placed in the hepatic vein close to the inferior vena cava junction[7]. The difference between wedged and free hepatic pressures corresponds to the hepatic venous pressure gradient. Normal values of hepatic venous pressure gradient range from 1 to 4 mmHg. The hepatic venous pressure gradient is normal in patients with extrahepatic portal hypertension. In patients with presinusoidal intrahepatic portal hypertension the hepatic venous pressure gradient is normal or moderately elevated. In patients with cirrhosis the hepatic venous pressure gradient is elevated but differs greatly from one patients to another, usually ranging from 8 to 30 mmHg.

Several studies have focused on determining the lowest hepatic venous pressure gradient necessary to reduce the risk of bleeding. A value of 12 mmHg was retrospectively determined[8].

Variceal pressure

The variceal pressure corresponding to the transmural pressure is the only value that can be measured in humans. Direct puncture of the variceal wall has been first proposed, but this technique is invasive and should be performed immediately before sclerotherapy, since bleeding occurs in 10% of cases[9].

Non-invasive measurement by endoscopic gauge has been shown to be well correlated with results obtained by direct variceal puncture[10]. Non-invasive measurement seems to have a low inter-observer variability and a good reproducibility in the same patient. Variceal pressure could provide additional information for standard haemodynamic measurements. Variceal pressure was approximately 15% lower than portal pressure measured by the hepatic venous pressure gradient[10], and there was no correlation between the hepatic venous pressure gradient and variceal pressure in patients with cirrhosis. On the other hand, variceal pressure may provide a useful reflection of collateral circulation, since a good correlation has been found between variceal pressure and azygos blood flow.

DOPPLER SONOGRAPHY

Portal vein

Enlargement of the portal vein is a sign of portal hypertension, but studies have shown that a diameter greater than 13 mm or 15 mm only have sensitivities of 40% and 12%, respectively[11].

In normal subjects the portal blood flow goes towards the liver and has a continuous spectrum, with mild waves. In patients with portal hypertension there is a continuous flow towards the liver. In some cases alterations of portal blood flow appear as an absence of end-diastolic, arterialized flow or bidirectional (back-and-forth) flow. Reversed flow is rarely observed in the portal vein (1.1%) and is associated with a significant reduction in portal vein diameter. Portal vein diameter and blood flow changes are not, however, correlated with the hepatic venous pressure gradient.

Splanchnic veins

One study has demonstrated that the diameters of the superior mesenteric and splenic veins were different in control subjects and patients with portal hypertension[12]. The best discriminant findings were expiration measurements.

A lack of variation in calibre of the superior mesenteric vein during breathing was first considered highly sensitive and specific for diagnosis.

In control subjects the diameter of the coronary vein measured up to 6 mm. In patients with portal hypertension dilation of the coronary vein was seen in 26% of cases, while hepatofugal flow in the coronary vein was seen in 78% of patients.

Collaterals

Detection of collaterals is a sensitive and specific sign for the diagnosis of portal hypertension at sonography[13]. The three most frequent collaterals detected are the gastro-oesophageal veins, the paraumbilical vein and the splenorenal or gastrorenal veins. A correlation was observed between the degree of portal hypertension and the number of portosystemic pathways.

COMPUTED TOMOGRAPHY (CT)

Improvements in CT technique, including the helical mode, allow excellent identification of portal venous structures. Especially in patients with portal hypertension due to portal venous obstruction with doubtful Doppler results, CT is a useful tool to determine the presence of an obstruction and to provide signs suggesting recent obstruction. Helical CT also allows the acquisition of consistent volumetric data of the upper abdomen during the peak of vascular enhancement. From these volumetric results, detailed three-dimensional images can be created, representing the portal venous system and the collaterals in patients with portal hypertension. However, the main limitation of CT is its incapacity to determine the direction of flow.

MAGNETIC RESONANCE IMAGING (MR)

For qualitative data, MR imaging is indicated when Doppler studies are inconclusive. MR imaging is especially useful for the detection of portosystemic collaterals[14], for the diagnosis of portal vein thrombosis, and for the diagnosis and evaluation of hepatic vein obstruction.

MR imaging is also an effective non-invasive method of visualization of surgical portosystemic shunts when Doppler sonography is effective. Moreover, MR imaging has also been used to measure blood flow in the portal vein. Correlation studies have shown that the mean portal velocities on MR were well correlated with Doppler sonography values. Calculations of the portal vein flow by phase-contrast MR imaging were significantly lower in patients with portal hypertension with hepatopetal flow.

TREATMENT OF PORTAL HYPERTENSION

Different treatments reduce portal pressure in patients with portal hypertension. Surgical portosystemic shunts are very effective in decreasing the degree of portal hypertension and thus in treating and preventing variceal bleeding and ascites, but significantly increase the risk of hepatic encephalopathy and have no beneficial effect on survival. Thus, surgical shunts have been abandoned in many centres. TIPS have similar effects as do surgical shunts on portal hypertension and its complications, and TIPS also induce hepatic encephalopathy. Pharmacological treatments reduce portal hypertension by only 1–4 mmHg (from 5% to 20%) and have beneficial effects only on variceal bleeding, but have no major side-effects. Moreover, it has been shown that two drugs (terlipressine and beta-blockers) significantly improve survival rate in patients with cirrhosis (see below). Vasoconstrictive drugs have, however, no major effects on the other complications of portal hypertension. Endoscopic treatments have no effect on portal hypertension but only affect the prevention and treatment of variceal bleeding.

Among more than 50 drugs that decrease portal hypertension[15], only four types of drug (non-selective beta-adrenergic antagonists, nitrates, terlipressine and somatostatin and its analogues) are used in the treatment of portal hypertension. The effects of these drugs in the prevention and treatment of variceal bleeding are reported.

Prevention of the first episode of bleeding

Patients with cirrhosis and portal hypertension should undergo oesophagogastric endoscopic examination to determine the presence, absence and size of oesophageal or gastric varices. When varices are small or absent the early administration of beta-adrenergic antagonists, which limits the development of portosystemic shunts in portal hypertensive rats[16] does not seem to prevent the development of large oesophageal varices. A first randomized double-blind trial evaluated propranolol in the prevention of the development of large oesophageal varices in patients without varices or with small varices[17]. At 2 years the size of varices estimated on video-recording was not significantly different between the two groups. In this trial there was also no significant difference in the proportion of patients who bled and died between the two groups. Preliminary results with timolol confirmed these findings[18]. A third trial with nadolol in the prevention of the worsening of oesophageal varices in patients with cirrhosis and small varices showed a significant difference between patients receiving nadolol and patients receiving a placebo[19]. Thus, other studies are needed in selected subgroups of patients.

In patients with large varices, non-selective beta-adrenoceptor antagonists (propranolol or nadolol) must be prescribed since several meta-analyses have shown that beta-blockers significantly reduce the relative risk of bleeding by approximately 50% at 2 years compared to a placebo[20–23]. Moreover, at 2 years the mortality rate was significantly lower in patients treated with beta-blockers than in control patients. These results were more marked in patients with cirrhosis and liver dysfunction, or in patients with cirrhosis and ascites, than in patients in good condition or without ascites[20]. Beta-blockers were well tolerated and were discontinued in less than 5% of the treated patients due to side-effects. Treatment should be continued as in patients treated for arterial hypertension.

It has been demonstrated that nitrate administration decreases portal pressure and may further decrease the hepatic venous pressure gradient in patients receiving beta-blockers, thus trials have compared the efficacy of isosorbide-5-mononitrate alone or in combination with beta-blockers versus beta-blockers alone in the prevention of first bleeding in patients with cirrhosis. The efficacy of isosorbide-5-mononitrate was compared to non-selective beta-blockers in three studies. In one trial isosorbide-5-mononitrate was found to be a safe and alternative treatment to propranolol in the prevention of a first episode of bleeding, but at 5 years the mortality rate in patients older than 50 receiving nitrates was significantly higher than in those receiving propranolol[24]. In two other trials[25,26], isosorbide-5-mononitrate was less effective with more side-effects than nadolol or propranolol administration. These trials suggest that nitrates alone must not be prescribed for preventing a first episode of bleeding in patients with cirrhosis and varices. The combination of beta-blockers and nitrates has been compared to beta-blockers alone in three studies. A first study showed that the combination was significantly more effective than nadolol alone[27], while results of two studies did not find any significant difference between the two groups, with more side-effects in patients receiving the combination of nitrates and beta-blockers[28,29]. These discrepant results indicate that further clinical studies are needed.

Treatment of acute gastrointestinal bleeding

Before emergency endoscopy and endoscopic treatment, pharmacological treatment should be begun as soon as possible[30]. At present, terlipressin administration is effective for acute variceal bleeding and improving survival. Somatostatin or its analogues are also effective. Vasopressin alone must not be used due its potential side-effects and, if it is used, it should be combined with nitroglycerine to decrease the side-effects. Recently it has been shown that terlipressin or somatostatin administration is as effective as endoscopic sclerotherapy for the treatment of acute variceal bleeding, but also for the prevention of early rebleeding. These findings must be confirmed by other trials. The combination of vasoactive drugs and endoscopic treatment should be considered in the treatment of acute gastrointestinal bleeding.

Finally, it has been shown that early administration of terlipressin plus glyceryl trinitrate was more effective than a placebo in patients with cirrhosis[31]. In this study a medical intensive-care team administered drugs within 1 h after an emergency call. Control of bleeding was significantly higher for terlipressin than for placebo groups; however, the rebleeding rate was not significantly different at 2 weeks. The mortality rate was significantly lower in the terlipressin group than in the placebo group at 2 weeks.

Prevention of recurrent gastrointestinal bleeding

Beta-blocker administration also significantly reduces the risk of rebleeding and improves survival rate compared to a placebo in patients with cirrhosis[21,32]. This beneficial effect was observed in patients who had had an episode of acute variceal bleeding, but also in patients who bled from portal hypertensive gastropathy. Certain factors were shown to be associated with the risk of rebleeding in patients treated with beta-blockers: lack of compliance, lack of a persistent decrease in heart rate, occurrence of hepatocellular carcinoma, lack of alcohol abstinence and a previous episode of bleeding[33]. Neither the dose of beta-blockers nor the cause or severity of cirrhosis was associated with rebleeding. The incidence of mild and transient hepatic encephalopathy was 0.025%, which was similar to that in patients receiving a placebo.

CONCLUSIONS

The diagnosis of portal hypertension might be difficult in patients with cirrhosis, particularly in patients without clinical manifestation ot this syndrome. Different drugs are effective in treating portal hypertension and gastrointestinal bleeding. New types of drugs or combinations of drugs should be tested. Finally, new ideas, hypotheses and approaches are needed to further our understanding of the mechanisms of portal hypertension and its complications.

References

1. Simpson KJ, Finlayson NDC. Clinical evaluation of liver disease. Clin Gastroenterol. 1995; 9:639–59.
2. Braillon JP, Calès P, Valla D, Gaudy D, Geoffroy P, Lebrec D. Influence of the degree of liver failure on systemic and splanchnic haemodynamis and on response to propranolol in patients with cirrhosis. Gut. 1986;27:1204–9.
3. Gressner AM, Tittor W, Kropf J. The predictive value of serum laminin for portal hypertension in chronic liver diseases. Hepatogastroenterology. 1988;235:95–100.
4. Gressner AM, Tittor W, Negwer A, Pick-Kober KH. Serum concentrations of laminin and aminoterminal propeptide of type III procollagen in relation to the portal venous pressure of fibrotic liver diseases. Clin Chim Acta. 1986;161:249–58.
5. Thabut D, Imbert-Bismuth F, Cazals-Hatem D et al. Diagnostic value of fibrosis biochemical markers (Fibrotes-fibrosure) for the prediction of severe portal hypertension in patients with and without cirrhosis. Hepatology. 2004;38 (Suppl. 1):202A.
6. Caletti GC, Brocchi E, Ferrari A, Fiorino S, Barbara L. Value of endoscopic ultrasonography in the management of portal hypertension. Endoscopy. 1992;24(Suppl. 1):342–6.
7. Valla D, Bercoff E, Menu Y, Bataille C, Lebrec D. Discrepancy between wedged hepatic venous pressure and portal venous pressure after acute propranolol administration in patients with alcoholic cirrhosis. Gastroenterology. 1984;86:1400–3.
8. Lebrec D, de Fleury P, Rueff B, Nahum H, Benhamou JP. Portal hypertension, size of esophageal varices, and risk of gastrointestinal bleeding in alcoholic cirrhosis. Gastroenterology. 1980;79:1139–44.
9. Gertsch P, Fischer G, Kleber G, Wheatley AM, Geigenberger G, Sauerbruch T. Manometry of esophageal varices: comparison of an endoscopic balloon technique with needle puncture. Gastroenterology. 1993;105:1159–66.

10. Bosch J, Bordas JM, Rigau J et al. Noninvasive measurement of the pressure of esophageal varices using an endoscopic gauge: comparison with measurements by variceal puncture in patients undergoing endoscopic sclerotherapy. Hepatology. 1986;6:667–72.
11. Bolondi L, Gandolfi L, Arienti V et al. Ultrasonography in the diagnosis of portal hypertension: diminished response of portal vessels to respiration. Radiology. 1982;142:167–72.
12. Zoli M, Dondi C, Marchesini G, Cordiani MR, Melli A, Pisi E. Splanchnic vein measurements in patients with liver cirrhosis: a case-control study. J Ultrasound Med. 1985;4:641–6.
13. Vilgrain V, Lebrec D, Menu Y, Scherrer A, Nahum H. Comparison between ultrasonographic signs and the degree of portal hypertension in patients with cirrhosis. Gastrointest Radiol. 1990;15:218–22.
14. Rafal RB, Kosovsky PA, Jennis R, Markisz JA. Magnetic resonance imaging evaluation of spontaneous portosystemic collaterals. Cardiovasc Intervent Radiol. 1990;13:40–3.
15. Lebrec D. Pharmacological treatment of portal hypertension: present and future. J Hepatol. 1998;28:896–907.
16. Lin HC, Soubrane O, Cailmail S, Lebrec D. Early chronic administration of propranolol reduces the severity of portal hypertension and portal-systemic shunts in conscious portal vein stenosed rats. J Hepatol. 199;13:213–19.
17. Calès P, Oberti F, Payen JL et al. and the French-Speaking Club for the Study of Portal Hypertension. Lack of effect of propranolol in the prevention of large oesophageal varices in patients with cirrhosis: a randomized trial. Eur J Gastroenterol Hepatol. 1999;11:741–5.
18. Groszmann RJ, Garcia-Tsao G, Makuch R et al. Multicenter randomized placebo-controlled trial of non-selective beta-blockers in the prevention of the complications of portal hypertension: final results and identification of a predictive factor. Hepatology. 2003;38 (Suppl. 1):206A.
19. Merkel C, Marin R, Angeli P et al. and the Gruppo Triveneto par l'Ipertensione Portale. A placebo-controlled clinical trial of nadolol in the prophylaxis of growth of small esophageal varices in cirrhosis. Gastroenterology. 2004;127:476–84.
20. Poynard T, Calès P, Pasta L et al. and the Franco-Italian Multicenter Study Group. Beta-adrenergic-antagonist drugs in the prevention of gastrointestinal bleeding in patients with cirrhosis and esophageal varices. An analysis of data and prognostic factors in 589 patients from four randomized clinical trials. N Engl J Med. 1991;324:1532–8.
21. Pagliaro L, D'Amico G, Sörensen TIA et al. Prevention of first bleeding in cirrhosis. A meta-analysis of randomized trials of nonsurgical treatment. Ann Intern Med. 1992;117:59–70.
22. Hayes PC, Davis IM, Lewis JA, Bouchier IA. Meta-analysis of value of propranolol in prevention of variceal haemorrhage. Lancet. 1990;336:153–6.
23. D'Amico G, Pagliaro L, Bosch J. The treatment of portal hypertension: a meta-analytic review. Hepatology. 1995;22:332–54.
24. Angelico M, Carli L, Piat C, Gentile S, Capocaccia L. Effects of isosorbide-5-mononitrate compared with propranolol on first bleeding and long-term survival in cirrhosis. Gastroenterology. 1997;113:1632–9.
25. Borroni G, Salerno F, Cazzaniga M et al. Nadolol is superior to isosorbide mononitrate for the prevention of the first variceal bleeding in cirrhotic patients with ascites. J Hepatol. 2002;37:315–21.
26. Lui HF, Stanley AJ, Forrest EH et al. Primary prophylaxis of variceal hemorrhage: a randomized controlled trial comparing band ligation, propranolol, and isosorbide mononitrate. Gastroenterology. 2002;123:735–44.
27. Merkel C, Marin R, Sacerdoti D et al. and the Gruppo Triveneto per l'Ipertensione portale (GTIP). Long-term results of a clinical trial of nadolol with or without isosorbide mononitrate for primary prophylaxis of variceal bleeding in cirrhosis. Hepatology. 2000;31:324–9.
28. D'Amico G, Pasta L, Politi F et al. Isosorbine mononitrate with nadolol compared to nadolol alone for prevention of the first bleeding in cirrhosis. A double-blind placebo-controlled randomised trial. Gastroenterol Intern. 2002;15:40–50.
29. Garcia-Pagan JC, Morillas R, Bañares R et al. and the Spanish Variceal Bleeding Study Group. Propranolol plus placebo versus propranolol plus isosorbide-5-mononitrate in the prevention of a first variceal bleed: a double-blind RCT. Hepatology. 2003;37:1260–6.

30. Groszmann RJ, Bendtsen F, Bosch J et al. II Consensus Statements: Drug Therapy for Portal Hypertension. In: De Franchis R, editor. Portal Hypertension II. Oxford: Blackwell, 1996;98–99.
31. Levacher S, Letoumelin P, Pateron D, Blaise M, Lapandry C, Pourriat JL. Early administration of terlipressin plus glyceryl-trinitrate to control active upper gastrointestinal bleeding in cirrhotic patients. Lancet. 1995;346:865–8.
32. Bernard B, Lebrec D, Mathurin P, Opolon P, Poynard T. Beta-adrenergic antagonists in the prevention of gastrointestinal rebleeding in patients with cirrhosis: a meta-analysis. Hepatology. 1997;25:63–70.
33. Poynard T, Lebrec D, Hillon P et al. Propranolol for prevention of recurrent gastrointestinal bleeding in patients with cirrhosis: a prospective study of factors associated with rebleeding. Hepatology. 1987;93:447–51.

10
Current therapy of hepatitis C

S. W. SCHALM

INTRODUCTION

Now that effective therapy for chronic hepatitis C is available, physicians face a considerable challenge to implement in practice this important progress in medical therapy. A recent assessment of the problem estimates that 20–25% of persons with chronic hepatitis C have been identified, 3–4% have received treatment and 1–2% have been cured. Awareness of the potential serious consequences of chronic hepatitis C and the realistic potential of cure by antiviral therapy is limited among general practitioners, public health officers, specialists other than hepatologists, government and insurance companies. How can we summarize what can be achieved?

ACHIEVEMENTS OF ANTIVIRAL THERAPY OF HEPATITIS C

Acute hepatitis C can be cured in more than 90% of cases with interferon-based therapy[1]. Chronic hepatitis C patients who reach a sustained virological response after antiviral therapy have a life expectancy similar to that of the normal population[2]. This might also be true for patients with cirrhosis; their survival is significantly higher than cirrhotics who do not respond to antiviral therapy.

WHAT IS THE MOST EFFECTIVE THERAPY FOR CHRONIC HEPATITIS C?

Combination therapy

Combination therapy using interferon and ribavirin results in better treatment responses than monotherapy in all subcategories investigated[3]. The highest response rates have been achieved with pegylated interferon in combination with ribavirin[4,5]. Currently the best indicator of effective treatment is a sustained virologic response (SVR), defined by the absence of detectable serum HCV RNA by a qualitative HCV RNA assay at 24 weeks after the end

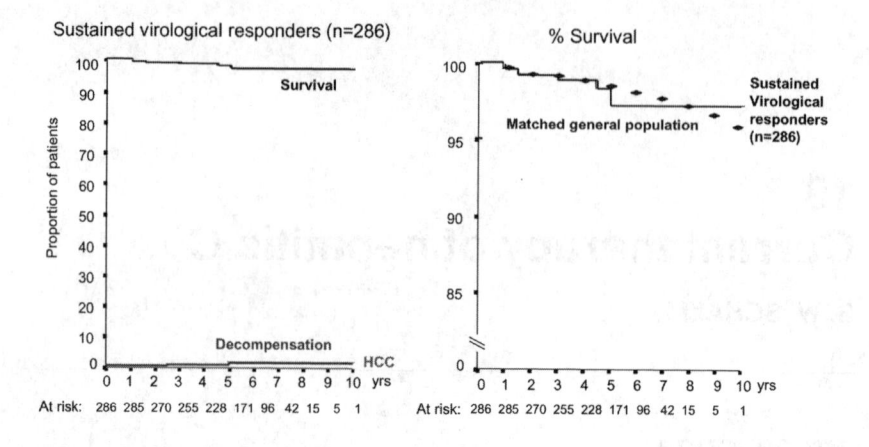

Figure 1 Based on current data, a sustained virological response reflects cure of chronic hepatitis C in Europe; the life expectancy returns to normal and the incidence of hepatocellular carcinoma is low

of treatment. In European patients such an endpoint virtually abolishes progression or complications of chronic hepatitis C infection[2]. Factors associated with successful therapy are mainly genotypes other than 1[4,5], and adherence to the doses and duration of therapy[6]. The presence of cirrhosis[7], HIV co-infection[8] or a previous non-response to therapy are unfavourable characteristics.

Patients with genotypes 2 or 3

Such patients should receive 24 weeks of pegylated interferon and ribavirin[4,5], and will achieve 95% SVR if adherent to therapy[6].

Patients with genotype 1 or 4

These patients need 48 weeks of treatment[4,5]. In genotype 1 SVR of 50–55% are to be expected if pegylated interferon is taken with ribavirin in adequate dosage (1000–1200 mg/day depending on weight)[6]. Responses are higher in genotype 4 and approach those of genotype 2 and 3.

Early viral response (EVR)

An EVR, defined as a minimum two-log decrease in viral load during the first 12 weeks of treatment, is predictive of SVR[5] and should be a routine part of genotype 1/4 patient monitoring. Patients who fail to achieve an EVR at week 12 have only a very small chance of achieving an SVR[5]; treatment should not be extended beyond 24 weeks in these patients[3].

Genotype 2 or 3

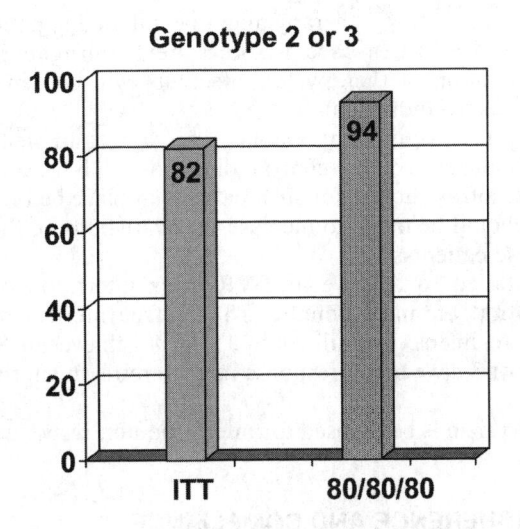

[Bar chart: ITT = 82, 80/80/80 = 94]

Figure 2 Pegylated interferon–ribavirin therapy cures almost all genotype 2/3 patients who take 80% of the dose of both drugs for 80% of the 6 months treatment duration (80/80/80); published results describe the cure rate in the intention-to-treat (ITT) population; i.e. all patients randomized

WHICH PATIENTS WITH CHRONIC HEPATITIS C SHOULD BE TREATED?

All patients with chronic hepatitis C are potential candidates for antiviral therapy. Treatment is recommended for patients with *(early) cirrhosis* and those with an *increased risk of developing cirrhosis*. Detectable HCV RNA levels and a liver biopsy with significant fibrosis or inflammation and necrosis characterize these patients. The majority also has persistently elevated ALT values[9,10].

Patients with *advanced cirrhosis* (no complications, but increased bilirubin or decreased platelets) have lower SVR rates and increased risks of severe side-effects. In those patients, as in patients with decompensated cirrhosis, liver transplantation may offer the primary treatment option.

Approximately 70% of patients with chronic HCV infection have normal or near-normal ALT levels (less than two times the upper limit of normal). Most of these patients have mild disease histologically; however, some may have advanced fibrosis or cirrhosis. Progression to cirrhosis is likely to be slow in patients who have minimal fibrosis and necroinflammatory changes. These patients need no treatment and should be monitored periodically for disease activity. However, decisions not to treat such patients should be individualized. If treated, results are similar to patients with elevated ALT[11].

Increasingly the desire to eliminate the HCV infection may influence decisions concerning therapy. In case of genotype 2/3, with its high chance of

SVR with 6 months of therapy, therapy might be initiated in patients with only minimal disease. In health-care workers performing exposure-prone procedures the duration of therapy for infectivity will be dependent on the genotype of the infected individual.

Injection drug use, significant alcohol use, age, and neuropsychiatric conditions are no longer absolute contraindications[9,10]; however, there should be a solid support infrastructure for such patients in place before commencing therapy. Efforts should be made to increase the availability of the best current treatments to these patients.

Patients who failed to achieve an SVR after interferon or interferon-ribavirin combination may benefit from retreatment with pegylated interferon-based regimens. Overall, only 15–20% achieve an SVR; patients with genotypes 2 or 3 have better response rates to retreatment than those with genotype 1[12].

In Japan glycyrrhizin is being used for interferon non-responders[13].

MAXIMIZING ADHERENCE AND COMPLIANCE

Cytopenias

Cytopenias, as currently defined by registration documents, are a frequent cause of dose reduction or even discontinuation. Dose reduction of pegylated interferon and/or ribavirin might be avoided by adaptation of time-tested toxicity rules, such as WHO toxicity grading as modified by the NCI. A study in Afro-Americans suggests that further lowering of the threshold for neutropenia is not associated with a detectable increase in the risk of severe infections[14]; the risk of severe infections appears restricted to patients with cirrhosis. Profound anaemia that requires dose reduction of ribavirin can be avoided by starting erythropoietin[15].

Neuropsychological side-effects

These are the other frequent cause of dose reduction. Difficulty in concentrating, loss of impulse control, and fear can be as troublesome as depression. Symptoms may appear after the second injection, justifying patient–doctor contact between 2 and 4 weeks after starting treatment; a low-dose serotonin uptake blocker (SSRI, such as paroxetine or citalopram) may be highly effective in reducing symptoms[16].

Dose reduction and/of discontinuation

This was shown to be more frequent in community hospitals than in referral hospitals participating in clinical trials (Table 1). Community hospitals, however, can have results similar to those in academic centres when the latter provide *expert support* to the former. Internet-based Doctor Online Consultation services are now in development[17].

Table 1 Early discontinuation of interferon–ribavirin therapy, by type of hospital (percentages)

	Referral hospitals in registration trials	Community-based practice
End treatment response	51	29
Sustained viral response	41	17
Early treatment discontinuation	20	51

Table 2 Genotype and infection: possible optimal duration of therapy, by early treatment response

HCV RNA PCR at week	4	12	24	Optimal treatment duration
Rapid responders	neg.	neg.	neg.	6 months
Intermediate responder	pos.	neg.	neg.	12 months
Slow responders	pos.	pos.	neg.	18 months

NEW DEVELOPMENTS

Evidence is accumulating that many genotype 2/3 patients need only 16 weeks of therapy[18]. Some patients with genotype 1 infection need only 24 weeks of therapy; others may achieve SVR only with extension of therapy until 72 weeks. Key to decision-making are HVC RNA PCR tests at 4 and 12 weeks, in addition to the generally accepted test at 24 weeks. (Table 2).

Doubling the dose of pegylated interferon, in genotype 1 patients who did not respond to a first course of therapy, can lead to a SVR rate of about 35%.

Clinical phase I–II studies with five to ten antiviral drugs that inhibit hepatitis C replication are under way. It is likely that one of those drugs will be successful in enhancing the effect of pegylated interferon, but it is difficult to predict which drug will be the winner.

References

1. Jäeckel E, Cornberg M, Wiedemeyer H et al. Treatment of acute hepatitis C with interferon alfa-2b. N Engl J Med. 2001;345:1452–7.
2. Veldt B, Saracco G, Boyer N et al. Long-term clinical outcome of chronic hepatitis C patients with sustained virological response to interferon monotherapy. Gut. 2004;53:1504–8.
3. Veldt B, Hansen B, Eijkemans M et al. Dynamic decision analysis to determine optimal treatment duration in chronic hepatitis C. Aliment Pharmacol Ther. 2005;21:539–47.
4. Manns MP, McHutchison JG, Gordon SC et al. Peginterferon alfa-2b plus ribavirin compared with interferon alfa-2b plus ribavirin for initial treatment of chronic hepatitis C: a randomised trial. Lancet. 2001;358:958–65.
5. Fried MW, Shiffman ML, Reddy KR et al. Peginterferon alfa-2a plus ribavirin for chronic hepatitis C virus infection. N Engl J Med. 2002;347:975–82.

6. McHutchison JG, Manns M, Patel K et al. Adherence to combination therapy enhances sustained response in genotype-1-infected patients with chronic hepatitis C. Gastroenterology. 2002;123:1061–9.
7. Lee S, Heathcote E, Reddy K et al. Prognostic factors and early predictability of sustained viral response with peginterferon alfa-2a (40KD). J Hepatol. 2002;37:500.
8. Carrat F, Bani-Sadr F, Pol S, et al. Pegylated interferon alfa-2b vs standard interferon alfa-2b, plus ribavirin, for chronic hepatitis C in HIV-infected patients: a randomized controlled trial. J Am Med Assoc. 2004;292:2839–48.
9. Lucidarme D. Hépatite C et Usage de drogues: Epidémiologie, dépistage, histoire naturelle et traitement. Gastroenterol Clin Biol. 2002;26:B112–20.
10. NIH Consensus Statement on Management of Hepatitis C: 2002. NIH Consens State Sci Statements. 2002;19:1–46.
11. Zeuzem S, Diago M, Gane E et al. Peginterferon alfa-2a (40 kilodaltons) and ribavirin in patients with chronic hepatitis C and normal aminotransferase levels. Gastroenterology. 2004; 127:1724–32.
12. Shiffman ML, Di Bisceglie AM, Lindsay KL et al. Peginterferon alfa-2a and ribavirin in patients with chronic hepatitis C who have failed prior treatment. Gastroenterology. 2004;126:1015–23.
13. Arase Y, Ikeda K, Murashima N et al. The long term efficacy of glycyrrhizin in chronic hepatitis C patients. Cancer. 1997;79:1494–500.
14. Soza A, Everhart JE, Ghany MG et al. Neutropenia during combination therapy of interferon alfa and ribavirin for chronic hepatitis C. Hepatology. 2002;36:1273–9.
15. Afdhal NH, Dieterich DT, Pockros PJ et al.Epoetin alfa maintains ribavirin dose in HCV-infected patients: a prospective, double-blind, randomized controlled study. Gastroenterology. 2004;126:1302–11.
16. Musselman DL, Lawson DH, Gumnick JF et al. Paroxetine for the prevention of depression induced by high-dose interferon alfa. N Engl J Med. 2001;344:961–6.
17. LiverDoc at www.liverdoc.nl, accessed 31 May 2005.
18. Dalgard O, Bjoro K, Hellum KB et al. Treatment with pegylated interferon and ribavarin in HCV infection with genotype 2 or 3 for 14 weeks: a pilot study. Hepatology. 2004;40:1260–5.

11
The role of mutation in drug resistance and pathogenesis of hepatitis B and hepatitis C

T. SHAW and S. A. LOCARNINI

HEPATITIS B AND HEPATITIS C: SIMILAR BUT DIFFERENT

HBV and HCV are the two most important causes of chronic viral hepatitis in humans. Human hepatitis B virus (HBV), the prototype member of the Hepadnaviridae family, is an enveloped DNA virus with a small ($\sim$3.2 kb) partially double-stranded genome which uses gene overlap to accommodate four genes. HCV is an enveloped single-stranded positive-sense RNA virus which is the sole member of the *Hepacivirus* genus in the Flaviviridae family. Its genome (approximately 9.6 kb) has a single open reading frame that encodes a polyprotein of about 3000 amino acids. Although they replicate using radically different strategies, they cause similar disease symptoms. Both are primarily hepatotrophic, but can infect lymphoid and other tissues and both can cause acute or chronic infection[1-4].

The outcome of infection in each case depends on the ability of viral gene products to suppress or subvert the host's normal immune responses. Neither HBV nor HCV is directly cytopathic, but chronic infection greatly increases the chance of development of serious, potentially terminal liver diseases including cirrhosis and hepatocellular carcinoma (HCC), which is one of the most common cancers worldwide, accounting for approximately 4% of all diagnosed malignancies. It has been estimated that 70–80% of deaths due to HCC can be attributed to prior infection with HBV or HCV. The fatality rate from HCC has been causing increasing numbers of deaths during the past two decades, mainly as a consequence of the increasing prevalence of HCV infection. Vaccines that effectively prevent HBV infection have been available for more than 20 years, but the global elimination of hepatitis B by universal vaccination has unfortunately been hindered by many economic and logistical problems. Effective anti-HCV vaccines have yet to be developed.

GLOBAL PREVALENCE

Recent estimates indicate that close to 400 million people are chronically infected with HBV and that nearly 80% of the infected population reside in Africa, Asia and the Western Pacific. The majority (70–80%) of chronic HBV infections are established neonatally or perinatally, with risk reducing to about 10% in adults.

It has been estimated that about 170 million people are chronically infected with HCV worldwide. It is the most common blood-borne infection and a major cause of chronic liver disease and liver transplantation in industrialized countries, where the prevalence of HCV infection is <5%. The prevalence of HCV infection is much greater (~20%) in some African and Asian countries. Although there are fewer people suffering from chronic hepatitis C than chronic hepatitis B, the risk of developing subsequent terminal liver disease is much higher (up to 85%) in all age groups.

CLINICAL COURSE

The clinical course of both hepatitis B and hepatitis C is extremely variable, influenced by numerous genetic and physiological factors which include viral genotype, host genotype, body mass index, specific genotypic polymorphisms, immune status and age at infection. Environmental factors such as exposure to promutagens and alcohol intake are also influential. The clinical presentation of acute HBV infection ranges from subclinical to acute symptomatic (or, rarely, fulminant) hepatitis. Presentation of chronic infection is similarly variable, ranging from inactive carrier states to chronic active hepatitis, fibrosis, cirrhosis and HCC, which occurs in up to 40% of chronic cases and is usually fatal. Similarly, initial infection by HCV is commonly asymptomatic or presents with non-specific flu-like prodromal symptoms, and acute symptomatic infections are infrequent. Although rarely detected, the most common type of HCV infections are probably those that spontaneously resolve. Up to 80% of cases in which HCV infection is detected eventually develop chronic hepatitis C which, like chronic hepatitis B, can progress to fibrosis, cirrhosis and HCC[1,2]. Difficulties in defining the natural histories of chronic hepatitis B and C infections are caused by the indolent course and heterogeneity of associated disease. In both cases liver damage is believed to result mainly from attempts by the host's immune system to eliminate infected cells; chronic infection is established when these attempts fail. By the time symptoms appear, viral replication, the target of the limited number of antiviral drugs available to treat hepatitis B and C, may either be established and stable, declining, or even undetectable, and initiating antiviral therapy at this stage may not alleviate disease. The limited chemotherapeutic options used for treatment of hepatitis B and hepatitis C are not available to a large proportion of the affected populations, and in any case are only about 50% effective in populations for whom they are available. Although much more detailed understanding is needed, the insidious nature of chronic viral hepatitis and the limited effectiveness of currently available treatments can be already partially explained in terms of viral and host genetics.

VIRAL REPLICATION STRATEGIES

HBV

The HBV genome contains four open reading frames (ORF), the longest of which encodes the viral polymerase (Pol). The envelope ORF is located within the Pol ORF, and the core (C) X ORFs also overlap partially the Pol ORF. Little is known about early events in HBV infection, which appears to be initiated by binding of the Pre-S1 domain to cellular receptor(s). HBV cores that gain entry to the cell disassemble and the partially double-stranded open circular DNA genome is translocated to the cell nucleus, where host cell enzymes convert it to a covalently closed circular (ccc) form. HBV ccc DNA associates with cellular histones to form viral minichromosomes, which function as a transcriptional template, generating four main RNA species of 3.5, 2.4, 2.1 and 0.7 kb, which are then translated to produce the viral proteins. The enhancer II/basal core, large surface antigen (L), major surface antigen (S), and enhancer I/X gene promoters, respectively, direct the expression of these transcripts. Translation of HBV mRNA produces: (1) the hepatitis B core antigen (HBcAg or nucleocapsid protein); (2) the soluble, secreted hepatitis B e antigen (HBeAg); (3) the HBV polymerase; (4) viral envelope proteins (HBsAg) and (5) the hepatitis B x protein (HBx). The 3.5 kb pregenomic RNA (pgRNA), which is the translational template for the nucleocapsid and Pol proteins, also acts as the template for reverse transcription of the viral genome. Currently available nucleosidic drugs (nucleoside and nucleotide analogues) inhibit HBV Pol, a multifunctional protein with RNA- and DNA-dependent DNA polymerase activity and RNase H activity, which also primes reverse transcription and coordinates nucleocapsid assembly[5].

HCV

The HCV genome encodes a single polyprotein precursor of approximately 3000 amino acid residues, which is co- and post-translationally processed by cellular and viral proteases to yield the mature structural and non-structural proteins[4]. These are, in order from the NH2 terminus: C, E1, E2, p7, NS2, NS3, NS4A, NS4B, NS5A, and NS5B. The structural proteins are the capsid protein (core; C) and the envelope glycoproteins E1 and E2, which are components of the virion. The p7 polypeptide, which is essential for infectivity, has been shown to oligomerize to form cation channels. The structural proteins are released from the polyprotein by host cell peptidases, but the non-structural proteins (NS2–NS5B) are generated by enzymatic action of the viral proteases NS2/3 and NS3/4A. NS3 has serine protease and helicase activity and NS5B is the viral RNA-dependent RNA polymerase. NS2 acts as a protease in complex with NS3 and is presumed to have other roles that have yet to be determined. An accumulating body of evidence suggests that the non-structural proteins mediate HCV immune evasion by perturbing cell signalling pathways. A second translation product, the F protein, is generated by ribosomal frameshift, but little is known about its function. Both NS3 and NS5B are essential components of the HCV replication complex and have been shown to be required for HCV replication in chimpanzees. Consequently, they have been the main targets for the development of specific small molecule inhibitors of HCV replication during the past decade[6].

SIGNIFICANCE OF VIRAL QUASISPECIES

RNA polymerases and reverse transcriptases are inherently error-prone because they lack associated proofreading functions, resulting in mutation rates of the order of 10^{-3} to 10^{-5} misincorporations per nucleotide copied. This has shown to be equivalent to between 0.1 and 10 mutations per RNA genome per replication cycle, and this led to the concept that RNA viruses exist as heterogeneous populations known as quasispecies. The quasispecies concept was originally developed as a formal mathematical model of early life forms based on chemical kinetics. It requires that equilibrium mutation–selection processes act to generate a heterogeneous distribution of whole genomes ordered around one or a small number of 'master' sequences, which are the fittest or 'strongest' in the existing environment. According to this model, despite the continuous generation of mutants resulting from low-fidelity replication, the master sequences maintain a stable frequency in the population rather than undergoing divergence and diffusion leading to genetic drift predicted by conventional population genetics. During *in-vivo* infections continual fluctuations in the environment caused by immune pressure, cellular tropism, or drug therapy make it unlikely that viral populations reach equilibrium, and whether they constitute quasispeces in the strictest sense has been questioned[7]. However, the quasispecies model has currently become the dominant paradigm for RNA virus evolution, and the term has been widely accepted to describe populations of HIV and HCV, among others[8,9]. Because their replication strategy requires reverse transcription, hepadnaviruses also have the potential to exist *in vivo* as quasispecies, although constraints imposed by overlapping reading frames probably restrict diversity and evolutionary potential.

It has been estimated that, in infected hosts with viral loads greater than about 10^8/ml, the viral quasispecies must include genomes with all possible single-point mutations as well as some with two or three point mutations. This can explain the great adaptive potential of some viral pathogens, evidenced by the need for combination antiviral therapy and polyvalent antiviral vaccines to control viral diseases (reviewed by Domingo et al.[9]). A variety of selective pressures, including host immune surveillance, antiviral therapies and virus–cell tropism, determine quasispecies composition and the outcome of infection. High quasispecies variability confers rapid but unpredictable evolutionary potential. Under some conditions variation may exceed the error threshold beyond which viral survival becomes impossible, a situation termed 'error catastrophe'[10]. The quasispecies theory predicts that viral variants will be retained as minor components of evolving populations during environmental changes that render them less fit (a phenomenon that has been named 'quasispecies memory') and that they should eventually be diluted to extinction[11]. These phenomena have important practical implications, as Briones and colleagues[12] showed recently for HIV. In addition to demonstrating retention of quasispecies replicative memory *in vivo*, they show that HIV quasispecies also retain 'cellular' memory; that is, minor quasispecies that have been 'hidden' in cellular or anatomical compartments for long periods of time.

QUASISPECIES, DRUG RESISTANCE AND IMMUNE ESCAPE

Quasispecies theory predicts that drug resistance and vaccine escape are likely to become problems that will eventually restrict the use of new drugs and vaccines at some time after they become available for clinical use. Indeed, the demonstration that specific mutations in the viral genomes can confer resistance to specific antiviral drugs is now regarded as evidence for specific antiviral activity, and frequently helps to confirm or elucidate mechanisms of action. This applies especially to nucleosidic drugs targeted at the viral nucleic acid polymerases and to peptidomimetic inhibitors of HCV proteases, as the following specific examples are intended to demonstrate. Space limitations prevent the inclusion of much recent evidence for the involvement of viral gene products in evading host immunity, a topic of increasing complexity, but a few examples relating to HCV are discussed separately.

TERMINOLOGY AND DEFINITIONS

A mutation is a heritable change in genetic information, a definition that seems deceptively simple. In some contexts the term 'mutation' implies disadvantageous change or one associated with loss of function or disease. By contrast 'polymorphism' (including single-nucleotide polymorphism [SNP], a synonym for point mutation) has often been used to refer to nucleotide sequence changes that are not associated with loss of function, observable phenotypic change or disease. 'Polymorphism' has also been used to describe a genetic change that occurs with a frequency of at least 1% in a population. Problems of definition are further compounded for viral genomes. For HBV, mutations are changes in the genomic deoxyribonucleotide sequence, but for HCV, which has an RNA genome, mutations are changes in ribonucleotide sequence – but which sequences and which populations? Because of the low copying fidelity and lack of proofreading activity of RNA-dependent nucleic acid polymerases, HBV and HCV populations are genetically heterogeneous. Currently, eight different HBV genotypes (A–H) can be distinguished on the basis of overall nucleotide sequence diversity of $>8\%$. For HCV the situation is even more complex: six clades and 11 major genotypes are currently distinguished on the basis of overall genetic diversity of 15–30%. For both HBV and HCV the individual genotypes have been found to differ in demographic and virological characteristics as well as clinical disease manifestations. Similarly, for both HBV and HCV, recombination between genotypes has been documented and substantial genetic dispersion also occurs within genotypes which, as noted above, are assumed to exist *in vivo* as quasispecies. It is very difficult to define what is meant by 'mutation' in this setting; consequently there has been a tendency to focus only on mutations that alter the function(s) of genes or their products. Different genotypes of HBV have genomes of different lengths, making it impossible to develop genotype-independent terminology for specific mutations. Confusingly, mutations in the HBV precore–core and X genes have been identified conventionally by nucleotide, whereas mutations in the polymerase and envelope genes have been identified by changes that they cause in the amino acid sequence of their respective protein products. Creation of a simple genotype-independent terminology for viral mutants with clinically important (eg, drug-resistant) phenotypes necessitated that they be distinguished by amino acid sequence changes[13]. Consequently, amino acid changes are now frequently, but incorrectly, referred to as 'mutations'. For simplicity, the now-accepted terminology 'pA$_{wt}$XA$_m$ mutant' (but not 'pA$_{wt}$XA$_m$ mutation') will be used here to refer to mutants that encode a different amino acid (A$_m$) in place of the amino acid found in the wild-type (A$_{wt}$) at position X in the sequence of expressed protein product (p).

VIRAL MUTATIONS AND DRUG RESISTANCE

The most obvious and easily studied viral mutations are those that are selected by exposure to specific antiviral drugs. In many cases the development of resistance provides evidence for, or confirms mechanism of drug action.

DRUG RESISTANCE IN HBV

Two safe and effective nucleosidic drugs, lamivudine and adefovir dipivoxil, are now available for treatment of chronic hepatitis B, and a third, entecavir, is likely to be licensed for use in the near future. Clinical use of lamivudine, in particular, is already limited by the developent of drug resistance, and resistance to adefovir dipivoxil and entecavir has also been observed. Several other new drugs, including non-nucleosidic inhibitors, have progressed to phase II/III clinical trials. Development of resistance to these agents is inevitable once they become available for clinical use, and long-term combination therapy analogous to HAART ('highly active antiretroviral therapy) will be almost certainly needed to suppress HBV replication *in vivo*[14,15]. This will require phenotypic and genotypic characterization of drug-resistant mutants and detailed information concerning mechanisms of drug resistance.

Lamivudine resistance

Lamivudine treatment produces a rapid 4–5 log$_{10}$ decrease in viraemia and reversal or arrest of existing liver disease in the majority of cases. Unfortunately, these improvements are rarely sustained due to development of drug resistance, which increases progressively at rates between 14% and 32% annually, approaching 100% after 4 years. This is a relatively slow rate of development of resistance (compared to the HIV rate) and is probably due to constraints imposed by overlapping reading frames in the HBV genome and by reduced opportunities for complementation and recombination imposed by genetic haploidy[14]. Factors known to increase the risk of development of resistance to lamivudine probably apply equally to other nucleosidic inhibitors. They include high pretherapy serum HBV DNA and ALT levels, incomplete suppression of viral replication, longer duration of therapy, infection with particular HBV serotypes and genotypes, HBeAg/anti-HBe status, and high body mass index. Lamivudine treatment selects for HBV quasispecies in which methionine (M) in the highly conserved tyrosine–methionine–aspartate–aspartate (YMDD) motif in the C (catalytic) domain of Pol is replaced by valine (V) or isoleucine (I), changes which have been designated rtM204V and rtM204I respectively. The former occurs only in association with rtL180M and other secondary changes that compensate for otherwise poor replication efficiency, but rtM204I has been detected both in isolation and in association with rtL180M. Lamivudine-resistant HBV mutants have been screened for cross-resistance to several other nucleosidic inhibitors: results are summarized in Table 1. Mutations that confer LMV resistance decrease *in-vitro* sensitivity to LMV from at least 20-fold to greater than 1000-fold, but do not confer cross-resistance to adefovir. Clinically, emergence of lamivudine resistance may be associated with biochemical and virological breakthroughs, frequently with hepatitic flares, sometimes hepatic decompensation, but rarely fatality. Management of lamivudine-resistant HBV has been a contentious issue, but current opinion indicates that any benefits of continuing lamivudine treatment after resistance emerges are negligible[16].

Adefovir resistance

Adefovir resistance emerges more slowly and less frequently (around 1% annually) than lamivudine resistance. Adefovir resistance is mainly due to substitution of threonine for asparagine 236 (rtN236T), which is located in the D motif[15], although other changes, notably rtA181V/T, have also been associated with clinical adefovir resistance. These changes increase adefovir resistance by only 5–10-fold, and they do not affect sensitivity to lamivudine[17] (Table 1).

Entecavir resistance

Resistance to entecavir has been observed in two patients who were infected with lamivudine-resistant mutants. Additional substitutions in the HBV rt associated with the emergence of entecavir resistance mapped to the B, C and D domains[18] (Table 1).

Table 1 Effects of HBV polymerase mutations on sensitivity to inhibitors

Drug: Wild-type (wt) EC_{50} (nM):	Lamivudine 2.0	Adefovir 200	Entecavir 0.02
Change in rt amino acid sequence	Log_{10} change in EC_{50} relative to wt		
None (wt)	0	0	0
rtL180M	0	−0.3	0
rtM204I	<1	−0.2	<0.7
rtM204V	<2	−0.2	<0.7
rtL180M/M204V	>3	−0.7	2
rtV173L/L180M/M204V	>3	1.3	1.5
rtI169T/V173L/L180M/M204V	>3	−0.4	2
rtI169T/V173L/L180M/M204V/M250V	>3	0.1	3.5
rtA181V	0	0.2	0
rtN236T	0.3	0.8	0

Relative sensitivity of HBV encoding mutations that alter the amino acid sequence of the reverse transcriptase (rt) region of the HBV polymerase gene. RtA181V and rtN236T mutants have been isolated from patients following treatment with adefovir. Other variants are selected *in vivo* by exposure to lamivudine or entecavir. WT EC_{50}s (first row of data) were estimated from *in-vitro* assays using the recombinant baculovirus-HBV system. The lower data are log_{10} values for the ratio mutant EC_{50}/wtEC_{50}. For example, no change in EC_{50} gives a ratio of 1.0 and a log_{10} value of 0; log_{10} values of 0.7, 1, 2 and 3 correspond to 5-, 10-, 100- and 1000-fold increases in EC_{50}, respectively. Note that EC_{50} values vary in different assay systems and are not directly indicative of relative *in-vivo* efficacy.

DRUG RESISTANCE IN HCV

Understanding of HCV replication has been advanced dramatically by structural analyses of viral enzymes and by the recent development of cell-based replicon systems. The latter rely on viral non-structural proteins to stably replicate subgenomic HCV RNA *in vitro* in Huh-7 cells. The original replicon system used an HCV genotype 1b-specific sequence co-expressed with a gene that conferred neomycin resistance. More recently, genotype 1b and 2a replicons have been described. Interestingly, in the course of development, the original replicon sequences have acquired 'adaptive' mutations that allow them to replicate more efficiently in specific cell lines[19]. Replicon systems have been successfully used to screen potential antiviral agents for activity. In particular, inhibitors of NS3/4A protease and NS5B polymerase activities have been identified. The latter include nucleoside derivatives targeted at the NS5B active site and structurally diverse inhibitors that bind to different allosteric sites[6,20]. Mutations that confer resistance to these agents have also been identified, confirming the sites and mechanisms of action. Some examples follow.

RESISTANCE TO NON-NUCLEOSIDE INHIBITORS OF HCV NS5B POLYMERASE

Many of the non-nucleoside inhibitors of the HCV replication complex are heterocyclic compounds[21,22]. They include benzimidazole, benzothiadiazine and thiophene derivatives. A benzothiadiazine derivative ('compound 4') was identified as a specific NS5B, as evidenced by the selection of antiviral resistance in an HCV replicon system. Several mutant replicon clones that encoded threonine instead of methionine at NS5B residue 414 (M414T) survived 28 days exposure to this inhibitor when present at a concentration ~20 times greater than the initial EC50 (50% effective concentration). A recombinant replicon engineered to encode the M414T substitution showed reduced susceptibility, and the expressed NS5B product was shown to be >125-fold less sensitive than the wild-type enzyme in cell-free polymerase assays, confirming that M414T alone was sufficient to confer resistance[21]. Studies aimed at establishing patterns of cross-resistance to the different types of non-nucleoside inhibitors, each of which has been shown to bind to different allosteric sites on NS5B, are currently in progress.

NS5B AND RESISTANCE TO RIBAVIRIN

Ribavirin (RBV), a guanosine analogue that has broad-spectrum antiviral activity, has been used as an antiviral agent for more than 30 years, but its mechanisms of action are still poorly understood. Recently, Crotty and co-workers showed that it could act as an RNA mutagen and induce error catastrophe in Poliovirus *in vitro*, proposing this as its primary mechanism of action against RNA viruses *in vivo*[23]. After intracellular phosphorylations, which generate ribavirin triphosphate (RTP), it can be incorporated internally, albeit with very low efficiency, into nascent viral RNA by the HCV RNA polymerase, which incorporates it opposite a pyrimidine (C or U), but not purine (A or G) residues. Conversely, HCV polymerase will incorporate a pyrimidine (but neither purine nor ribavirin) monophosphate opposite internal ribavirin residues, again with low catalytic efficiency compared to the efficiencies of incorporation templated by A or G residues. Consequently, efficiency of RNA polymerization on ribavirin-containing templates is very low, indicating that ribavirin is not only mutagenic for HCV, but also inhibits viral RNA synthesis. To test whether these mechanisms operate *in vivo*, Young and colleagues[24] studied the evolution of the nucleotide sequences of HCV RNA in the NS5B region in patients receiving RBV, placebo, or interferon-α (IFN-α) monotherapy. The rate of HCV quasispecies change was found to be faster in the ribavirin-treated group than in either the IFN-α or placebo group. RBV caused preferentially A-to-G and U-to-A mutations. In addition, a mutation which caused a phenylalanine to tyrosine substitution at amino acid residue 415 of NS5B (F415Y) was observed in all (five of five) patients infected with HCV genotype 1a during treatment with ribavirin. Furthermore, the parental (415F) strain re-emerged in some patients after ribavirin treatment was stopped. Assays using an HCV subgenomic replicon system demonstrated that ribavirin caused dose-dependent inhibition of viral RNA synthesis by the F415 replicon, but not the F415Y replicon, confirming that F415Y confers ribavirin resistance. Three-dimensional modelling revealed that the NS5B residue 415 is located in the 'thumb' subdomain of the viral polymerase, which has been proposed to be involved in binding the HCV template–primer duplex.

These results not only confirm that ribavirin can act as a weak viral mutagen *in vivo* in HCV-infected patients, but also confirm that ribavirin can inhibit the HCV polymerase directly. Confirmation that ribavirin can act as a viral mutagen *in vivo* raises an intriguing question: how will this affect the evolution of drug resistance when ribavirin is used in combination with other antiviral drugs?

MUTATIONS THAT CONFER RESISTANCE TO INHIBITORS OF THE NS3/4A PROTEASE

The HCV NS3/4A protease is an essential component of the HCV replication complex and has been shown to be required for HCV replication in chimpanzees. It is responsible for cleavage at four sites within the HCV polyprotein, which generates the N termini of the NS4A, NS4B, NS5A, and NS5B proteins. Consequently, it has been a target for development of small molecule inhibitors, most of which have been modified peptide substrate mimetics. The central region (amino acids 21–30) of the 54-residue NS4A protein is essential and sufficient for the enhancement of proteolytic activity of the NS3 serine protease. The central region of NS4A has been shown to form a tight heterodimer with the NS3 protein and the structure of the complex has been solved by X-ray crystallography.

BILN 2061 was the first HCV serine protease inhibitor to progress to clinical trials against hepatitis C. During phase I trials, 2 days treatment with BILN 2061 produced 2–3 $\log_{10}$ reductions in viral load, providing the first evidence that the clinical use of HCV NS3/4A protease inhibitors is feasible. More recently, another HCV NS3/4A protease inhibitor, VX-950, has also progressed to clinical trials. Mutations in NS3/NS4A that confer resistance to BILN 2061 and VX-950 have been independently identified using HCV subgenomic replicon systems. Substitution of serine for alanine at residue156 in the HCV NS3 protease domain (A156S) conferred resistance to VX-950. The mutations that conferred resistance to BILN 2061 caused replacement of aspartate 168 by glutamate or glutamine (D168E/Q). A GenBank search showed that A156 is absolutely conserved in sequences of all 437/437 HCV isolates from all six major genotypes. The lack of polymorphism suggests that substitution at this position decreases viral replication efficiency. Although a large majority (>96%) of the 437 recorded isolates had aspartic acid at residue 168, three naturally occurring HCV variants were identified. Glutamate was substituted for aspartate (D168G) in 10 isolates of genotypes 1b or genotype 5 and six isolates of genotype 3 had glutamine at this position (D168Q). Molecular modelling predicted that the genotype 1b and 5 isolates would remain susceptible to both HCV protease inhibitors but that the genotype 3 HCV strains would be resistant because of steric hindrance which would prevent binding of the inhibitors[25,26].

HCV NS3/4A PROTEASE AND DISRUPTION OF HOST IMMUNE RESPONSES

Disruption of the host's immune responses by viral gene products is known to play an important part in establishment of many persistent viral infections, including chronic hepatitis B and C. Although details of the molecular mechanisms involved are largely unknown, recent work has revealed how some HCV NS proteins contribute to establishing persistent infection. Production of cytokines and other cellular gene products that stimulate and amplify further immune responses and/or directly inhibit viral replication is the result of activation of multiple signalling cascades in response to viral antigens. For example, induction of IFN expression in response to viral infection depends on post-translational modification of a variety of transcription factors, which include nuclear factor κB (NF-κB), ATF/c-Jun and the IFN regulatory factors (IRF). IRF are activated by phosphorylation of their C-terminal domains, which triggers dimerization and translocation to the cell nucleus where they induce transcription of antiviral genes including type I IFN. Phosphorylation of IRF-3, an important mediator of the early antiviral response, is catalysed by a cellular virus-activated kinase (VAK) which is activated by dsRNA and other viral replication products.

Foy and colleagues[27] recently demonstrated that HCV NS3/4A can block the phosphorylation, nuclear translocation and effector action of IRF-3. Ablation of the serine protease activity of NS3/4A, either by specific mutation that affected the catalytic site, or by treatment with a peptidomimetic inhibitor, prevented the blockade, but ablation of its helicase activity did not. Moreover, dominant negative or constitutively active IRF-3 mutants, respectively, enhanced or suppressed HCV replicon replication in Huh-7 cells. These observations have several important implications. First, they show that HCV NS3/4A can directly inhibit IRF-3 activation, most likely by proteolysis of VAK or other cellular proteins that control its phosphorylation. Secondly, inhibition of IRF-3 activation may not only promote persistent infection but may also reduce the effectiveness of IFN-based therapies, because many IFN-stimulated genes contain IRF-3 target sites. Thirdly, HCV variants that encode NS3/4A proteases with different enzymatic properties are likely to differ correspondingly in resistance to host immunity and in their immunosuppressive potential. Conversely, polymorphisms in genes encoding cellular substrates for the NS3/4A complex are likely to influence the outcome of infection. Finally, inhibitors of HCV NS3/4A protease may act by two distinct mechanisms: prevention of proteolytic processing of the HCV polyprotein as well as restoration of responsiveness of the IRF-3 pathway.

MUTATIONS IMPLICATE NS4B AND NS5A IN IFN RESISTANCE

Ample evidence indicates involvement of both viral and host factors in failure of HCV infection to respond to treatment with endogenous IFN. The induction of cellular production of IFN and cellular responses to IFN involve complex, interacting signalling pathways and hundreds of cellular genes, many of which have been identified by microarray analyses[28-30]. Mechanisms for virally mediated resistance to IFN therapy have been intensively studied, usually with inconclusive results. Infection with HCV genotype 1, high baseline viral loads, or both, are associated with poor response to IFN therapy, but molecular mechanisms which underlie failure to respond to IFN treatment remain largely unknown. Recently, Namba and co-workers[31] reported that they have successfully generated IFN-resistant HCV replicons by exposing IFN-sensitive replicons to a low concentration of IFN-α for prolonged periods. They obtained four clones of HCV replicon cells that survived treatment with 200 IU/ml IFN-α. These were then treated with gradually increasing concentrations of IFN-α or IFN-β (up to 2000 or 1000 IU/ml, respectively), producing subclones with corresponding resistance phenotypes. Two additional subclones were found to be partly resistant to both IFN-α and IFN-β. Genetic analysis of corresponding HCV replicons found a single amino acid substitution in NS4B common to all clones as well as several additional amino acid substitutions in NS5A in the IFN-β resistant clones, suggesting that they may be involved in IFN resistance. Girard and colleagues[32] further investigated the effects of NS5A expression on gene expression in Huh-7 cells. By using microarray analyses they identified 103 genes (43 up- and 60 down-regulated, and belonging to various functional groups) whose expression was affected at least 2-fold by co-expression of NS5A. Genes encoding the receptors for lymphotoxin-β and tumour necrosis factor (TNF) were among those down-regulated. Computational analysis revealed that 39 of the 43 up-regulated genes contained at least 1 NF-κB binding site in their promoter regions, and activation of NF-κB was subsequently demonstrated in luciferase reporter assays. Furthermore, adenovirus-mediated expression of IkBa reversed NS5A mediated up-regulation of gene expression. However, similar effects on gene expression were observed following expression of mutant NS5A genes derived from clinical HCV isolates regardless of whether they were IFN-sensitive or resistant *in vivo*.

THE INFLUENCE OF HOST GENOTYPE

Differences in host susceptibility to infection cannot be attributed solely to the virulence of individual pathogens, and a large body of accumulated epidemiological evidence supports the case for a strong genetic component to individual susceptibility and resistance to infectious disease. Although, to date, no single allele(s) that determine the response to infection with HBV or HCV have been identified, the great variability in severity and the close interplay between viral gene products and the host's immune system imply that host genetic background is important. In addition, the limited coding capacity of the genomes of both HBV and HCV indicates that viral replication must rely on numerous cellular functions that will be subject to genetic variability. Lines of evidence for individual and ethnic differences in response to infection can be briefly summarized as follows:

1. Infection with the same virus has been found to cause various clinical outcomes in different individuals.
2. Long-term studies show that some individuals in high-risk groups do not develop disease, and in some cases may not even acquire infection, suggesting the existence of individual-specific resistance factors.
3. Overall infection rate, prevalence and response to infection varies between different ethnic groups, regardless of their geographic location.
4. There is a wide variation in response to treatment with the antiviral drugs currently available.
5. A minority ($\sim 15\%$) of healthy vaccinees fail to produce protective antibody in response to vaccination against HBV. (Vaccines against HCV have not yet been developed.)

These observations suggest that identifying host genetic factors that determine response to HBV and HCV infection will provide clues to the diversity of disease manifestations and reasons for the disparities in response to therapy and vaccination. The complexity of the disease process suggests that numerous genes and genetic interactions are likely to be involved. Approximately 35 000 genes have been identified by the human genome project, along with an estimated 3.5 million single-nucleotide polymorphisms (SNP) within their encoding or flanking regions. If specific polymorphisms in genetic alleles are associated with low risk of infection or disease progression, they can be considered to be 'resistant' alleles; conversely if they are associated with high risk of infection and rapid disease progression, they may be considered as conferring susceptibility. Intensive research is currently directed at identifying these alleles, a formerly impossible task that is now approaching possibility as a result of recent technical advances, such the development of microarray technology.

Two different strategies have been employed to identify disease associations of genetic markers. The first involves a search for variation in flanking regions of genes known or suspected to be associated with disease susceptibility or resistance. Genes that play important roles in the development or resolution of viral hepatitis can be provisionally identified from knowledge of host responses. These include production of specific cytokines and antibodies as well as cell-mediated responses. The genes responsible for these responses, together with linked or neighbouring genes, become candidates for examination for possible polymorphisms. This approach, although still in its infancy, has already been productive. An alternative and complementary approach involves screening entire genomes or large parts of the genome to identify SNP and mutational hotspots, which may be correlated by more detailed studies with function and phenotype. For recent reviews of this topic see refs 33–35.

Cytokine and human lymphocyte antigen (HLA) genes were among the first and most obvious candidate genes, since they are primary modulators of the host immune response. Most studies have concentrated on HLA associations. Genes for HLA class I and class II products are located on the short arm of

Table 2 Examples of association between host genotype and response to infection

Host gene, gene product or other characteristic	Observations and suggested mechanisms
IL-10	High serum IL-10 concentrations correlate with poor response to IFN-α. Inheritance of IL-10 promoter alleles which reduce or increase IL-10 production are associated with better or poorer prognoses. IL-10 inhibits IFN-mediated responses and increases Th2 T cell responses.
CCR5	CCR5 promoter 59029A allele associated with better response to IFN-α.
HLA class II	DQB1*0301 and DRB1*11 alleles are associated with self-limiting HBV and HCV infection, mainly in Caucasian populations. Other class II alleles appear to reduce susceptibility to HCV infection or to affect rate of development of fibrosis.
TNF-α	TNF-α can inhibit HBV gene expression. A promoter variant that results in decreased production of TNF-α found to be associated with HBV persistence.
Mannose-binding protein (MBP) complement.	MBP acts as opsonin. Mutations in gene or its promoter that reduce its expression reduce ability to activate MBP polymorphisms association with symptomatic persistent HBV infection in some populations; may depend on ethnic background.
Vitamin D receptor	Active form of vitamin D is an immunomodulator which inhibits Th1 response and activates Th2 response. Association of receptor polymorphisms demonstrated for other infectious diseases. Association between genotype tt and HBV clearance.

For further examples and detailed discussion and specific references see reviews by Thio et al.[33], Wang[34] and Lee[35].

chromosome 6 with other genes of the major histocompatibility complex (MHC). Their products are glycoproteins that are expressed on the surface of lymphocytes where they present antigens to both CD4$^+$ helper T cells and CD8$^+$ cytolytic T cells. Various MHC allelles that appear to be correlated with more favourable outcomes in cases of viral hepatitis have been identified in diverse populations. Many correlations between class II alleles and viral clearance or persistence have been reported, but convincing correlations between class I alleles, if they exist, have yet to be identified (see refs 33–35 and references therein) (see Table 2).

Proinflammatory Th1 cytokines including interleukin-2 (IL-2), interferon-γ (IFN-γ) and tumour necrosis factor-α (TNF-α) have been shown to participate in resolution of HBV infection. TNF-α and IFN-γ are involved in non-cytotoxic clearance of viral infection. The TNF-α gene is located in the class III region of the MHC complex. To date five SNP, which presumably influence its expression, have been identified in its promoter region. Two of these (–G308A and –G238A, where – signifies location upstream from the transcription initiation site) have been found to be significantly associated with HBV or HCV persistence. Similarly, it has been reported that genetic variants associated with low expression of IFN-γ are more prevalent in Asian than Caucasian populations, suggesting a basis for the susceptibility of the former to persistent infection. The Th2 cytokine IL-10, which inhibits Th1 responses, provides a further example. Three SNPs (–A1082G, –T819C and –A592C, which assort into three different haplotypes) have been identified in its promoter region. In a Japanese population the wild type allelles –819T and –592A were significantly over-represented in asymptomatic carriers of HBV compared to those with chronic progressive liver disease, suggesting that the –819T/–592A haplotype affected IL-10 expression in a way that favoured chronic infection. Other host SNP that have been associated with altered susceptibility to HBV or HCV infection include those affecting genes that encode mannose-binding protein (MBP) and the vitamin D receptor (Table 2).

CONCLUSION

The complexity of the interactions between host and virus following infection makes it very likely that the combinatorial interaction between large numbers of genes and their products will influence susceptibility and resistance to infection with HBV and HCV. Future studies of the genetics of host response will have the benefit of expanding genetic databases and rapidly developing technology for gene identification and analysis. More data derived from larger study populations will be required, which will require global collaboration and cooperation. In future it will be necessary, and should be possible, to accumulate libraries of sequences of genes of interest and to functionally characterize their products. It may eventually be possible to unravel the interactions between products of virus and host genes, which would not only provide insights into the pathogenesis of viral hepatitis but also suggest strategies by which it can be controlled and prevented.

References

1. Poynard T, Yuen MF, Ratziu V, Lai CL. Viral hepatitis C. Lancet. 2003;362:2095–100.
2. Lai CL, Ratziu V, Yuen MF, Poynard T. Viral hepatitis B. Lancet. 2003;362:2089–94.
3. Lavanchy D. Hepatitis B virus epidemiology, disease burden, treatment, and current and emerging prevention and control measures. J Viral Hepatol. 2004;11:97–107.
4. Penin F, Dubuisson J, Rey FA, Moradpour D, Pawlotsky JM. Structural biology of hepatitis C virus. Hepatology. 2004;39:5–19.
5. Locarnini S. Molecular virology of hepatitis B virus. Semin Liver Dis. 2004;24(Suppl. 1):3–10.
6. Ni ZJ, Wagman AS. Progress and development of small molecule HCV antivirals. Curr Opin Drug Discov Devel. 2004;7:446–59.
7. Holmes EC, Moya A. Is the quasispecies concept relevant to RNA viruses? J Virol. 2002;76:460–5.
8. Kamp C. A quasispecies approach to viral evolution in the context of an adaptive immune system. Microbes Infect. 2003;5:1397–405.
9. Domingo E. Quasispecies and the development of new antiviral strategies. Prog Drug Res. 2003;60:133–58.
10. Graci JD, Cameron CE. Challenges for the development of ribonucleoside analogues as inducers of error catastrophe. Antivir Chem Chemother. 2004;15:1–13.
11. Wilke CO, Novella IS. Phenotypic mixing and hiding may contribute to memory in viral quasispecies. BMC Microbiol. 2003;3:11.
12. Briones C, Domingo E, Molina-Paris C. Memory in retroviral quasispecies: experimental evidence and theoretical model for human immunodeficiency virus. J Mol Biol. 2003;331:213–29.
13. Stuyver LJ, Locarnini SA, Lok A et al. Nomenclature for antiviral-resistant human hepatitis B virus mutations in the polymerase region. Hepatology. 2001;33:751–7.
14. Lewin S, Walters T, Locarnini S. Hepatitis B treatment: rational combination chemotherapy based on viral kinetic and animal model studies. Antiviral Res. 2002;55:381–96.
15. Locarnini S, McMillan J, Bartholomeusz A. The hepatitis B virus and common mutants. Semin Liver Dis. 2003;23:5–20.
16. Angus P, Locarnini S. Lamivudine-resistant hepatitis B virus and ongoing lamivudine therapy: stop the merry-go-round, it's time to get off! Antivir Ther. 2004;9:145–8.
17. Werle B, Cinquin K, Marcellin P et al. Evolution of hepatitis B viral load and viral genome sequence during adefovir dipivoxil therapy. J Viral Hepatol. 2004;11:74–83.
18. Tenney DJ, Levine SM, Rose RE et al. Clinical emergence of entecavir-resistant hepatitis B virus requires additional substitutions in virus already resistant to lamivudine. Antimicrob Agents Chemother. 2004;48:3498–507.
19. Yi M, Lemon SM. Adaptive mutations producing efficient replication of genotype 1a hepatitis C virus RNA in normal Huh7 cells. J Virol. 2004;78:7904–15.
20. Sarisky RT. Non-nucleoside inhibitors of the HCV polymerase. J Antimicrob Chemother. 2004;54:14–16.
21. Nguyen TT, Gates AT, Gutshall LL et al. Resistance profile of a hepatitis C virus RNA-dependent RNA polymerase benzothiadiazine inhibitor. Antimicrob Agents Chemother. 2003;47:3525–30.
22. Tomei L, Altamura S, Bartholomew L et al. Characterization of the inhibition of hepatitis C virus RNA replication by nonnucleosides. J Virol. 2004;78:938–46.
23. Crotty S, Cameron CE, Andino R. RNA virus error catastrophe: direct molecular test by using ribavirin. Proc Natl Acad Sci USA. 2001;98:6895–900.
24. Young KC, Lindsay KL, Lee KJ et al. Identification of a ribavirin-resistant NS5B mutation of hepatitis C virus during ribavirin monotherapy. Hepatology. 2003;38:869–78.
25. Trozzi C, Bartholomew L, Ceccacci A et al. In vitro selection and characterization of hepatitis C virus serine protease variants resistant to an active-site peptide inhibitor. J Virol. 2003;77:3669–79.
26. Lin C, Lin K, Luong YP et al. In vitro resistance studies of hepatitis C virus serine protease inhibitors, VX-950 and BILN 2061: structural analysis indicates different resistance mechanisms. J Biol Chem. 2004;279:17508–14.

27. Foy E, Li K, Wang C et al. Regulation of interferon regulatory factor-3 by the hepatitis C virus serine protease. Science. 2003;300:1145-8.
28. Zhu H, Zhao H, Collins CD et al. Gene expression associated with interferon alfa antiviral activity in an HCV replicon cell line. Hepatology. 2003;37:1180-8.
29. Daiba A, Inaba N, Ando S et al. A low-density cDNA microarray with a unique reference RNA: pattern recognition analysis for IFN efficacy prediction to HCV as a model. Biochem Biophys Res Commun. 2004;315:1088-96.
30. Scholle F, Li K, Bodola F, Ikeda M, Luxon BA, Lemon SM. Virus–host cell interactions during hepatitis C virus RNA replication: impact of polyprotein expression on the cellular transcriptome and cell cycle association with viral RNA synthesis. J Virol. 2004;78:1513-24.
31. Namba K, Naka K, Dansako H et al. Establishment of hepatitis C virus replicon cell lines possessing interferon-resistant phenotype. Biochem Biophys Res Commun. 2004;323:299-309.
32. Girard S, Vossman E, Misek DE et al. Hepatitis C virus NS5A-regulated gene expression and signaling revealed via microarray and comparative promoter analyses. Hepatology. 2004;40:708-18.
33. Thio CL, Thomas DL, Carrington M. Chronic viral hepatitis and the human genome. Hepatology. 2000;31:819-27.
34. Wang FS. Current status and prospects of studies on human genetic alleles associated with hepatitis B virus infection. World J Gastroenterol. 2003;9:641-4.
35. Yee LJ. Host genetic determinants in hepatitis C virus infection. Genes Immun. 2004;5:237-45.

Section IV
Liver II

Chair: W. GEROK and M.P. MANNS

12
Aetiology, pathogenesis and treatment of haemochromatosis

L. W. POWELL

REGULATION OF IRON HOMEOSTASIS

Iron is essential for many biochemical pathways but in excess it is highly cytotoxic due to its propensity to catalyse the formation of reactive oxygen radicals. To cater for this cells and organisms have developed elaborate mechanisms for regulating iron intake and efflux. The pathways of normal iron homeostasis and the major molecules and transporters involved are discussed in detail by Anderson[1].

Iron is absorbed from the diet across the epithelial cells of the proximal small intestine. The major protein facilitating the uptake of non-haem iron across the apical brush border is the protein-coupled divalent metal transporter DMT1. Once within the epithelial cell, iron is either directed immediately across the basolateral membrane if it is required to meet body iron demands or, if not, is stored within ferritin in the cytoplasm. The passage of iron across the basolateral membrane is mediated by the recently identified integral membrane protein IREG1 (also known as ferroportin or MTP1). The caeruloplasmin homologue, hephaestin, is also required for efficient basolateral transport, but whether it interacts with IREG1 or operates independently is unknown[1].

The liver plays a particularly important role in iron storage. Transferrin delivers iron to cells by interacting with cell surface transferrin receptors (TfR). The Tf/TfR complex is internalized by receptor-mediated endocytosis and iron is released from Tf following endosomal acidification. Iron is then transported across the endosomal membrane via DMT1 where it can be utilized for metabolic processes or stored within ferritin.

Iron uptake and release by cells are tightly regulated processes. The best-characterized mode of regulation of molecules of iron homeostasis is the post-transcriptional control of the expression of ferritin, TfR, DMT1, IREG1, and several others genes including the recently described haemojuvelin. The HFE protein, which is defective in haemochromatosis, appears to play an important role in determining how the intestine responds to body iron needs, but the mechanism by which this is achieved has yet to be resolved.

HFE is widely expressed in body tissues and encodes an MHC class I-like molecule[2,3]. Like other class I molecules, HFE is able to bind to β_2-microglobulin and this complex is expressed on the cell surface. The C282Y common missense mutation disrupts the association of HFE and β_2-microglobulin and thus the correct trafficking of the complex. While the precise function of HFE is unknown, the demonstration that the HFE/β_2-microglobulin heterodimer is able to bind to transferrin receptor 1 (TfR1) (an abundant cell surface protein required for the uptake of transferrin-bound iron) provides a strong link to iron metabolism[2]. HFE carrying the C282Y mutation is unable to interact with TfR1. Major advance has come with the demonstration that the expression of the liver-derived antimicrobial peptide hepcidin is greatly reduced in haemochromatosis individuals. Hepcidin has recently emerged as a critical molecule in the control of body iron homeostasis and it appears to act as a repressor of iron absorption[1]. Thus reduced hepcidin expression in haemochromatosis can explain the increased iron absorption associated with this disorder. These findings suggest that the major site of the basic metabolic defect in haemochromatosis is in the liver, a conclusion supported by the observation that the liver is the strongest site of HFE expression. Whether HFE has additional roles in other cell types has yet to be determined.

In 2000, ferroportin (IREG1/MTP1) protein was identified independently by three different laboratories and was shown to play a role in the export of iron from enterocytes, hepatocytes and RE macrophages[1]. In the human intestine this protein is expressed strongly under conditions of enhanced iron absorption, such as anaemia or haemochromatosis. It is involved in the pathogenesis of the hypoferraemia associated with anaemia of chronic disease, characterized by iron trapping in reticuloendothelial (RE) cells and reduced intestinal iron transfer. Mutations in the ferroportin gene lead to iron overload in parenchymal cells and RE macrophages and the full clinical syndrome of haemochromatosis (see later).

The precise functions of transferrin receptor 2 and haemojuvelin have yet to be determined. However, there is increasing evidence for a complex interplay between HFE, hepcidin, TfR2 and haemojuvelin in the regulation of intestinal iron absorption and the maintenance of body iron homeostasis.

NOMENCLATURE AND PATHOGENESIS

The term 'genetic' or 'hereditary haemochromatosis' (HHC) is generally used to describe an inherited disorder of iron metabolism leading to progressive iron loading of parenchymal cells of the liver, pancreas, and heart. In its fully developed form, organ structure and function are impaired with the classic findings of diabetes, bronze pigmentation of the skin and cirrhosis of the liver – the classical triad described over 100 years ago. Arthritis, hypogonadism and cardiomyopathy are additional features of advanced disease[2]. However, with the recent cloning of the HFE gene and the mutations responsible for iron overload, the majority of cases are diagnosed at an earlier stage in the disease and often before clinical and/or biochemical evidence of the disease has developed. Thus, four stages of the disorder have been described[4]:

1. Genetic predisposition with no abnormality other than possibly a raised serum transferrin saturation as the sole finding.
2. Iron overload (2–5 g) but without symptoms.
3. Iron overload with early symptoms, e.g. lethargy, arthralgia.
4. Iron overload with organ damage, particularly cirrhosis.

With such a serial progression the importance of adequate diagnostic and screening strategies to ensure early case detection in stages 1–3 prior to the development of irreversible end-organ damage becomes evident.

Until recently it was thought that hereditary haemochromatosis was a single entity due to an inherited disorder of iron metabolism although a more severe form of the disease in young subjects in the second and third decade of life (called juvenile haemochromatosis) was recognized and considered to be a more severe variant of the disease[5]. However, following identification (the cloning) of the *HFE* gene remarkable developments have occurred in our understanding of iron transport and storage molecules with the description of ferroportin, hephaestin, hepcidin and haemojuvelin[6]. Mutations in each of the relevant genes can cause similar forms of iron overload and the Online Mendelian Inheritance in Man (OMIM) database[7] lists four types of hereditary haemochromatosis resulting from mutations in these genes (Table 1).

Table 1 Classification of haemochromatosis

Primary hereditary haemochromatosis
HFE-associated hereditary haemochromatosis (type 1)
   C282Y homozygosity
   C282Y/H63D compound heterozygosity

Non-HFE associated hereditary haemochromatosis
   Juvenile haemochromatosis (type 2) (2A hepcidin mutations; 2B haemojuvelin mutations)
   Type 3 haemochromatosis (transferrin receptor 2 mutations)
   Type 4 ferroportin mutations (autosomal dominant haemochromatosis)

However, this chapter will be confined primarily to the common HFE-associated form which is responsible for approximately 90% of cases of haemochromatosis in Caucasian subjects. A more detailed account of the less common forms of haemochromatosis – including their molecular basis, inheritance and clinicopathological manifestations – can be found in the excellent review article by Pietrangelo[8].

PREVALENCE

HFE-associated haemochromatosis (now commonly referred to as hereditary haemochromatosis type 1 (HHC) is one of the most common genetic diseases, although its prevalence varies in different ethnic groups. It is most common in populations of northern European extraction in whom approximately 1 in 10 persons are heterozygous carriers and 0.3–0.5% are homozygotes for the C282Y mutation in the *HFE*. However, expression of the disease is modified by several factors, especially dietary iron intake, alcohol consumption, blood loss, menstruation and pregnancy, and blood donation. The clinical expression of overt disease is 5–10 times more frequent in men than in women[9–11]. Nearly 70% of affected patients develop the first symptoms between ages 40 and 60. The disease is rarely evident before age 30, although with family screening (see below) and periodic health examinations, asymptomatic patients with iron overload can be identified, including young menstruating women. The penetrance of the mutations is variable (see another chapter in this book). Recent population studies have indicated that the clinical penetrance of HHC is lower than previously thought, especially since many subjects are now detected with elevated biochemical markers (transferrin saturation or serum ferritin levels) without any apparent clinical disease. Population screening of Norwegian and Australian adults has revealed the presence of hepatic fibrosis or cirrhosis in 25% and 10% respectively of homozygous subjects[12,13]. In contrast a screening programme performed in a health appraisal clinic in California revealed classical multiorgan HHC in only 1 of 152 homozygous subjects[14]. However, this was on the basis of a self-administered questionnaire, laboratory results and physical examination without liver biopsy or radiological assessment. It is of interest that in this study some 70% of homozygous subjects had an elevated serum ferritin level, and 25% had elevated levels of collagen type IV, a surrogate marker for hepatic fibrosis. Nevertheless, several additional recent population studies have suggested that the clinical expression of HHC is lower than previously thought, with many homozygous subjects living to the ninth decade or beyond[15].

Several studies have confirmed that heavy alcohol consumption accentuates the clinical expression of haemochromatosis[16–18]. The reason is unclear. Increased dietary iron or increased iron absorption is unlikely. The most likely explanation would seem to be the added co-factor effect of iron and alcohol, both of which cause oxidative stress, hepatic stellate cell activation, and hepatic fibrogenesis. In addition, the cumulative effects of other forms of liver injury may result when iron and alcohol are present concurrently.

The clinical features of HHC have been described in detail elsewhere[19]. Clinical symptomatology is directly related to the degree of body iron overload[20]. In the fully established form, several symptoms classical of the disorder may occur, especially fatigue (the most common), malaise, abdominal pain, arthralgia and impotence with clinical findings of hepatomegaly, skin pigmentation, diabetes, and cardiomegaly. Abnormal liver enzymes are common, but are not always present[21].

GENETICS OF CLASSICAL HFE-ASSOCIATED HEREDITARY HAEMOCHROMATOSIS

Classical hereditary haemochromatosis is an autosomal recessive iron-overload disorder associated with mutation of the *HFE* gene, which is located in the MHC region on chromosome 6; in most cases the mutation is a single-base change that results in the substitution of tyrosine for cysteine at position 282 of the HFE protein (C282Y). C282Y seems to have originated by chance in a single Celtic or Viking ancestor in northwestern Europe some 2000 years ago. The genetic defect, which caused no serious obstacle to reproduction and may even have conferred some selective advantage (e.g. resistance to dietary iron deficiency and certain infectious diseases), was spread by population migration[22-24]. Homozygosity for the C282Y mutation is now found in approximately 5 of every 1000 persons of northern European descent – a prevalence 10 times that of cystic fibrosis genotypes.

The inheritance of the disease follows classical Mendelian genetics. Thus, the most common scenario is where two parents are heterozygous for the C282Y mutation and thus 25% of offspring are either normal or homozygous and 50% are heterozygous. A not-uncommon situation, however, in view of the high frequency of the mutation in the population, is for a homozygous–heterozygous mating to occur. In this case 50% of offspring will be homozygous for the mutation.

DIAGNOSIS OF HEREDITARY HAEMOCHROMATOSIS

The diagnosis of established symptomatic HHC will be addressed briefly first, and then the diagnosis in first-degree relatives of known cases and in individuals detected during clinical evaluation at health checks will be addressed. The insidious onset and high prevalence of non-specific symptoms in the early stages of the disease requires the clinician to have a high index of suspicion and careful clinicopathological correlation to arrive at a correct diagnosis of HHC.

The criteria for the diagnosis of established HHC include at least one of the following in the absence of other known causes of iron overload[25,26]:

1. Stainable hepatic iron grade 3 or 4.

2. Hepatic iron concentration > 80 µmol/L per gram (dry weight).

3. Hepatic iron index (hepatic iron concentration ÷ age) > 1.9.

4. Removal of 5 g or more of iron by therapeutic venesection without inducing iron deficiency.

The diagnosis of HFE-associated haemochromatosis is confirmed by the demonstration of homozygosity for the C282Y mutation.

Subjects found to be carrying the C282Y mutation in the homozygous state but without evidence of iron overload are best characterized as non-expressing homozygotes. Factors that determine whether they progress to develop significant iron overload and clinical disease are both environmental and genetic. The environmental ones are well characterized and have been discussed earlier; the genetic factors are currently poorly understood but of much current interest. They include co-inheritance of known genetic mutations but also modifying genes and molecules such as hepcidin (HAMP) TNF-α[27,28].

The serum iron level and percentage saturation of transferrin are elevated early in homozygous subjects as the first phenotypic manifestations (analogous to familial hypercholesterolaemia where an elevated serum cholesterol level is manifested in the first decade of life). However, their specificity is reduced by significant false-positive and false-negative rates. For example, serum iron concentration may be increased in patients with alcoholic liver disease without iron overload: in this situation, however, the hepatic iron index is usually not increased as in haemochromatosis[25,29]. In otherwise healthy persons a fasting serum transferrin saturation greater than 50% is abnormal, and suggests homozygosity for haemochromatosis.

The serum ferritin concentration is usually a good index of body iron stores, whether decreased or increased. An increase of 1 µg/L in serum ferritin level reflects an increase of about 7 mg in body stores[20,30]. In most untreated patients with haemochromatosis the serum ferritin level is greatly increased. However, in patients with inflammation and hepatocellular necrosis, serum ferritin levels may be elevated out of proportion to body iron stores due to increased release from tissues. Levels can be abnormal in approximately 50% of patients with alcoholic liver disease, non-alcoholic steatohepatitis or chronic hepatitis C virus infection in the absence of HHC. In other inflammatory disorders, e.g. rheumatoid arthritis and various neoplastic diseases, serum ferritin levels can be elevated; however, importantly in these situations, the transferrin saturation is usually normal whereas the level is usually increased in cases of HHC. Indeed, as mentioned above, an elevated transferrin saturation is a characteristic early biochemical finding in HFE-associated HHC, and probably related to the basic pathophysiological defect. Thus, an elevated transferrin-iron saturation is an early phenotypic marker of the genetic disorder, whereas the serum ferritin in the absence of inflammation is a good guide to the degree of iron overload. A repeat determination of serum ferritin should therefore be carried out after acute hepatocellular damage has subsided, e.g. alcoholic liver disease. Ordinarily, the combined measurements of the percentage transferrin saturation and serum ferritin level provide a simple and reliable screening test for haemochromatosis, including the precirrhotic phase of the disease. If either of these tests is abnormal, genetic testing for haemochromatosis should be performed (Figure 1).

Although the use of liver biopsy has long been the gold standard for diagnosis of haemochromatosis, its role has been changed after the introduction of the genetic test to one of prognostic value; however, this is still important[31]. Previously, liver biopsy was performed after detection of an elevated fasting transferrin saturation and serum ferritin level. Biopsy aimed to establish or exclude a diagnosis using histochemical iron stains (Perls' Prussian blue stain) and biochemical determination of hepatic iron concentration (HIC) with calculation of the hepatic iron index (HII) (HII = HIC ÷ age). Characteristically the iron is found predominantly in a periportal

HAEMOCHROMATOSIS

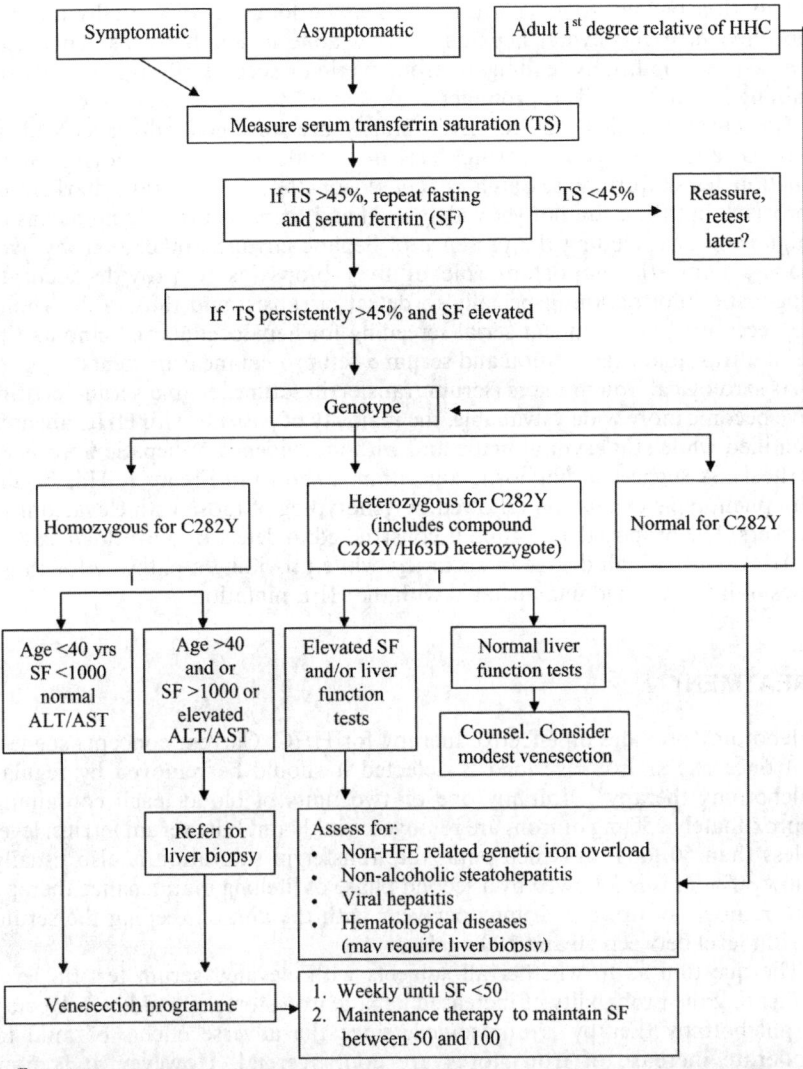

```
   ┌─────────────┐    ┌─────────────┐    ┌──────────────────────────┐
   │ Symptomatic │    │Asymptomatic │    │Adult 1st degree relative │
   └──────┬──────┘    └──────┬──────┘    │        of HHC            │
          │                  │           └────────────┬─────────────┘
          └──────────┬───────┘                        │
                     ▼                                │
   ┌──────────────────────────────────────┐          │
   │ Measure serum transferrin saturation │          │
   │                (TS)                  │          │
   └──────────────────┬───────────────────┘          │
                      ▼                               │
   ┌──────────────────────────┐   TS <45%   ┌───────────────┐
   │ If TS >45%, repeat fasting│────────────▶│   Reassure,   │
   │  and serum ferritin (SF) │              │ retest later? │
   └──────────────┬───────────┘              └───────────────┘
                  ▼
   ┌──────────────────────────────────┐
   │ If TS persistently >45% and SF    │
   │           elevated                │
   └──────────────┬───────────────────┘
                  ▼
            ┌──────────┐◀──────────────────────────────┐
            │ Genotype │                                │
            └────┬─────┘                                │
    ┌────────────┼───────────────────┐                  │
    ▼            ▼                   ▼                  │
┌─────────┐ ┌────────────────┐  ┌─────────────┐         │
│Homozygous│ │ Heterozygous   │  │  Normal for │         │
│for C282Y│ │ for C282Y       │  │    C282Y    │         │
│         │ │(includes compound│  │             │         │
│         │ │C282Y/H63D        │  │             │         │
│         │ │heterozygote)    │  │             │         │
└────┬────┘ └────────┬───────┘  └─────────────┘         │
     │               │                                   │
  ┌──┴──┐      ┌─────┴─────┐                             │
  ▼     ▼      ▼           ▼                             │
┌─────┐┌─────┐┌────────┐┌──────────┐                     │
│Age  ││Age  ││Elevated││  Normal  │                     │
│<40  ││>40  ││SF and/ ││  liver   │                     │
│yrs  ││and  ││or liver││ function │                     │
│SF   ││or SF││function││  tests   │                     │
│<1000││>1000││  tests ││          │                     │
│norm ││or   ││        │└────┬─────┘                     │
│ALT/ ││elev ││        │     ▼                           │
│AST  ││ALT/ ││        │┌──────────────┐                 │
│     ││AST  ││        ││Counsel.      │                 │
└──┬──┘└──┬──┘└────────┘│Consider      │                 │
   │      ▼             │modest        │                 │
   │  ┌────────┐        │venesection   │                 │
   │  │Refer   │        └──────────────┘                 │
   │  │for     │                                         │
   │  │liver   │  ┌──────────────────────────────────┐   │
   │  │biopsy  │  │ Assess for:                      │   │
   │  └───┬────┘  │  • Non-HFE related genetic iron  │   │
   │      │      │    overload                      │───┘
   │      │      │  • Non-alcoholic steatohepatitis │
   │      │      │  • Viral hepatitis               │
   │      │      │  • Hematological diseases        │
   │      │      │    (may require liver biopsy)    │
   │      │      └──────────────────────────────────┘
   ▼      │
┌─────────────┐   ┌──────────────────────────────────┐
│ Venesection │   │ 1. Weekly until SF <50           │
│  programme  │   │ 2. Maintenance therapy to        │
└─────────────┘   │    maintain SF between 50 and 100│
                  └──────────────────────────────────┘
```

Footnotes:
1. An isolated elevation of TS with normal SF may indicate early (non-expressing) HHC and annual checks of SF may be indicated.
2. H63D +/+ or +/- does not itself lead to significant iron overload for practical purposes (see text).
3. The metabolic syndrome is a common cause of elevated SF with normal TS.

Figure 1 Algorithm for screening for haemochromatosis. SF, serum ferritin; TS, transferrin saturation. (Adapted with permission from the *Canadian Journal of Gastroenterology*)

distribution (acinar zone 1) within the hepatic lobule with virtually all iron deposited in parenchymal hepatocytes and none in Kupffer cells. This is in contrast to conditions leading to iron overload secondarily, in which iron staining in Kupffer cells is prominent[32].

The current indications for liver biopsy are now generally accepted as follows: age >40 years, serum ferritin >1000 µg/L or abnormal liver function tests. Current research is focused on the use of serum markers of fibrosis[33], but these are not yet widely used and there is currently no means of diagnosing or excluding the presence of hepatic cirrhosis other than by liver biopsy. Thus, the important role of liver biopsy is to provide accurate prognostic information (especially to detect cirrhosis) and thus to determine the necessity for subsequent serial screening for hepatocellular carcinoma (by serial ultrasound examination and serum α-fetoprotein measurements).

As serological iron markers (serum transferrin saturation and serum ferritin) have become more widely available, the majority of patients with HHC are now identified while still asymptomatic and without evidence of hepatic fibrosis or cirrhosis. A suggested diagnostic algorithm is shown in Figure 1. This begins with phenotypic evaluation followed by genotyping of those with elevated iron markers. The proposed algorithm is constructed to detect iron overload caused by HHC with a high degree of accuracy, while providing a pathway for those cases of iron overload unassociated with the HFE mutation.

TREATMENT

Phlebotomy provides an effective therapy for HHC. Current concepts suggest that once excess iron overload is detected it should be removed by regular phlebotomy therapy[34]. Initially one or two units of blood (each containing approximately 250 mg of iron) are removed weekly until the serum ferritin level is less than 50 µg/L at which point the transferrin saturation is also usually below 30%. This is followed by a second phase of lifelong maintenance therapy with removal of up to 3–4 units per year with the aim of keeping the serum ferritin level between 50 and 100 µg/L.

The question as to whether all subjects with elevated serum ferritin level (indicating the probability of increased hepatic iron stores) should be subjected to phlebotomy therapy is unresolved, since the adverse effects of mild to moderate increase of iron stores are controversial. However, it is now established that once the serum ferritin level reaches 1000 µg/L there is a significant risk of underlying hepatic fibrosis or cirrhosis and phlebotomy therapy is indicated[31,35].

Subjects homozygous for the C282Y mutation with elevated transferrin saturation levels but normal serum ferritin, do not need therapy, but the serum ferritin should be checked at periodic intervals, e.g. every 2 years.

SCREENING STRATEGIES FOR HEREDITARY HAEMOCHROMATOSIS

Diagnostic screening strategies should target high-risk groups such as those with likely organ involvement, a family history of HHC or those with a chance detection of biochemical or radiological abnormalities suggestive of the possibility of iron overload. Thus, there are three possible methods of screening for HHC: (a) population screening targeting subjects over 30 years of age, for example using large employer groups such as banks, insurance companies, etc.[36-39]; (b) relatives of index cases diagnosed with classical symptomatic HHC[40] (see below); (c) primary-care subjects, i.e. subjects who present to primary-care physicians for a health check. In such circumstances a standard check of plasma lipid profile is commonplace. The available evidence in terms of mutation frequency and expression for HHC would warrant the inclusion of transferrin saturation with or without serum ferritin levels to be included in such tests performed at that time.

Clearly the efficacy of each of these methods needs to be evaluated. At the present time the available evidence suggests that general population screening is probably not warranted because, as stated above, the clinical expressivity of HHC appears to be much lower than previously thought and the cost-effectiveness of population screening has been challenged[14]. However, screening of relatives of known cases (cascade screening) has a significant yield[40].

FAMILY SCREENING FOR HEREDITARY HAEMOCHROMATOSIS

This method of detection of subjects in the preclinical or presymptomatic phase of HHC is widely used. Once a patient with HHC has been identified (proband), family screening is recommended for all first-degree relatives (genotypic followed by phenotypic evaluation). Where there are two or more children, HFE testing of the spouse is recommended because if normal the children can only be obligate heterozygotes and need not undergo further testing[41]. If C282Y homozygosity or compound heterozygosity (C282Y/H63D) is found in adult relatives of the proband, serum iron indices should be performed. If serum ferritin levels are increased therapeutic phlebotomy should be undertaken. In addition, as indicated earlier, if liver function tests are abnormal or the serum ferritin is >1000 µg/L liver biopsy should be performed.

Thus, all first-degree relatives of patients with HFE-associated haemochromatosis should be tested for the C282Y and H63D mutations and counselled appropriately. In affected individuals it is important to confirm or exclude the presence of cirrhosis, and begin therapy as early as possible. When all children of a proband are affected, a homozygote–homozygote mating is most likely.

Bulaj et al.[40] studied the prevalence of haemochromatosis-related conditions among 214 unselected homozygous relatives of 291 probands with the disease. Disease-related conditions were defined as hepatic fibrosis and cirrhosis, haemochromatotic arthropathy and abnormal liver enzymes, and were sought in homozygous relatives identified without reference to health status. Iron overload in male homozygous relatives became prominent after age 20, and after 50 years in women, and was present in 90% of men over 40 years and 88% of women over 50 years. Disease-related conditions occurred in 43 (38%) of the 113 homozygous male relatives (mean age 41), and in 52% of those men over 40 years of age. Of the 101 female homozygous relatives (mean age 44), 10 (10%) had at least one disease-related condition, and of the 43 women over 50 years of age, 7 (16%) had at least one disease-related condition. This study emphasized the important role of family screening in facilitating the detection of a significant number of patients with haemochromatosis-related conditions yet to be detected clinically.

RELATIVES WHO CARRY ONLY ONE COPY OF THE C282Y MUTATION

The obvious question arises as to the clinical significance of the finding in relatives of other mutations in *HFE*. Simple heterozygosity for C282Y does not lead to iron overload, and for practical purposes can be ignored – with one exception. Where there is other liver disease present, mild iron overload associated with C282Y heterozygosity may act as a cofactor for significant liver disease[42,43]. This is most clearly established for non-alcoholic steatohepatitis[44,45] and porphyria cutanea tarda[46]. Its role as a factor for other liver disease such as hepatitis C and alcoholic liver disease is controversial. Subjects who carry one or two copies of the H63D mutation may have an elevated transferrin saturation but do not manifest clinically significant iron overload[47].

The clinical relevance of compound heterozygosity (C282Y/H63D) has been less clear and several authors have suggested that it may lead to significant iron overload and indeed haemochromatosis. However, the available evidence suggests that compound heterozygosity does not lead to progressive iron overload and clinical disease. The only exception is where cofactors are present such as alcoholic liver disease, porphyria cutanea tarda or steatohepatitis[48].

OPTIMAL AGE FOR SCREENING OF RELATIVES

An important practical issue relates to the optimal age at which to screen relatives of known HFE C282Y homozygous subjects. Several studies have indicated that in HFE-associated haemochromatosis significant clinical disease rarely occurs under the age of 30 years[20,49]. In one large study of 120 relatives under the age of 35 years the serum ferritin concentration was an accurate predictor of body iron stores as assessed by phlebotomy ('mobilized body iron')[20]. Of those subjects submitted to liver biopsy all showed normal architecture except three with hepatic fibrosis and four with cirrhosis. However, in these subjects steatohepatitis or heavy alcohol consumption were common confounding factors. The authors of this study concluded that the combination of serum ferritin and transferrin saturation is a reliable screening regimen for the detection of haemochromatosis and for predicting the level of body iron stores in young subjects with haemochromatosis.

Since the discovery of hepcidin[50,51] and haemojuvelin[52] as key molecules involved in iron metabolism, there has been at least one report of severe HFE-associated haemochromatosis modified by the co-inheritance of a mutation in hepcidin[27]. We have recently studied a young woman with severe iron overload and cirrhosis who was heterozygous for C282Y but who was also homozygous for a haemojuvelin mutation (Wallace et al., unpublished). However, such cases are rare, and for practical purposes screening for HFE-associated HHC need not be performed until 20 or even 30 years of age unless there is a strong family history of severe disease or cofactors such as heavy alcohol consumption are present.

OTHER FORMS OF HAEMOCHROMATOSIS

Since the discovery of hepcidin and haemojuvelin as key molecules involved in iron metabolism, there have been reports of severe HFE-associated haemochromatosis modified by the co-inheritance of a mutation in hepcidin or haemojuvelin. However, such cases are rare and for practical purposes screening for HFE-associated HHC need not be performed until 20 or even 30 years of age unless there is a strong family history of severe disease or cofactors such as heavy alcohol consumption are present.

Ferroportin-associated iron overload is an autosomal dominant inherited disorder of iron metabolism that results from pathogenic mutation of the SLC40A1 gene[8]. The first description of the disease was published in 1999, when an autosomal dominant form of hereditary iron overload similar to classic haemochromatosis but not linked to chromosome 6p was reported. Distinctive features included tissue iron accumulation predominantly in reticuloendothelial (RE) cells, very high increasing serum ferritin levels, disproportionate compared with transferrin saturation, marginal anaemia, and mild organ disease. Although phlebotomy is an effective therapeutic tool, in some individuals, a weekly phlebotomy programme is not tolerated, and slight anaemia and low transferrin saturation rapidly occur despite still-elevated serum ferritin levels. With a less aggressive phlebotomy regimen these patients also can become iron depleted. Adjuvant therapy with erythropoietin may be beneficial.

Acknowledgements

This work was supported in part by funding from the National Health and Medical Research Council of Australia and the National Institutes of Health, USA, Grant 5R01DK057648-02.

References

1. Anderson GJ. Ironing out disease: inherited disorders of iron homeostasis. IUBMB Life. 2001;51:11–17.
2. Bacon BR, Powell LW, Adams PC, Kresina TF, Hoofnagle JH. Molecular medicine and hemochromatosis: at the crossroads. Gastroenterology. 1999;116:193–207.

3. Feder JN, Gnirke A, Thomas W et al. A novel MHC class I-like gene is mutated in patients with hereditary haemochromatosis. Nat Genet. 1996;13:399–408.
4. Tavill AS. Diagnosis and management of hemochromatosis. Hepatology. 2001;33:1321–8.
5. Perkins KW, McInnes IW, Blackburn CR, Beal RW. Idiopathic haemochromatosis in children; report of a family. Am J Med. 1965;39:118–26.
6. Hentze MW, Muckenthaler MU, Andrews NC. Balancing acts: molecular control of mammalian iron metabolism. Cell. 2004;117:285–97.
7. OMIM. Hemochromatosis. In: Online Mendelian Inheritance in Man, OMIM, Baltimore. McKusick-Nathans Institute for Genetic Medicine; 2000.
8. Pietrangelo A. Hereditary hemochromatosis – a new look at an old disease. N Engl J Med. 2004;350:2383–97.
9. Adams PC, Deugnier Y, Moirand R, Brissot P. The relationship between iron overload, clinical symptoms, and age in 410 patients with genetic hemochromatosis. Hepatology. 1997;25:162–6.
10. Niederau C, Fischer R, Purschel A, Stremmel W, Haussinger D, Strohmeyer G. Long-term survival in patients with hereditary hemochromatosis. Gastroenterology. 1996;110:1107–19.
11. Adams PC, Valberg LS. Evolving expression of hereditary hemochromatosis. Semin Liver Dis. 1996;16:47–54.
12. Asberg A, Hveem K, Thorstensen K et al. Screening for hemochromatosis: high prevalence and low morbidity in an unselected population of 65,238 persons. Scand J Gastroenterol. 2001;36:1108–15.
13. Olynyk JK, Cullen DJ, Aquilia S, Rossi E, Summerville L, Powell LW. A population-based study of the clinical expression of the hemochromatosis gene. N Engl J Med. 1999;341:718–24.
14. Beutler E, Felitti VJ, Koziol JA, Ngoc J Ho, Gelbart T. Penetrance of 845G – a (C282Y) *HFE* hereditary haemochromatosis mutation in the USA. Lancet. 2002;359:211–18.
15. Milman N, Pedersen P, Ovesen L, Melsen GV, Fenger K. Frequency of the C282Y and H63D mutations of the hemochromatosis gene (HFE) in 2501 ethnic Danes. Ann Hematol. 2004;13:13.
16. Fletcher LM, Dixon JL, Purdie DM, Powell LW, Crawford DH. Excess alcohol greatly increases the prevalence of cirrhosis in hereditary hemochromatosis. Gastroenterology. 2002;122:281–9.
17. Fletcher LM, Powell LW. Hemochromatosis and alcoholic liver disease. Alcohol. 2003;30:131–6.
18. Powell LW. The role of alcoholism in hepatic iron storage disease. Ann NY Acad Sci. 1975;252:124–34.
19. Bacon BR, Sadiq SA. Hereditary hemochromatosis: presentation and diagnosis in the 1990s. Am J Gastroenterol. 1997;92:784–9.
20. Bassett ML, Halliday JW, Ferris RA, Powell LW. Diagnosis of hemochromatosis in young subjects: predictive accuracy of biochemical screening tests. Gastroenterology. 1984;87:628–33.
21. George DK, Powell LW, Losowsky MS. The haemochromatosis gene: a co-factor for chronic liver diseases? J Gastroenterol Hepatol. 1999;14:745–9.
22. Simon M. Genetics of hemochromatosis. N Engl J Med. 1979;301:1291–2.
23. Simon M, Alexandre JL, Fauchet R, Genetet B, Bourel M. The genetics of hemochromatosis. Prog Med Genet. 1980;4:135–68.
24. Merryweather-Clarke AT, Pointon JJ, Shearman JD, Robson KJ. Global prevalence of putative haemochromatosis mutations. J Med Genet. 1997;34:275–8.
25. Bassett ML, Halliday JW, Powell LW. Value of hepatic iron measurements in early hemochromatosis and determination of the critical iron level associated with fibrosis. Hepatology. 1986;6:24–9.
26. Bassett ML, Halliday JW, Powell LW. Genetic hemochromatosis. Semin Liver Dis. 1984;4:217–27.
27. Merryweather-Clarke AT, Cadet E, Bomford A et al. Digenic inheritance of mutations in HAMP and HFE results in different types of haemochromatosis. Hum Mol Genet. 2003;12:2241–7.
28. Fargion S, Valenti L, Dongiovanni P, Fracanzani AL. TNFalpha promoter polymorphisms. Methods Mol Med. 2004;98:47–58.

29. Summers KM, Halliday JW, Powell LW. Identification of homozygous hemochromatosis subjects by measurement of hepatic iron index. Hepatology. 1990;12:20–5.
30. Walters GO, Miller FM, Worwood M. Serum ferritin concentration and iron stores in normal subjects. J Clin Pathol. 1973;26:770–2.
31. Guyader D, Jacquelinet C, Moirand R et al. Noninvasive prediction of fibrosis in C282Y homozygous hemochromatosis. Gastroenterology. 1998;115:929–36.
32. Powell LW, Kerr JF. The pathology of the liver in hemochromatosis. Pathobiol Annu. 1975; 5:317–37.
33. George DK, Ramm GA, Walker NI, Powell LW, Crawford DH. Elevated serum type IV collagen: a sensitive indicator of the presence of cirrhosis in haemochromatosis. J Hepatol. 1999;31:47–52.
34. Tavill AS, Bacon BR. Hemochromatosis: how much iron is too much? Hepatology. 1986;6: 142–5.
35. Morrison ED, Brandhagen DJ, Phatak PD et al. Serum ferritin level predicts advanced hepatic fibrosis among U.S. patients with phenotypic hemochromatosis. Ann Intern Med. 2003;138:627–33.
36. Leggett BA, Halliday JW, Brown NN, Bryant S, Powell LW. Prevalence of haemochromatosis amongst asymptomatic Australians. Br J Haematol. 1990;74:525–30.
37. Nisselle AE, Delatycki MB, Collins V et al. Implementation of HaemScreen, a workplace-based genetic screening program for hemochromatosis. Clin Genet. 2004;65:358–67.
38. Allen K, Williamson R. Screening for hereditary haemochromatosis should be implemented now. Br Med J. 2000;320:183–4.
39. Allen K, Williamson R. Should we genetically test everyone for haemochromatosis? J Med Ethics. 1999;25:209–14.
40. Bulaj ZJ, Ajioka RS, Phillips JD et al. Disease-related conditions in relatives of patients with hemochromatosis. N Engl J Med. 2000;343:1529–35.
41. Adams PC. Implications of genotyping of spouses to limit investigation of children in genetic hemochromatosis. Clin Genet. 1998;53:176–8.
42. Powell LW, Dixon JL, Ramm GA et al. Phenotypic expression of HFE-associated hemochromatosis in C282Y homozygous relatives: implications for screening. Hepatology. 2002;36:307A.
43. Leggett BA, Brown NN, Bryant SJ, Duplock L, Powell LW, Halliday JW. Factors affecting the concentrations of ferritin in serum in a healthy Australian population. Clin Chem. 1990;36:1350–5.
44. George DK, Goldwurm S, MacDonald GA et al. Increased hepatic iron concentration in nonalcoholic steatohepatitis is associated with increased fibrosis. Gastroenterology. 1998; 114:311–18.
45. Bonkovsky HL, Jawaid Q, Tortorelli K et al. Non-alcoholic steatohepatitis and iron: increased prevalence of mutations of the HFE gene in non-alcoholic steatohepatitis. J Hepatol. 1999;31:421–9.
46. Stuart KA, Busfield F, Jazwinska EC et al. The C282Y mutation in the haemochromatosis gene (HFE) and hepatitis C virus infection are independent cofactors for porphyria cutanea tarda in Australian patients. J Hepatol. 1998;28:404–9.
47. Gochee PA, Powell LW, Cullen DJ, Du Sart D, Rossi E, Olynyk JK. A population-based study of the biochemical and clinical expression of the H63D hemochromatosis mutation. Gastroenterology. 2002;122:646–51.
48. Hewett DG, Dixon JL, Purdie DM, Ramm GA, Anderon GJ, Subramaniam VN, et al. The clinical relevance of compound heterozygosity for the hemochromatosis mutations (C282Y/H63D). Hepatology. 2003;38(Suppl. 1):666A.
49. Yapp TR, Eijkelkamp EJ, Powell LW. Population screening for HFE-associated haemochromatosis: should we have to pay for our genes? Intern Med J. 2001;31:48–52.
50. Krause A, Neitz S, Magert HJ et al. LEAP-1, a novel highly disulfide-bonded human peptide, exhibits antimicrobial activity. FEBS Lett. 2000;480:147–50.
51. Park CH, Valore EV, Waring AJ, Ganz T. Hepcidin, a urinary antimicrobial peptide synthesized in the liver. J Biol Chem. 2001;276:7806–10.
52. Papanikolaou G, Samuels ME, Ludwig EH et al. Mutations in HFE2 cause iron overload in chromosome 1q-linked juvenile hemochromatosis. Nat Genet. 2004;36:77–82.

13
Wilson disease: from gene to patient

D. W. COX

INTRODUCTION

Copper is an essential component of the diet, required in enzymes involved in connective tissue development, neurological function, and tissue defence from oxidation. Since dietary intake of copper generally exceeds the trace amount required, homeostatic mechanisms are essential to effectively eliminate excess copper from the body. The copper storage disorder, Wilson disease (WND) or hepatolenticular degeneration, results when the excretory mechanisms for copper are defective. WND was first described in 1912 by Kinnear Wilson, who reported the combination of neurological and hepatic disease. WND is inherited as an autosomal recessive disorder. The incidence in most populations is approximately one in 30 000. Certain regions, for example Sardinia, China, and Japan, appear to have higher frequencies, in the order of one in seven to 10 000.

WND presents with a wide variety of symptoms. Classical features include liver disease with or without neurological disease, Kayser–Fleischer rings, formed by copper deposits in Descemet's membrane of the cornea (but frequently absent), and biochemical evidence of copper storage. Liver disease can be acute or chronic. Neurological disease can manifest as ataxia or tremors. Psychiatric abnormalities with abnormal behaviour can be another mode of presentation. Age of onset ranges from 3 to over 50 years. Because of this wide clinical variability, diagnosis can often be challenging.

THE COPPER TRANSPORT PATHWAY

Approximately 3 mg of copper is ingested in the average diet. Absorption of copper in the intestine and transfer into the circulating plasma involves a membrane copper-transporting ATPase, ATP7A, which is found in a variety of tissues, and particularly in the intestinal epithelial cells. Copper is then transported to the liver, where it is incorporated into a variety of essential copper-containing enzymes, and mainly into the plasma protein, caeruloplasmin, now known to be critical for the mobilization of iron from cells[1]. This incorporation requires the action of a second copper-transporting

ATPase, ATP7B. ATP7B is also involved in transporting the majority of copper out of the hepatocyte via the bile. Copper is not free in the cell. Specific low molecular weight chaperones shuttle copper to specific protein targets[2]. ATOX1 is the intracellular copper chaperone for ATP7A and B. The pathway is shown in Figure 1.

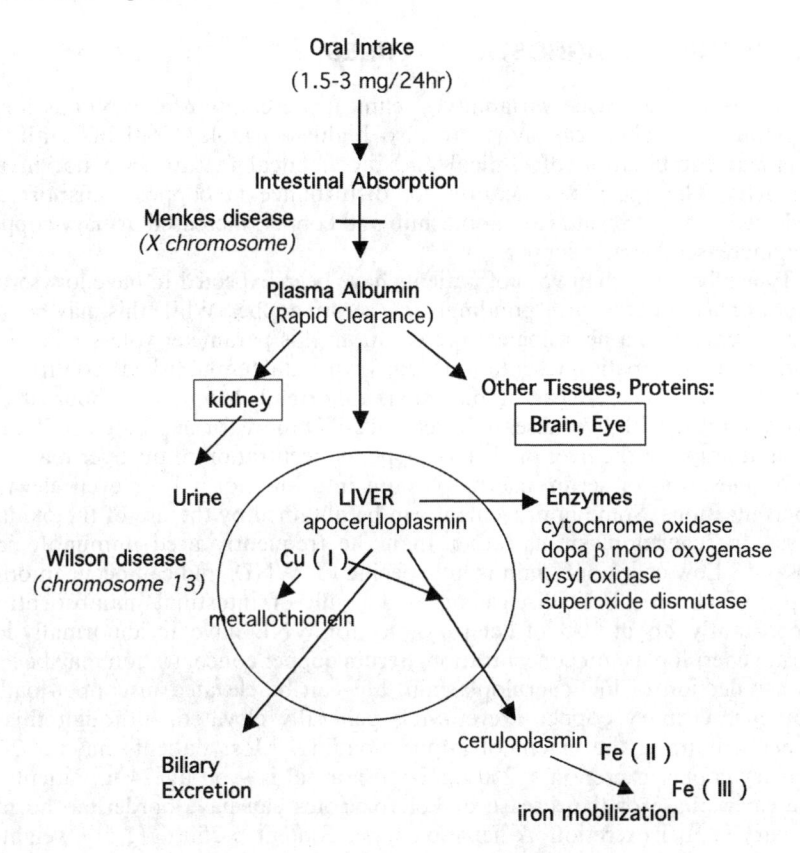

Figure 1 Copper transport pathway from oral ingestion to excretion, mainly from the liver via bile, small amount from urine. Excess copper is stored in metallothionein. Caeruloplasmin is essential for normal iron transport

The basic defect in the gene encoding the intestinal copper transporter, ATP7A, results in the X-linked disorder, Menkes disease. The consequences of this disease reflect a widespread copper deficiency due to the inability to transfer copper absorbed in the intestinal epithelial cell. WND results from a defect in the gene, *ATP7B,* on human chromosome 13. It has now been 12 years since the discovery, in 1993, of the gene defective in Wilson disease[3,4], an exciting highlight in our laboratory. This chapter focuses particularly on the subsequent knowledge we have gained about WND, and practical applications, since discovery of the causative gene.

The gene product is a P-type ATPase, with six copper-binding domains, eight transmembrane domains, an ATP-binding domain with a conserved aspartate residue at which phosphorylation takes place, and a transduction domain for the transfer of energy[3].

BIOCHEMICAL DIAGNOSTIC FEATURES

In addition to the wide variability in clinical presentation of WND as noted previously, biochemical signs are also highly variable[5]. Patients with the classical combination of clinical and biochemical features are not in the majority. The specific indications of disturbance in copper transport are reflected in a low serum caeruloplasmin and copper, increased urinary copper, and increased hepatic copper.

Typically, more than 95% of patients have been expected to have low serum caeruloplasmin and correspondingly low serum copper. While this may be true for patients with a neurological presentation, this parameter is less reliable in patients with hepatic presentation. Our own data (unpublished) confirm the observation that serum caeruloplasmin is abnormally low in only about 60% of cases of those with liver disease onset[6], possibly more for neurological disease. Inflammation of the liver or a high copper concentration in the liver may lead to an elevation of serum caeruloplasmin into low normal, or even elevated concentrations. Some improvement can be obtained by the use of the oxidase assay for caeruloplasmin, rather than the frequently used immunological assay[7,8]. Low caeruloplasmin is not specific for WND, and can occur in other types of chronic liver disease or as a result of intestinal malabsorption. Importantly, about 10% of heterozygotes for WND have an abnormally low serum caeruloplasmin concentration. Serum copper concentration may be low, as a reflection of low caeruloplasmin, but can be elevated in copper-loaded patients. Urinary copper excretion is generally elevated, although this is dependent upon the extent of copper loading. Most patients have a 24-h urinary copper excretion >250 µg/24 h; normal is <50 µg/24 h. Patients in the early phase of the disease or heterozygotes can have borderline normal urinary copper excretion. A hepatic copper content >250 µg/g dry weight is considered diagnostic of WND, although elevations can occur in clinically distinguishable disorders of bile excretion. Hepatic copper may not be elevated to this degree in patients with neurological disease, in early phases of the disease, or because of biopsy sampling error. Also, some heterozygotes have moderate elevations of liver tissue copper concentration.

A diagnostic scale has been proposed, but has not yet been validated[9]. Detailed information on diagnosis has been published in the AASLD Practice Guidelines[10].

DIAGNOSIS BY MUTATION ANALYSIS

Although typical biochemical parameters can sometimes provide a firm diagnosis for WND, gene mutation analysis has led us to conclude that the

Table 1 Distribution of types of mutations in *ATP7B**

Deletion	56
Insertion	21
Nonsense	19
Missense	155
Splice site	22
Total	271

*Mutations are described in the Wilson Disease Mutation Database::
http://www.uofa-medical-genetics.org/wilson/index.php

established diagnostic criteria need further consideration. Diagnosis by mutation analysis of DNA has an important role.

The WND gene (*ATP7B*) consists of 21 exons. Reported mutations now numbering more than 260, are listed in the Wilson disease database (http://www.uofa-medical-genetics.org/wilson/index.php). The distribution of types of mutations in *ATP7B* is shown in Table 1. Nonsense, missense, and splice-site mutations are located throughout all parts of the gene. Missense mutations, as predicted, lie predominantly within functional domains. Deletions, duplications and nonsense mutations can be predicted to severely affect the production of the ATP7B transporter. Missense mutations, the most common form of mutation, have effects that are difficult to predict.

For mutation analysis, each of the 21 exons and the 5′ promoter region must be considered as possible sites for disease-causing mutations. While mutation analysis seems to be a daunting task, high-speed methods of analysis will make mutation analysis considerably easier and faster. Furthermore, certain mutations in a limited number of exons are often characteristic of specific populations, so feasible methods for mutation analysis can be devised. In our laboratory we typically test for the most common mutation(s) in the population under study, sequence the six exons most likely to carry mutations, and complete the remainder of exons by sequencing or by single-strand conformation polymorphism (SSCP) analysis as needed.

The specific mutations present are dependent upon the ethnic origin of the patient. Each population has its own spectrum of mutations concentrated in specific exons. The most common mutation, histidine1069glutamine (His1069Gln or H1069Q), is present at least in the heterozygous state (i.e. one of the two mutations) in 35–75% of affected patients of European origin, particularly those from Eastern Europe[11]. This mutation is not found in Asian populations, where arginine 778 leucine (Arg778Leu, R778L)[12] is common in patients of Chinese origin. Patients from the Mediterranean regions and Japan have a large number of mutations, with none in a particularly high frequency. One of the exceptions is the island of Sardinia, where the majority of patients have a 15 base-pair deletion in the promoter region[13]. This is the only population in which a promoter mutation has been identified to date[14]. In some populations feasible mutation identification schemes can be developed for rapid mutation assessment for 90% of patients, as in Sardinia[15]. The difference in mutation distribution is illustrated between two populations, one from Sardinia and one from patients of French origin, mostly in Canada (Figure 2).

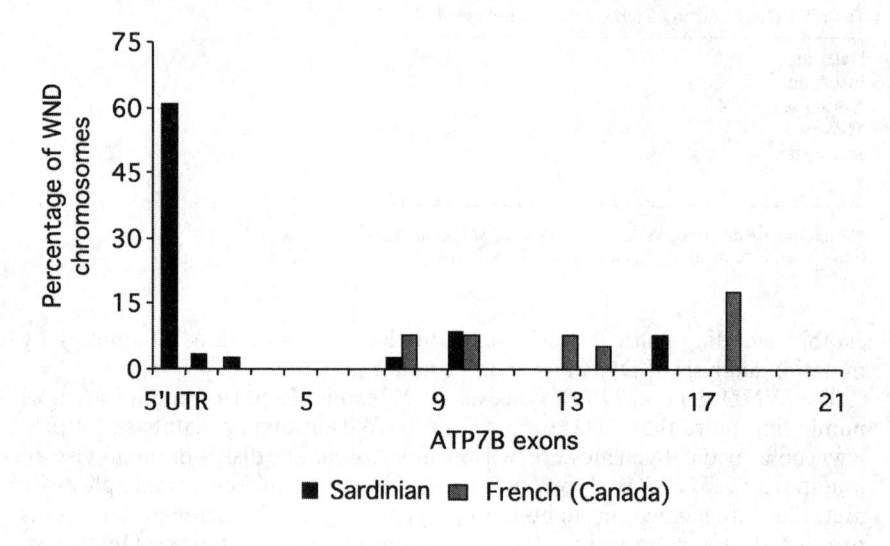

Figure 2 Distribution of most common mutations in Sardinian and French (Canadian) WND patients. Sardinian figures are from Loudianos[13]; French samples are from patients with French ancestry, from Canada, USA and UK (Cox et al., unpublished, 2004)

In addition to complete sequencing of the gene, new technologies are being developed for rapid mutation analysis. Denaturing high-performance liquid chromatography (e.g. WAVE) is also effective for mutation identification[16]. The identification of only one of the two mutations is usually adequate to confirm the diagnosis, in the presence of definite clinical symptoms and some evidence of disturbance of copper transport. Identification of only one mutation is inadequate for a patient with atypical or no symptoms, as this could reflect the heterozygous state. Mutation identification is very likely to become the diagnostic aid of choice, in the presence of clinical features and biochemical tests that arouse suspicion.

DISEASE-CAUSING MUTANT VERSUS NORMAL VARIANT

Care must be taken to distinguish normal variation from disease-causing mutations. Prediction of the disruption of the molecule, conservation of the specific residue between species, and absence in at least 50 controls are among the features examined to attempt to identify which mutations are disease-causing. This can be done by examination of changes in size, shape and hydrophobicity. We have carried out modelling experiments for the ATPase domain, using a model of the calcium transporter SERCA1, which has been crystallized and for which the structure is identified. Modelling helps us to assess which mutations lie in critical regions of the protein. Functional assays are also useful. We carry out functional assays in two different ways. The components of the copper transport system are completely conserved between yeast and humans. Therefore a yeast assay is useful to determine if the mutant ATP7B is capable of transporting copper, the requirement for its normal function[17]. Secondly, we use a cell culture assay, in CHO cells to determine if ATP7B can traffic normally within the cell[18]. Normal ATP7B trafficks in the cell from its location in the *trans* Golgi network to cytoplasmic vesicles, as a requirement for biliary excretion. For certain mutations this trafficking does not occur. Functional evidence for causing disease has been demonstrated for only a few of these missense variants.

One of the greatest challenges will be to ensure that mutations identified within ATP7B are actually responsible for defective function causing WND.

PHENOTYPE AND GENOTYPE

Data from a number of laboratories indicate that there is not a high correlation between clinical symptoms (phenotype) and specific mutations (genotype). However, generally the more severe mutations result in an earlier age of onset, which tends also to be associated with an onset of hepatic symptoms. For the most common His1069Gln mutation, age of onset in various studies ranges from 9 or 10 years of age to 50 years of age (mean of about 20 years), for homozygous individuals with this specific mutation[19]. Clearly other modifiers, which could be both genetic and environmental, are involved.

Most patients are compound heterozygotes; that is, they carry two different mutations of the *ATP7B* gene. This makes correlation of clinical features with specific mutations difficult. Homozygosity for a single mutation is most useful for phenotype–genotype correlations. For patients who are clinically normal, or have only slight clinical evidence of disease, the possibility exists that the patient is actually a heterozygote. Up to now heterozygotes have not been known to become clinically affected or require treatment. Heterozygotes can have a very low level of serum caeruloplasmin, borderline 24-h urinary copper, and increased liver copper. However, there is no evidence that such individuals develop clinical symptoms.

SIB DIAGNOSIS IN FAMILIES

Because of the recessive nature of the disease, the sibs (brothers and sisters) of a patient have a 25% risk of also being affected, and a 50% risk of being a heterozygote. Because of the variability of biochemical tests, diagnosis in the early stages before obvious symptoms develop is often difficult. Since lifetime treatment is required, unnecessary treatment of a heterozygote must be avoided. The only certain way to diagnose presymptomatic sibs, when the patient has a confirmed diagnosis of WND, is by direct mutation analysis or by the use of markers flanking the gene[5]. Marker analysis can be used without identification of the specific mutations, providing that the initial patient (proband) has definitely been confirmed as having WND. Markers are variable regions in the DNA within the gene or in regions just flanking the gene. The specific markers indicate which parental chromosome a sib has

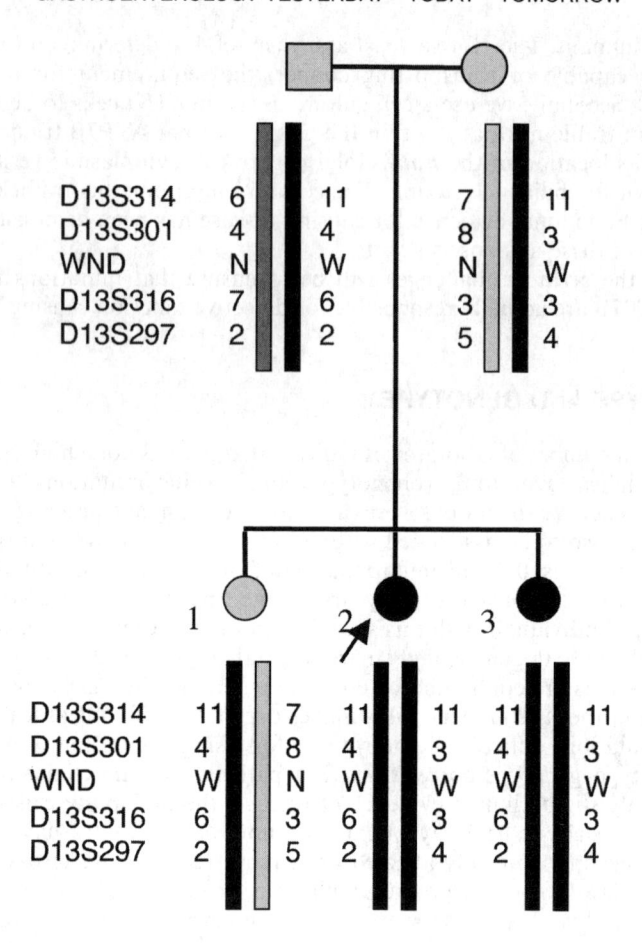

Figure 3 Pedigree showing inheritance of microsatellite markers flanking the WND gene (*ATP7B*). Even if the specific mutations are not identified, the status of sibs of the patient can be determined reliably. The initial patient (proband) is indicated by the arrow. Sib 1 is a heterozygote. Sib 3 is affected

inherited. This is indicated in the example in Figure 3. In order to diagnose presymptomatic sibs or unnecessary treatment of heterozygotes, this use of marker analysis is highly recommended, if not essential.

MURR1: A NEW COMPONENT OF THE COPPER TRANSPORT SYSTEM?

Some Bedlington terriers develop a recessively inherited copper toxicosis [20]. This disorder can be variable, with death after 2–3 years of age, or can have a more chronic disease course. Some affected dogs appear to show few symptoms from their very high levels of hepatic copper, which can range from 600 to several thousand micrograms/gram dry weight (normal < 300 µg/g). Normal dogs have a considerably higher hepatic copper content than do humans (normal human concentration is < 50 µg/g). The proposed defective canine gene was identified by positional cloning, a technique in which the disease locus was identified on a specific chromosome (dog chromosome 10) and markers were used to identify the specific region in which the gene lies. This led to the identification of *MURR1*, in which an exon deletion occurred in the affected dogs[21]. However, we have identified affected dogs that do not have the deletion[22]. This raises the question of whether *MURR1* is truly the defective gene responsible for canine copper toxicosis. The protein itself is interesting. It has been shown to interact with the copper-binding region of ATP7B[23], and has also been shown to affect the activity of the human delta epithelial sodium channel[24].

The question then arises as to whether a defect in *MURR1* could cause copper storage in humans. This is an important question, since the use of markers for the accurate diagnosis of sibs depends upon the fact that copper storage is always due to mutations in *ATP7B* on human chromosome 13. We have examined a series of patients with definite symptoms of WND but no mutation identified, and also patients with at least one biochemical assay indicative of disturbed copper transport. Of 27 patients studied, none has been identified with a disease-causing change in *MURR1* (Coronado and Cox, unpublished). Two common genetic variants, or polymorphisms, were identified. In another study of 63 patients diagnosed with WND, a polymorphic codon change, with no change of amino acid, was suggested to influence age at onset[25]. At the present time we can conclude that *MURR1*, if associated with disease in humans, must be exceedingly rare or does not manifest with signs and symptoms clinically similar to that of WND.

TREATMENT OF WND

The prognosis for patients with WND is excellent, when treatment begins sufficiently early to avoid excessive tissue damage. The liver is often able to recover exceedingly well, but neurological damage remains when treatment is not initiated sufficiently early. Treatment rationale and options have been presented[10].

Penicillamine and trientene have been used as effective chelators of copper. Many thousands of patients have been effectively treated since 1956, when J. M. Walshe first described penicillamine. A high incidence of side-effects from the long-term use of penicillamine has led to trientene as another agent for chelation. Oral administration of zinc is also effective, acting through another mechanism by preventing absorption of copper. Metallothionein is induced in the intestinal cells by the ingestion of zinc. Copper in the diet replaces zinc and the metallothionein copper complex is eliminated through normal shedding of the intestinal epithelium. Treatment with a combination of chelating agents and zinc is being tested. Extensive clinical trials are not yet reported for this more complex treatment regime. Ammonium tetrathiolmolybdate appears to be particularly useful as the initial treatment for patients with a neurological onset[26] and is the only known oral agent that effectively removes copper from the liver. This is an experimental drug, and caution will be required to ensure that the rapid removal of high concentrations of copper from the liver will not be harmful for erythrocytes or brain. This treatment may be used as a short-term way to remove copper from the liver, followed by more conventional treatment. Further research is required before this becomes an established mode of treatment. For patients with fulminant hepatic failure or decompensated liver disease not responding to therapy, liver transplantation is the only life-saving option.

The use of antioxidant supplementation, such as vitamin E, should be useful in counteracting the free radical production of copper. Patients have been found to be vitamin E deficient[27], compatible with the mitochondrial injury observed in copper overload[28]. These findings and others suggest a need for vitamin E replacement, along with use of other standard therapy.

With improved means of early diagnosis, transplantation, with its lifetime of immune suppression, should seldom be required.

CONCLUSIONS

The discovery of the gene for the copper transporter, *ATP7B*, has identified an important aspect of the copper transport pathway. This has led to the possibility of accurate diagnosis by mutation analysis. The early diagnosis of affected sibs is more reliable with the use of genetic markers, and does not require knowledge of the specific mutation present in the confirmed patient. Future new treatments must be carefully evaluated before the long-established treatments are replaced.

Acknowledgements

Mutation analysis for our studies was carried out by Lisa Prat, computer molecular modelling by Georgina Macintyre, *MURR1* studies by Veronica Coronado, ATP7B functional assays by Gloria Hsi, sequencing by Susan Kenney and Lynn Podemski. Our copper studies are supported by CIHR (Canadian Institutes for Health Research) and NSERC (National Science and Engineering Research Council of Canada).

References

1. Harris ZL, Takahashi Y, Miyajima H, Serizawa M, MacGillivray RT, Gitlin JD. Aceruloplasminemia: molecular characterization of this disorder of iron metabolism. Proc Natl Acad Sci USA. 1995;92:2539–43.
2. Field LS, Luk E, Culotta VC. Copper chaperones: personal escorts for metal ions. J Bioenerg Biomembr. 2002;34:373–9.
3. Bull PC, Thomas GR, Rommens JM, Forbes JR, Cox DW. The Wilson disease gene is a putative copper transporting P-type ATPase similar to the Menkes gene. Nat Genet. 1993; 5:327–37.
4. Tanzi RE, Petrukhin KE, Chernov I et al. The Wilson disease gene is a copper transporting ATPase with homology to the Menkes disease gene. Nat Genet. 1993;5:344–50.

5. Cox DW, Roberts EA. Wilson disease. In: Feldman M, Scharschmidt B, Sleisinger MH, editors. Sleisinger and Fordtrans Gastrointestinal Disease: Pathophysiology, Diagnosis, Management. Philadelphia: WB Saunders, 2002:1104–12.
6. Steindl P, Ferenci P, Dienes HP, Grimm G, Pabinger I, Madl C, et al. Wilson's disease in patients with liver disease: a diagnostic challenge. Gastroenterology. 1998;113:212–18.
7. Walshe JM. Wilson's disease: the importance of measuring serum caeruloplasmin non-immunologically. Ann Clin Biochem. 2003;40:115–21.
8. Macintyre G, Gutfreund K, Cammicioli N, Martin W, Cox DW. The enzymatic assay for serum ceruloplasmin. J Lab Clin Med. 2004;144:294–301.
9. Ferenci P, Caca K, Loudianos G et al. Diagnosis and phenotypic classification of Wilson disease. Liver Int. 2003;23:139–42.
10. Roberts EA, Schilsky ML. A practice guideline on Wilson disease. Hepatology. 2003;37: 1475–92.
11. Caca K, Ferenci P, Kuhn HJ et al. High prevalence of the H1069Q mutation in East German patients with Wilson disease: rapid detection of mutations by limited sequencing and phenotype-genotype analysis. J Hepatol. 2001;35:575–81.
12. Thomas GR, Forbes JR, Roberts EA, Walsh JM, Cox DW. The Wilson disease gene: spectrum of mutations and their consequences. Nat. Genet. 1995;9:217.
13. Loudianos G, Dessi V, Lovicu M et al. Molecular characterization of Wilson disease in the Sardinian population – evidence of a founder effect. Hum Mutat. 1999;14:294–303.
14. Cullen LM, Prat L Cox DW. Genetic variation in the promoter and 5' UTR of ATP7B in patients with Wilson disease. Clin Genet. 2003;64:429–32.
15. Lovicu M, Dessi V, Zappu A, De Virgiliis S, Cao A, Loudianos G. Efficient strategy for molecular diagnosis of Wilson disease in the. Clin Chem 2003;49:496–8.
16. Weirich G, Cabras AD, Serra S, Conni PP, Nurchi AM, Faa G, Hofler H. Rapid identification of Wilson's disease carriers by denaturing high-performance liquid chromatography. Prev Med. 2002;35:278–84.
17. Forbes JR, Cox DW. Functional characterization of missense mutations in ATP7B: Wilson disease mutation or normal variant? Am J Hum Genet. 1998;63:1663–74.
18. Forbes JR, Cox DW. Copper-dependent trafficking of Wilson disease mutant ATP7B proteins. Hum Mol Genet. 2000;9:1927–35.
19. Stapelbroek JM, Bollen CW, van Amstel JK et al. The H1069Q mutation in ATP7B is associated with late and neurologic presentation in Wilson disease: results of a meta-analysis. J Hepatol. 2004;41:758–63.
20. Twedt DC, Sternlieb I, Gibertson SR. Clinical, morphologic, and chemical studies on copper toxicosis of Bedlington terriers. J Am Vet Med Assoc. 1979;175:269–73.
21. van de Sluis B, Rothuizen J, Pearson PL, Van Oost BA, Wijmenga C. Identification of a new copper metabolism gene by positional cloning in a purebred dog population. Hum Mol Genet. 2002;11:165–73.
22. Coronado VA, Damaraju D, Kohijoki R, Cox DW. New haplotypes in the Bedlington terrier indicate complexity in copper toxicosis. Mamm Genome. 2003;14:483–91.
23. Tao TY, Liu F, Klomp L, Wijmenga C, Gitlin JD. The copper toxicosis gene product Murr1 directly interacts with the Wilson disease protein. J Biol Chem. 2003;278:41953–6.
24. Biasio W, Chang T, McIntosh CJ, McDonald FJ. Identification of Murr1 as a regulator of the human delta epithelial sodium channel. J Biol Chem. 2003;279:5429–34.
25. Stuehler B, Reichert J, Stremmel W, Schaefer M. Analysis of the human homologue of the canine copper toxicosis gene MURR1 in Wilson disease patients. J Mol Med. 2004;82:629–34.
26. Brewer GJ, Hedera P, Kluin KJ et al. Treatment of Wilson disease with ammonium tetrathiomolybdate: III. Initial therapy in a total of 55 neurologically affected patients and follow-up with zinc therapy. Arch Neurol. 2003;60:379–85.
27. von Herbay A, de Groot H, Hegi U, Stremmel W, Strohmeyer G, Sies H. Low vitamin E content in plasma of patients with alcoholic liver disease, hemochromatosis and Wilson's disease. J Hepatol. 1994;20:41–6.
28. Sokol RJ, Devereaux M, Mier GW, Hambidge KM, Shikes RH. Oxidant injury to hepatic mitochondrial lipids in rats with dietary copper overload. Modification by vitamin E deficiency. Gastroenterology. 1990;99:1061–71.

14
Hepatic stem cells and hepatocyte transplantation: future therapeutic applications

S. GUPTA and M. INADA

INTRODUCTION

The most effective treatments for a variety of diseases involve the possibility of organ replacement with cells which, at least in principle, has enormous potential and has generated corresponding, perhaps far greater, excitement than borne out by the current clinical results. Nevertheless, reasonable hype is often allowed in contemplating visions that require some time for realization, although sowing pure hype will only yield the crop of superhype! Discussion of stem cell potential generates optimism and excitement – of exploring new frontiers and chancing upon unimagined treasures, as well as pessimism and negativity – of anxieties driven by unresolved socio-ethical considerations, especially in respect of the derivation and use of embryonic stem cells (hESC). The questions of how, where and when should (or could) we apply stem cells in treating people then acquire lives far beyond the scientific community. To have a certain degree of scepticism always portends well for good science. To have too much scepticism for the principles of scientific discovery will not be good for science and history teaches us that to have only godly scepticism drive science may paralyse scientific inquiry, which cannot be good at all.

Therefore, the unresolved debate at present in various ways colours the way we think about the potential and challenge of stem cells in modern medicine. It goes without saying that the good, the bad and the ugly of stem cells must be balanced for making suitable progress. The task on hand is learning which is which, because uncertainties abound. The focused discussion below is based on work done yesterday and today, to consider what we may hold in our hands tomorrow, particularly from the clinical perspective.

WHAT DEFINES STEM CELLS, WHERE STEM CELLS COME FROM AND WHAT CAN STEM CELLS DO?

The existence of stem cells was recognized over 40 years ago with work concerning analysis of haematopoietic stem cells. The early operational definition of Till and McCulloch indicated that stem cells are 'clonogenic cells capable of both self-renewal and differentiation to lineage-restricted progenitors and/or functionally specialized mature cells'[1]. This remains an excellent definition to date, albeit with some enhancements, in view of further insights and complexities in stem cell biology. From an ontogenetic perspective it is useful to talk about the potency of stem cells, which can vary from totipotent stem cells to stem cells with lower orders of potency (Table 1). Undifferentiated embryonic stem cells constitute the best example of totipotent or pluripotent stem cells since these cells can produce an entire animal or all germlayers in a given animal.

Similarly, stem cells could be classified on the basis of their state of differentiation, e.g. whether stem cells are completely undifferentiated or committed in some way along specific lineages to turn into progenitor, facultative or lineage-restricted cells. These terms refer to specific changes in stem cell behaviour, where undifferentiated stem cells constitute rare subsets of non-cycling cells, particularly in healthy adult organs, whereas lineage-committed or facultative progenitor cells might be more obvious, as typically encountered in the bone marrow, skin and gastrointestinal tract, as well as other organs during periods of injury associated with accelerated cell turnover. A good example of this process within the liver concerns cell types populating the fetal liver, where extensive cell proliferation is characteristic of 'undifferentiated' parenchymal cells with multilineage gene expression, including markers of hepatocytes and bile duct cells, as well as additional

Table 1 Stem cell potency

Terminology	Characteristic features	Representative cell type
Totipotent	Capable of originating an entire animal; undifferentiated in native state	Embryonic stem cells
Pluripotent	Retain capacity for generating all germlayers	Embryonic stem cell subsets; some organ resident stem cells
Multipotent	Capable of generating more than two differentiated cell types	Multipotent adult progenitor cells (MAPC), haematopoietic stem cells, neuronal stem cells
Bipotent	Could generate two cellular lineages	Hepatic oval cells; pancreatic ductal cells; many other cell types
Stem-like	Differentiated cells capable of extensive replication and organ repopulation	Hepatocytes

| Cell loss | Hepatic homeostasis | Cell gain |

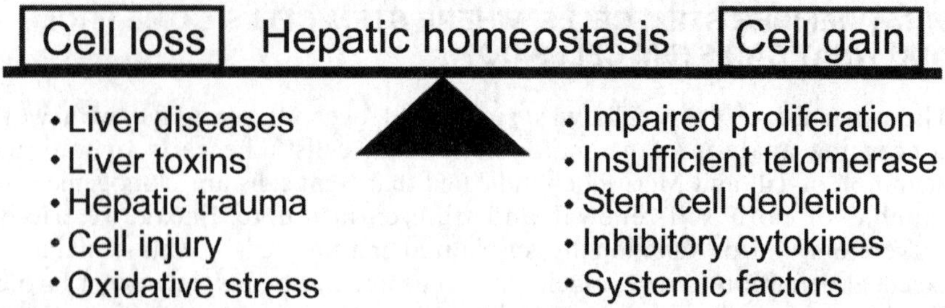

- Liver diseases
- Liver toxins
- Hepatic trauma
- Cell injury
- Oxidative stress

- Impaired proliferation
- Insufficient telomerase
- Stem cell depletion
- Inhibitory cytokines
- Systemic factors

Figure 1 Mechanisms of hepatic homeostasis and stem cell recruitment. The model shown indicates that hepatic homeostasis requires an appropriate balance between physiological cell losses and replenishment of lost cells. In the normal adult liver this balance is maintained by virtually invisible liver cell apoptosis and proliferation. However, in the setting of various perturbations listed on the left-hand side, that accelerate liver cell loss, the physiological balance between cell losses and gains could be perturbed, leading to recruitment of either hepatocytes and corresponding additional cell types alone, or additionally of stem/progenitor cells, e.g. oval cells, for liver repair. On the other hand, perturbations listed on the right-hand side may impair the liver repair capacity with progression toward organ failure

lineages[2,3]. In contrast with the adult liver, the fetal liver contains large numbers of such hepatoblasts with the capacity to generate mature hepatocytes and other lineages. This situation changes markedly in the adult liver, where cells are no longer in a cycling state, although progenitor cells can be activated during various types of liver injury[4,5]. The presence of few stem/progenitor cells in the adult human liver is consistent with an age-dependent decline in stem cell numbers and restriction of stem cells to unique niches in adult organs[6,7]. Whether specific cell compartments will be perturbed sufficiently for recruitment of stem/progenitor cells in the adult liver becomes a matter of homeostatic mechanisms (Figure 1). Among various types of hepatic perturbations, oncogenetic or toxic liver injury leads to the activation of so-called oval cells, which are facultative stem/progenitor cells, and emanate from the canals of Hering in the liver[8,9]. In general these types of stem/progenitor cells, which are resident in specific organ compartments constituting the equivalent of stem cell niches, are of interest because analysis of such cells offers insights into mechanisms regulating stem cell trafficking, cellular replenishment and life span of cells under various circumstances.

On the other hand it is imperative to reiterate the unique regenerative capacity of the liver, which has been a concept in ancient knowledge, as indicated by the Greek myth of Prometheus[10]. There is ample evidence to indicate that mature hepatocytes themselves can restore the liver in many situations, including after partial hepatectomy, without requiring the assistance of other, more classically defined, stem cells. Although the capacity of hepatocytes to proliferate in cell culture is markedly restricted, in studies involving serial transplantation in a mouse model, where transplanted cells can proliferate extensively, hepatocytes exhibited an indefinite replication potential with >90 estimated divisions per cell across several generations of animals[11]. In these studies the limits of the patience and resources of the investigators were reached, but not of the replication capacity of transplanted hepatocytes! This then raises another operational definition of stemness, i.e. the capacity of cells to proliferate extensively *in vivo* and to repopulate organs with functionally intact progeny. From a practical standpoint of translational activity this stem cell property cannot be emphasized enough.

Obviously, organogenesis will require regulated cell growth and differentiation, during which multiple intrinsic cellular, as well as extrinsic membrane-bound and soluble, signals come into play[12]. In the embryonic liver cell differentiation is regulated by signals from other cell types, particularly embryonic endothelial cells. This process has been defined most effectively in the context of the mouse liver, although information concerning development of the human liver is quite limited at present. Nonetheless, recent studies have begun to demonstrate that rapidly proliferating parenchymal cells in the fetal human liver demonstrate unique profiles of adhesion molecule expression, especially epithelial cell adhesion molecule (Ep-CAM), which begins to identify hepatoblasts with expression of albumin, α-fetoprotein, cytokeratin (CK)-19 and vimentin, and additional genes. On the other hand, mature hepatocytes in the adult liver do not express CK-19, which is restricted to biliary cells, or vimentin, which is expressed in hepatic stellate cells that are of mesenchymal origin. These findings raise the possibility of naturally occurring epithelial–mesenchymal transitions in the fetal liver, which has recently been observed during health and disease in adult organs, and gained considerable interest for studies of mechanisms in cellular transdifferentiation[13,14].

An assumption has been made that not only could specific lineages be cross-derived from cells resident within a given organ, but that cells entering from outside could contribute to organ repair during physiological and pathophysiological processes[15] (Figure 2). The idea that circulating stem/progenitor cells could thus be involved in surveillance and repair of organ damage gained interest following early demonstrations of multilineage differentiation potential of specific stem cells, in particular, haematopoietic stem cells, which could generate liver cells[16-20]. The capacity of stem cells derived from one organ or lineage to generate differentiated cells of another germlayer or lineage has been repeatedly demonstrated and critically reviewed[4,5]. Certainly, if stem cells could be conveniently harvested, as is the case with haematopoietic or mesenchymal stem cells from the bone marrow, peripherally circulating mononuclear cells, umbilical cord blood, etc., one could envision utilizing autologous cells for organ repair. After the initial demonstration of the possibility that haematopoietic stem cells could generate cells of additional lineages, much work has been performed. Indeed, a variety of evidence has now been gathered to substantiate that such cells can produce mature hepatocytes, both *in vitro* and *in vivo*[16-23]. The most convincing demonstration of the potential of haematopoietic cells was provided by studies utilizing a mouse model of hereditary tyrosinaemia type 1, in which fumaryl acetoacetate hydrolase (FAH) enzyme activity is deficient. Transplantation of healthy bone marrow-derived stem cell subpopulations in FAH knockout mice resulted in liver repopulation with healthy hepatocytes

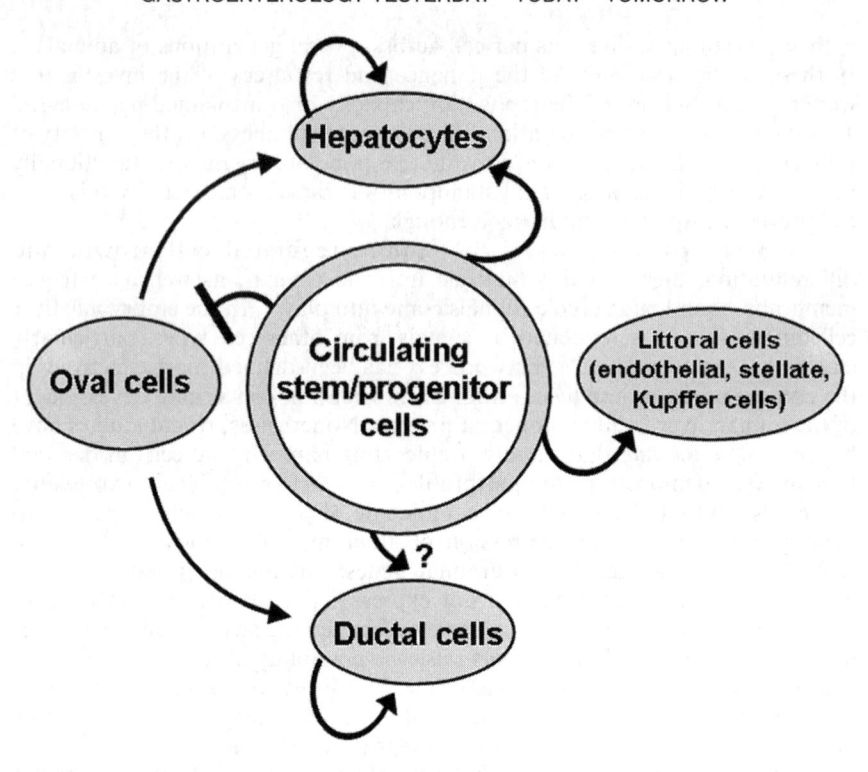

Figure 2 Potential sources of stem/progenitor cells for restoring the adult liver. Under many circumstances hepatocytes and bile duct cells can proliferate extensively, e.g. as observed in the partial hepatectomy or bile duct ligation models. In addition, resident stem/progenitor cells, e.g. the oval cell compartment, are thought to contribute in generating hepatocytes, as well as bile duct cells. Experimental evidence has been provided for the capacity of bile duct cells in generating mature hepatocytes. Circulating stem/progenitor cells do not contribute significantly in producing parenchymal liver cells under physiological circumstances although, following liver injury, sinusoidal liver endothelial cells, hepatic stellate cells and Kupffer cells, as well as some hepatocytes, may be derived from circulating stem/progenitor cells. Whether bone marrow-derived haematopoietic stem cells can produce mature bile duct cells is unclear, although these cells seem incapable of generating hepatic oval cells

and correction of metabolic abnormalities[19]. However, the overall frequency by which transplanted bone marrow-derived cells produced hepatocytes was extremely limited, perhaps not more than a handful of cells in an entire mouse liver[24]. While extreme selection pressure in the FAH mouse resulted in extensive expansion of these healthy cells in the mouse liver, other less robust cell selection strategies have not been as successful, and results of transplantation studies in mice with healthy livers have generated considerable scepticism with respect to the liver repopulation potential of haematopoietic stem cells[5].

Additional studies have also demonstrated that haematopoietic stem cells generated mature hepatocytes by a process involving nuclear fusion of transplanted and native cells, including generation of aneuploid cells[25], which will be undesirable due to obvious genetic instability and cancer risk in the long term. Nonetheless, whether bone marrow-derived haematopoietic cells will or will not fuse with native hepatocytes is a subject of controversy, because this phenomenon has not always been encountered, including in animals where human haematopoietic stem cells were transplanted[26–28]. Possible explanations to account for these discrepancies in various laboratories include intrinsic differences in the stem cell subsets analysed, as well as the nature of animal models used for analysis, with the existence of greater or lesser fusogenic pressure. At the same time, whether haematopoeitic stem cells are more capable of producing non-parenchymal liver cells, such as Kupffer cells, endothelial cells or hepatic stellate cells, is a possibility[29,30]. Whether such cell differentiation along non-hepatocyte lineages, if not properly recognized, might well confound analysis of cell differentiation in some studies is not excluded. Nonetheless, it does seem to be resolved for now that bone marrow-derived stem cells do not replenish the oval cell compartment of the liver[31,32]. On the other hand, examples of the success of bone marrow-derived stem cells in reconstituting the injured liver keep accumulating[33–35], which makes it difficult to place the true potential of haematopoietic stem cells into an appropriate perspective. The issue of whether correct methods are being employed to assess the magnitude of liver replacement by bone marrow cells becomes especially relevant, as emphasized recently[5]. Therefore, the bottom line at present is that while hamatopoietic stem cells may give rise to hepatocytes on occasion, this process is probably too random and inefficient to be of great value in cell therapy efforts in the near future. Similarly, while the potential of organ-resident stem cells, such as hepatic oval cells, has long been of interest, isolation of these cells in large enough numbers for clinical applications is problematic, and not particularly realistic.

How about the role of mesenchymal stem cells, especially the so-called multipotent adult progenitor cells (MAPC)[36,37], which can also be obtained from the bone marrow or circulating blood? MAPC have been capable of producing multiple lineages, including endodermal lineages – hepatocytes, as well as pancreatic beta cells – to generate hopes of developing appropriate cell therapy substrates. The demonstrations of the potential of MAPC extend to *in-vitro* studies, as well as blastocystic reconstitution in intact animals with generation of mature cells in all three germlayers[37]. However, MAPC require cumbersome methods for culture, and obtaining large numbers of cultured MAPC is also apparently difficult. Moreover, no studies have yet been reported to indicate that transplanted MAPC will be capable of reconstituting specific adult organs, including the liver, although studies aimed at understanding the full potential of MAPC appear to be in progress.

Coming back to the potential of hESC, it would be wonderful if these cells could be tailor-made for specific applications in given individuals with avoidance of allograft rejection. For instance, if one could initiate the processes of hepatic differentiation in hESC, without inducing terminal differentiation, such that cells could still be expanded in culture to a desired mass, it will become possible to contemplate serious clinical applications. In early studies hESC have been shown to differentiate into suitable cell types following transplantation into animals[38]. However, a variety of uncertainties exist at present in our knowledge of basic hESC biology, including relevant differentiation signals, appropriate culture conditions to help avoid feeder cells of animal origin, oncogenetic potential of fully or incompletely differentiated cells, etc. While differentiation of hESC along certain lineages, especially neuronal and cardiomyocyte lineages, is readily achieved, cell differentiation along other lineages, particularly hepatic and pancreatic beta cells, has been generally unyielding, except for modest successes in achieving limited gene expression at the transcriptional level[39,40]. This summary judgement is not a denouément of investigative efforts in this area; it only recognizes the uncertainties that position other cell types in a different place, so far as the practical realm of clinical therapeutics is concerned.

WHAT ARE ALTERNATIVE SOURCES OF CELLS FOR CLINICAL APPLICATIONS?

Liver-directed cell therapy has gained significant numbers of devotees and approximately 50–100 patients have been treated worldwide with hepatocyte transplantation. However, some of the difficulties have been commonly recognized, including the need for better donor organs, the supply of which has rapidly dwindled owing to increasing use of organs that might previously have been rejected for orthotopic transplantation; difficulties in cryopreserving mature hepatocytes, although some progress has been made[41,42]; and lack of protocol-driven trials utilizing similar disease targets, immunosuppression, cell number, route of transplantation, and other issues. The impasse could potentially be resolved by concerted efforts to generate alternative sources of donor cells. Some investigators have begun to consider isolating cells from liver tissue resected from living-related donors with the hope that cell viability will be superior, although this obviously poses risks for the donor. Similarly, whether sufficient numbers of cells could be isolated from healthy liver resected during removal of metastatic deposits or other lesions has been entertained, although diseased or cancerous cells in such specimens may cause problems, and this will need careful examination. Others have considered that cadaveric livers may yield significant numbers of viable cells, particularly because liver is relatively resistant to hypoxia, and cells isolated under these conditions might represent the most robust cell populations anyway. The potential of xenogeneic cells, e.g. from genetically modified pigs bred under specific pathogen-free conditions, has interested yet other investigators. Although use of porcine cells carries the risk of zoonotic disease transmission, e.g. porcine endogenous retrovirus might become activated in recipients, this has not yet been observed in people treated with bioartificial livers using pig hepatocytes[43].

Our own bias concerns use of fetal human liver cells, which can be isolated from cadaveric donor organs, obtained after elective terminations of pregnancy[2]. In our and other laboratories, fetal human liver cells show extensive replication capacity, cryopreserve very well, are amenable to genetic manipulation, engraft in immunodeficient animals and produce mature hepatocytes. Moreover, it is possible to overcome the naturally restricted proliferation potential of somatic cells, including fetal human liver cells, e.g. following genetic reconstitution of telomerase activity[44]. In recent studies fetal human liver cells were manipulated further with the introduction of Pdx-1, a homeobox regulator of pancreatic development, which led to the conversion of these cells into pancreatic beta-like cells, including insulin expression[45]. Such capacity of fetal liver stem/progenitor cells offers exciting possibilities for pursuing multidisciplinary cell therapy research across traditional boundaries of specialist care, consistent with the general vision of regenerative medicine.

Fetal human liver cells have previously been transplanted into people with acute liver failure, although the therapeutic value of such cell therapy was unclear, since only a few patients were studied[46]. Nonetheless, these findings are in line with studies in syngeneic recipients of rodent fetal liver cells, which have been demonstrated to engraft well, produce multiple liver cell types and proliferate in a superior fashion compared with adult hepatocytes[47–49]. Therefore, programmes aimed at harvesting, characterizing, cryopreserving and utilizing fetal liver cells probably offer some of the best opportunities in the near future of setting up a series of clinical studies.

WHAT WILL HELP ACHIEVE THE POTENTIAL OF LIVER-DIRECTED CELL THERAPY?

The potential targets of such studies are many, including acquired and genetic disorders (Table 2). The fundamental principles of cell therapy concern identification of a suitable disease target, transplantation of healthy or disease-resistant cells and repopulation of the liver to a therapeutically relevant extent. This calls for insights into the biology of various candidate cell types, as discussed above, as well as knowledge of the processes by which transplanted cells can engraft and proliferate in the diseased liver. While much information has been obtained in multiple laboratories to establish the biology of transplanted hepatocytes, significant gaps remain in critical areas involving clinical strategies to induce proliferation in transplanted cells, minimize the consequences of allograft rejection and assess the presence, as well as function, of transplanted cells[50]. The recent clinical experience and limitations with current studies have recently been reviewed[51].

Among areas where significant progress has recently been made are the steps by which transplanted cells engraft and proliferate in the recipient liver. These mechanisms have previously been discussed in Falk symposia, as well as in other recent reviews[50]; therefore the discussion below will present key concepts without attempting a comprehensive overview of the relevant processes. First, it is clear that cell engraftment in the liver is driven by the unique anatomy and physiology of liver sinusoids. Transplanted cells engraft after deposition into liver sinusoids via the portal vein, whereas injection of cells into the hepatic artery is associated with cell destruction. After reaching liver sinusoids, transplanted cells must breach the endothelial barrier to enter the space of

Table 2 Potential targets of liver-directed cell therapy

Metabolic or genetic deficiency states
α_1-antitrypsin deficiency
Congenital hyperbilirubinaemia, e.g. Crigler–Najjar syndrome
Coagulation defects
Cholestasis syndromes
Defects of carbohydrate metabolism
Erythropoietic protoporphyria
Familial hypercholesterolaemia
Hyperammonaemia syndromes
Lipidoses, e.g. Niemann–Pick disease
Tyrosinaemia, type 1
Wilson disease
Oxalosis

Acquired disorders
Acute liver failure
Chronic viral hepatitis
Cirrhosis and liver failure
Fatty degeneration of liver
Liver cancer

Disse followed by insinuation between native hepatocytes in the liver parenchyma and remodelling of plasma membrane structures. These processes are associated with multiple events, including release of specific soluble factors, e.g. vascular endothelial growth factor, to permeabilize endothelial cells, as well as activation of matrix-type metalloproteinases and other proteins to facilitate parenchymal remodelling[52]. On the other hand, deleterious changes are also encountered, such as Kupffer cell activation during mechanovascular perturbations of sinusoidal blood flow and disruption of the hepatic microcirculation by transplanted cell emboli[53,54]. The latter process is associated with transient and self-limited portal hypertension since transplanted cells eventually clear the sinusoidal spaces. Fortunately, this process of cell engraftment offers several pharmacological opportunities for intervention and enhancement of transplanted cell engraftment. For instance, the vasomotor tone of the liver sinusoids can be manipulated, Kupffer cells can be depleted and the endothelial barrier can be disrupted before cell transplantation[53–55]. This results not only in superior engraftment of transplanted cells, but also in acceleration of the kinetics of liver repopulation under specific situations.

Subsequent to the completion of cell engraftment, transplanted cells do not proliferate in the normal healthy liver because cell turnover in this situation is extremely limited[56]. To induce proliferation in transplanted cells an essential principle has evolved, in which damage in native liver cells that leaves transplanted cells unaffected, results in extensive liver repopulation. Initial studies demonstrating this principle utilized toxic transgenes[57–59]. Later, animals were preconditioned with genotoxic hepatic injury using the combination of chemicals, partial hepatectomy and liver radiation[60,61]. The manipulations were especially effective in repopulating the rodent liver without prior liver disease. More recently, the principle of genotoxic liver damage for inducing transplanted cell proliferation was extended to the use of radiation and warm ischaemia–reperfusion[62], which is particularly relevant because these modalities are used routinely in clinical practice. Therefore, it is now possible to repopulate the healthy rodent liver virtually completely with transplanted cells, and to demonstrate that transplanted cells survive throughout the life of animals. If similar findings are reproduced in humans, cell therapy results could certainly be very effective.

A variety of mechanisms need to be defined in contemplating therapies of specific disorders. Although discrete enzyme deficiency states constitute outstanding examples of suitable experimental models for establishing principles of cell therapy, it will perhaps be much more fulfilling to develop therapies for chronic hepatitis, which afflicts some 500 million people worldwide. However, this will require transplantation of cells that could resist disease; otherwise circulating hepatitis viruses will probably infect transplanted cells with eventual cell clearance. Therefore, efforts have been made to identify whether established disease could be overcome in surrogate models. One such system is provided by Wilson disease (WD), which is an excellent example of a genetically determined toxic liver and brain disease. This disorder is transmitted in an autosomal recessive fashion due to mutations in the *ATP7B* gene located on chromosome 13[63]. The *ATP7B* gene product is normally localized in the trans-Golgi apparatus and transports copper into the secretory pathway after its incorporation into apocaeruloplasmin, as well as into bile. Without functionally intact ATP7B protein, copper accumulates to toxic levels, first in the liver and then in the brain, cornea and other organs and tissues. Copper toxicosis is the central pathophysiological mechanism in WD, and drugs capable of removing copper, e.g. penicillamine, trientine, or interference with copper handling, e.g. zinc, are helpful. However, these drugs are not always effective. Development of novel therapies in WD has been facilitated by the availability of the Long-Evans Cinnamon (LEC) rat model[64]. More recently, a knockout mouse model of WD was obtained by targeted disruption of the *atp7b* gene[65]. Additional animal models are also available for studying WD, e.g. the toxic milk mouse, in which copper accumulates in the liver[66]. The LEC rat exhibits a deletion in the 3' region of the *atp7b* gene, which leads to the absence of atp7b mRNA or protein, hypocaeruloplasminaemia, virtually no biliary copper excretion, and progressive hepatic copper accumulation[64,67]. This results in extensive liver injury, although neurological disease is not obvious in LEC rats.

The LEC rat has been utilized in our laboratory over the past several years to develop suitable assays for demonstrating correction of pathophysiological perturbations in LEC rats, as well as mechanisms concerning survival, proliferation and function of hepatocytes isolated from healthy syngeneic LEA donor rats. Cell transplantation in LEC rats preconditioned with retrorsine and partial hepatectomy resulted in extensive liver repopulation with transplanted cells, removal of liver copper and restoration of liver histology to normal[68]. On the other hand, cell transplantation in unmanipulated adult LEC recipients was essentially ineffective. However, transplantation of healthy LEA hepatocytes into 1-week-old LEC pups resulted in gradual liver repopulation over several months, leading to the restoration of biliary copper excretion, liver repopulation with transplanted cells and correction of liver disease[69]. Further studies showed that hepatocyte survival was impaired by copper-induced oxidative perturbation of extracellular matrix components[70], which could be one explanation for delayed proliferation of transplanted cells in LEC rats. Finally, in additional cell transplantation studies, hepatic radiation before cell transplantation significantly accelerated therapeutic liver repopulation with correction of the WD phenotype in LEC rats[71]. A remarkable feature of these successful efforts in correcting copper toxicosis was that established liver fibrosis and structural perturbations reverted, and the restored liver following copper removal was histologically indistinguishable from normal healthy liver!

These findings establish the paradigm concerning the boundaries of liver-directed cell therapy, stretching from the restoration of deficient function to correction of morphological abnormalities and reversal of disease. If similar results could be achieved in patients with chronic hepatitis, the lives of a very large number of people could be saved or beneficially affected, and the odyssey for liver-directed cell therapy will become even more compelling.

Acknowledgements

Some of the work discussed above was supported in part by NIH grants R01 DK46952, P01 DK052956, P30 DK41296, and P30 CA13330. The contribution of many of our colleagues in generating our own data is gratefully acknowledged.

References

1. Till JE, McCulloch EA. A direct measurement of the radiation sensitivity of normal mouse bone marrow cells. Radiat Res. 1961;14:213–22.
2. Malhi H, Irani AN, Gagandeep S, Gupta S. Isolation of human progenitor liver epithelial cells with extensive replication capacity and differentiation into mature hepatocytes. J Cell Sci. 2002;115:2679–88.
3. Lazaro CA, Croager EJ, Mitchell C et al. Establishment, characterization, and long-term maintenance of cultures of human fetal hepatocytes. Hepatology. 2003;38:1095–106.
4. Burra P, Samuel D, Wendon J, Pietrangelo A, Gupta S. Strategies for liver support: from stem cells to xenotransplantation. J Hepatol. 2004;41:1050–9.
5. Fausto N. Liver regeneration and repair: hepatocytes, progenitor cells, and stem cells. Hepatology. 2004;39:1477–87.
6. Sigal SH, Gupta S, Gebhard DF Jr, Holst P, Neufeld D, Reid LM. Evidence for a terminal differentiation process in the rat liver. Differentiation. 1995;59:35–42.
7. Hackney JA, Charbord P, Brunk BP, Stoeckert CJ, Lemischka IR, Moore KA. A molecular profile of a hematopoietic stem cell niche. Proc Natl Acad Sci USA. 2002;99:13061–6.
8. Crawford JM. Development of the intrahepatic biliary tree. Semin Liver Dis. 2002;22:213–26.
9. Saxena R, Theise N. Canals of Hering: recent insights and current knowledge. Semin Liver Dis. 2004;24:43–8.
10. Michalopoulos GK, Khan Z. Liver regeneration, growth factors, and amphiregulin. Gastroenterology. 2005;128:503–6.

11. Overturf K, Al-Dhalimy M, Ou C-N, Finegold M, Grompe M. Serial transplantation reveals the stem-cell-like regenerative potential of adult mouse hepatocytes. Am J Pathol. 1997;151:1273–80.
12. Zaret KS. Regulatory phases of early liver development: paradigms of organogenesis. Nat Rev Genet. 2002;3:499–512.
13. Kalluri R, Neilson EG. Epithelial–mesenchymal transition and its implications for fibrosis. J Clin Invest. 2003;112:1776–84.
14. Gershengorn MC, Hardikar AA, Wei C, Geras-Raaka E, Marcus-Samuels B, Raaka BM. Epithelial-to-mesenchymal transition generates proliferative human islet precursor cells. Science. 2004;306:2261–4.
15. Blau HM, Brazelton TR, Weimann JM. The evolving concept of a stem cell: entity or function? Cell. 2001;105:829–41.
16. Petersen BE, Bowen WC, Patrene KD et al. Bone marrow as a potential source of hepatic oval cells. Science. 1999;284:1168–70.
17. Theise ND, Badve S, Saxena R et al. Derivation of hepatocytes from bone marrow cells in mice after radiation-induced myeloablation. Hepatology. 2000;31:235–40.
18. Alison MR, Poulsom R, Jeffery R et al. Hepatocytes from non-hepatic adult stem cells. Nature. 2000;406:257.
19. Lagasse E, Connors H, Al Dhalimy M et al. Purified hematopoietic stem cells can differentiate into hepatocytes *in vivo*. Nat Med. 2000;6:1229–34.
20. Korbling M, Katz RL, Khanna A et al. Hepatocytes and epithelial cells of donor origin in recipients of peripheral-blood stem cells. N Engl J Med. 2002;346:738–46.
21. Avital I, Inderbitzin D, Aoki T et al. Isolation, characterization, and transplantation of bone marrow-derived hepatocyte stem cells. Biochem Biophys Res Commun. 2001;288:156–64.
22. Fiegel HC, Lioznov MV, Cortes-Dericks L et al. Liver-specific gene expression in cultured human hematopoietic stem cells. Stem Cells. 2003;21:98–104.
23. Kakinuma S, Tanaka Y, Chinzei R et al. Human umbilical cord blood as a source of transplantable hepatic progenitor cells. Stem Cells. 2003;21:217–27.
24. Wagers AJ, Sherwood RI, Christensen JL, Weissman IL. Little evidence for developmental plasticity of adult hematopoietic stem cells. Science. 2002;297:2256–9.
25. Vassilopoulos G, Wang PR, Russell DW. Transplanted bone marrow regenerates liver by cell fusion. Nature. 2003;422:901–4.
26. Newsome PN, Johannessen I, Boyle S et al. Human cord blood-derived cells can differentiate into hepatocytes in the mouse liver with no evidence of cellular fusion. Gastroenterology. 2003;124:1891–900.
27. Willenbring H, Bailey AS, Foster M et al. Myelomonocytic cells are sufficient for therapeutic cell fusion in liver. Nat Med. 2004;10:744–8.
28. Jang YY, Collector MI, Baylin SB, Diehl AM, Sharkis SJ. Hematopoietic stem cells convert into liver cells within days without fusion. Nat Cell Biol. 2004;6:532–9.
29. Bailey AS, Jiang S, Afentoulis M et al. Transplanted adult hematopoietic stems cells differentiate into functional endothelial cells. Blood. 2004;103:13–19.
30. Jiang S, Walker L, Afentoulis M et al. Transplanted human bone marrow contributes to vascular endothelium. Proc Natl Acad Sci USA. 2004;101:16891–6.
31. Wang X, Foster M, Al-Dhalimy M, Lagasse E, Finegold M, Grompe M. The origin and liver repopulating capacity of murine oval cells. Proc Natl Acad Sci USA. 2003;100(Suppl. 1):11881–8.
32. Menthena A, Deb N, Oertel M et al. Bone marrow progenitors are not the source of expanding oval cells in injured liver. Stem Cells. 2004;22:1049–61.
33. Theise ND, Nimmakayalu M, Gardner R et al. Liver from bone marrow in humans. Hepatology. 2000;32:11–16.
34. Sakaida I, Terai S, Yamamoto N et al. Transplantation of bone marrow cells reduces CCl_4-induced liver fibrosis in mice. Hepatology. 2004;40:1304–11.
35. Yamamoto N, Terai S, Ohata S et al. A subpopulation of bone marrow cells depleted by a novel antibody, anti-Liv8, is useful for cell therapy to repair damaged liver. Biochem Biophys Res Commun. 2004;313:1110–18.
36. Jiang Y, Jahagirdar BN, Reinhardt RL et al. Pluripotency of mesenchymal stem cells derived from adult marrow. Nature. 2002;418:41–9.

37. Keene CD, Ortiz-Gonzalez XR, Jiang Y, Largaespada DA, Verfaillie CM, Low WC. Neural differentiation and incorporation of bone marrow-derived multipotent adult progenitor cells after single cell transplantation into blastocyst stage mouse embryos. Cell Transplant. 2003;12:201–13.
38. Shirahashi H, Wu J, Yamamoto N et al. Differentiation of human and mouse embryonic stem cells along a hepatocyte lineage. Cell Transplant. 2004;13:197–211.
39. Ku HT, Zhang N, Kubo A et al. Committing embryonic stem cells to early endocrine pancreas *in vitro*. Stem Cells. 2004;22:1205–17.
40. Kania G, Blyszczuk P, Jochheim A, Ott M, Wobus AM. Generation of glycogen- and albumin-producing hepatocyte-like cells from embryonic stem cells. Biol Chem. 2004;385: 943–53.
41. Mitry RR, Hughes RD, Dhawan A. Progress in human hepatocytes: isolation, culture and cryopreservation. Semin Cell Dev Biol. 2002;13:463–7.
42. Cho J, Joseph B, Sappal BS et al. Analysis of the functional integrity of cryopreserved human liver cells including xenografting in immunodeficient mice to address suitability for clinical applications. Liver Int. 2004;4:361–70.
43. Irgang M, Sauer IM, Karlas A et al. Porcine endogenous retroviruses: no infection in patients treated with a bioreactor based on porcine liver cells. J Clin Virol. 2003;28:141–54.
44. Wege H, Le HT, Chui MS et al. Telomerase reconstitution immortalizes human fetal hepatocytes without disrupting their differentiation potential. Gastroenterology. 2003;124: 432–44.
45. Zalzman M, Gupta S, Giri RK et al. Reversal of hyperglycemia in mice using human expandable insulin-producing cells differentiated from fetal liver progenitor cells. Proc Natl Acad Sci USA. 2003;100:7253–8.
46. Habibullah CM. Hepatocyte transplantation: need for liver cell bank. Trop Gastroenterol. 1992;13:129–31.
47. Sigal S, Rajvanshi P, Reid LM, Gupta S. Demonstration of differentiation in hepatocyte progenitor cells using dipeptidyl peptidase IV deficient mutant rats. Cell Mol Biol Res. 1995;41:39–47.
48. Dabeva MD, Petkov PM, Sandhu J et al. Proliferation and differentiation of fetal liver epithelial progenitor cells after transplantation into adult rat liver. Am J Pathol. 2000;156: 2017–31.
49. Sandhu, JS, Petkov PM, Dabeva MD, Shafritz DA. Stem cell properties and repopulation of the rat liver by fetal liver epithelial progenitor cells. Am J Pathol. 2001;159:1323–34.
50. Gupta S, Inada M, Joseph B, Kumaran V, Benten D. Emerging insights into liver-directed cell therapy for genetic and acquired disorders. Transplant Immunol. 2004;12:289–302.
51. Fox IJ, Chowdhury JR. Hepatocyte transplantation. Am J Transplant. 2004;4(Suppl. 6):7–13.
52. Gupta S, Rajvanshi P, Sokhi RP et al. Entry and integration of transplanted hepatocytes in liver plates occur by disruption of hepatic sinusoidal endothelium. Hepatology. 1999;29: 509–19.
53. Joseph B, Malhi H, Bhargava KK, Palestro CJ, McCuskey RS, Gupta S. Kupffer cells participate in early clearance of syngeneic hepatocytes transplanted in the rat liver. Gastroenterology. 2002;123:1677–85.
54. Slehria S, Rajvanshi P, Ito Y et al. Hepatic sinusoidal vasodilators improve transplanted cell engraftment and ameliorate microcirculatory perturbations in the liver. Hepatology. 2002; 35:1320–8.
55. Malhi H, Annamaneni P, Slehria S et al. Cyclophosphamide disrupts hepatic sinusoidal endothelium and improves transplanted cell engraftment in rat liver. Hepatology. 2002;36: 112–21.
56. Sokhi RP, Rajvanshi P, Gupta S. Transplanted reporter cells help in defining onset of hepatocyte proliferation during the life of F344 rats. Am J Physiol Gastroint Liver Physiol. 2000;279:G631–40.
57. Rhim JA, Sandgren EP, Degen JL, Palmiter RD, Brinster RL. Replacement of diseased mouse liver by hepatic cell transplantation. Science. 1994;263:1149–52.
58. Overturf K, Muhsen A-D, Tanguay R et al. Hepatocytes corrected by gene therapy are selected *in vivo* in a murine model of hereditary tyrosinemia type 1. Nat Genet. 1996;12: 266–73.

59. Mignon A, Guidotti JE, Mitchell C et al. Selective repopulation of normal mouse liver by Fas/CD95-resistant hepatocytes. Nat Med. 1998;10:1185-8.
60. Laconi E, Oren R, Mukhopadhyay DK et al. Long-term, near-total liver replacement by transplantation of isolated hepatocytes in rats treated with retrorsine. Am J Pathol. 1998; 153:319-29.
61. Guha C, Sharma A, Gupta S et al. Amelioration of radiation-induced liver damage in partially hepatectomized rats by hepatocyte transplantation. Cancer Res. 1999;59:5871-4.
62. Malhi H, Gorla GR, Irani AN, Annamaneni P, Gupta S. Cell transplantation after oxidative hepatic preconditioning with radiation and ischemia-reperfusion leads to extensive liver repopulation. Proc Natl Acad Sci USA. 2002;99:13114-19.
63. Ferenci P. Pathophysiology and clinical features of Wilson disease. Metab Brain Dis. 2004; 19:229-39.
64. Schilsky ML, Quintana N, Volenberg I, Kabishcher V, Sternlieb I. Spontaneous cholangiofibrosis in Long-Evans Cinnamon rats: a rodent model for Wilson's disease. Lab Anim Sci. 1998;48:156-61.
65. Buiakova OI, Xu J, Lutsenko S et al. Null mutation of the murine ATP7B (Wilson disease) gene results in intracellular copper accumulation and late-onset hepatic nodular transformation. Hum Mol Genet. 1999;8:1665-71.
66. Allen KJ, Cheah DM, Wright PF et al. Liver cell transplantation leads to repopulation and functional correction in a mouse model of Wilson's disease. J Gastroenterol Hepatol. 2004; 19:1283-90.
67. Wu J, Forbes JR, Chen HS, Cox DW. The LEC rat has a deletion in the copper transporting ATPase gene homologous to the Wilson disease gene. Nat Genet. 1994;7:541-5.
68. Irani AN, Malhi H, Slehria S, Gorla GR, Volenberg I, Schilsky ML, Gupta S. Correction of liver disease following transplantation of normal hepatocytes in LEC rats modeling Wilson's disease. Mol Ther. 2001;3:302-9.
69. Malhi H, Irani AN, Volenberg I, Schilsky ML, Gupta S. Early cell transplantation in LEC rats modeling Wilson's disease eliminates hepatic copper with reversal of liver disease. Gastroenterology. 2002;122:438-447.
70. Giri RK, Malhi H, Joseph B, Kandimalla J, Gupta S. Metal catalyzed oxidation of extracellular matrix components perturbs hepatocyte survival with activation of intracellular signaling pathways. Exp Cell Res. 2003;291:451-62.
71. Joseph B, Kumaran V, Volenberg I, Schilsky M, Gupta S. Wilson's disease in the LEC rat model is corrected by cell transplantation with hepatic preconditioning using radiation and bile salt administration. Hepatology. 2004;40:577A.

Section V
Bilary tract

Chair: A.F. HOFMANN and U. LEUSCHNER

15
Pathomechanisms of cholestasis: targets for medical treatment

G. PAUMGARTNER

INTRODUCTION

Much progress has been made in the understanding and treatment of cholestasis since the first Falk Symposium in Freiburg in 1971. In this chapter a brief overview concerning present concepts of bile formation and its disturbances in cholestasis will be given, and targets for medical treatment will be identified. Finally, some aspects related to treatment will be illustrated using primary biliary cirrhosis (PBC), the model disease for chronic cholestatic liver disease, as an example.

Cholestasis can be defined as an impairment of bile flow. The consequences are a retention of bile acids, bilirubin and other cholephils in the liver and in the blood and a deficiency of bile acids in the intestine[1]. All forms of cholestasis have in common an impairment of bile secretion or an obstruction of bile flow or a combination of the two (Figure 1). The impairment of bile secretion can be inborn, for instance in progressive familial intrahepatic cholestasis (PFIC) types 1–3, benign recurrent intrahepatic cholestasis (BRIC) types 1 and 2[2] or cystic fibrosis, or it can be acquired, caused by inflammation, toxins, drugs or hormones. Obstruction of bile flow can also be inborn, for instance in PFIC3 or cystic fibrosis or acquired, for instance in PBC, primary sclerosing cholangitis (PSC) or the vanishing bile duct syndrome (VBDS), and more often by stones and tumours[3].

Bile flow is driven by active transport of solutes into the bile canaliculi. For instance, bile acids are transported into the bile canaliculi by the bile salt export pump (BSEP). Water then follows passively through the tight junctions according to the osmotic gradient[1] (Figure 2).

PATHOMECHANISMS

As mentioned, bile secretion can be impaired by genetic defects (Figure 2). If BSEP is defective because of a gene mutation, PFIC2 or BRIC2[2] can occur. Mutations of the multidrug resistance-associated protein 2 (MRP2), the

Impaired Bile Secretion
- Inborn
   PFIC 1-3, BRIC 1-2,
   cystic fibrosis
- Acquired
   Inflammation, toxins,
   drugs, hormones

Obstruction of Bile Flow
- Inborn
   PFIC 3, cystic fibrosis
- Acquired
   Small bile ducts:
   PBC, PSC, VBDS

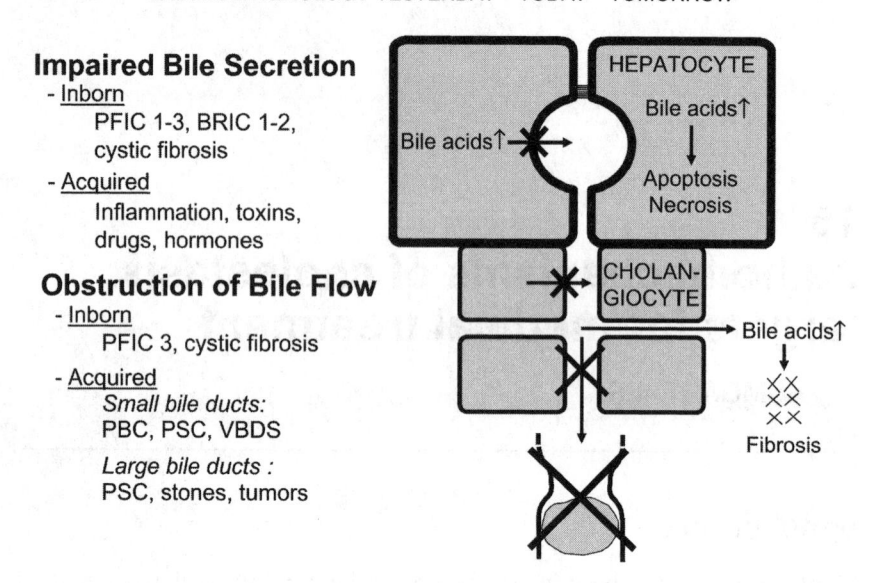

   Large bile ducts :
   PSC, stones, tumors

Figure 1 Causes of cholestasis. PBC: primary biliary cirrhosis; PFIC: progressive familial intrahepatic cholestasis; BRIC: benign recurrent intrahepatic cholestasis; PSC: primary sclerosing cholangitis; VBDS: vanishing bile duct syndrome

canalicular transporter for conjugated bilirubin, glutathione and many, mostly conjugated anionic compounds, which is also called conjugate export pump, cause the Dubin Johnson syndrome which, strictly speaking, is not a complete cholestasis, but a more selective defect of biliary secretion. Mutations of the multidrug resistance P-glycoprotein (MDR3), also called the phospholipid export pump, cause PFIC3. Mutations of the cystic fibrosis transmembrane regulator (CFTR) gene cause cystic fibrosis. Today these inborn forms of cholestasis can be detected, for instance by immunostaining of the transporters in liver biopsies[4].

Impairment of canalicular transport function can also be acquired, for instance by drugs. Some drugs act on the bile salt export pump (BSEP) from the inside of the cell; this is called *cis*-inhibition. Examples are bosentan, cyclosporin A, glibenclamid and troglitazone. Other drugs, such as oestradiol 17β-D-glucuronide, must first be transported into the canalicular lumen by the conjugate export pump, MRP2, and then act on BSEP from the luminal side; this is called *trans*-inhibition[5,6].

In sepsis, bacterial infections, viral hepatitis as well as toxin- or drug-induced hepatitis, cytokines can impair bile secretion. Thus, TNF-α and IL-1β down-regulate the sodium taurocholate co-transporting polypeptide (NTCP) and BSEP which are responsible for bile acid transport, as well as the organic anion transporting polypeptide (OATP2) and MRP2 which are responsible for bilirubin transport[7,8].

PATHOMECHANISMS OF CHOLESTASIS

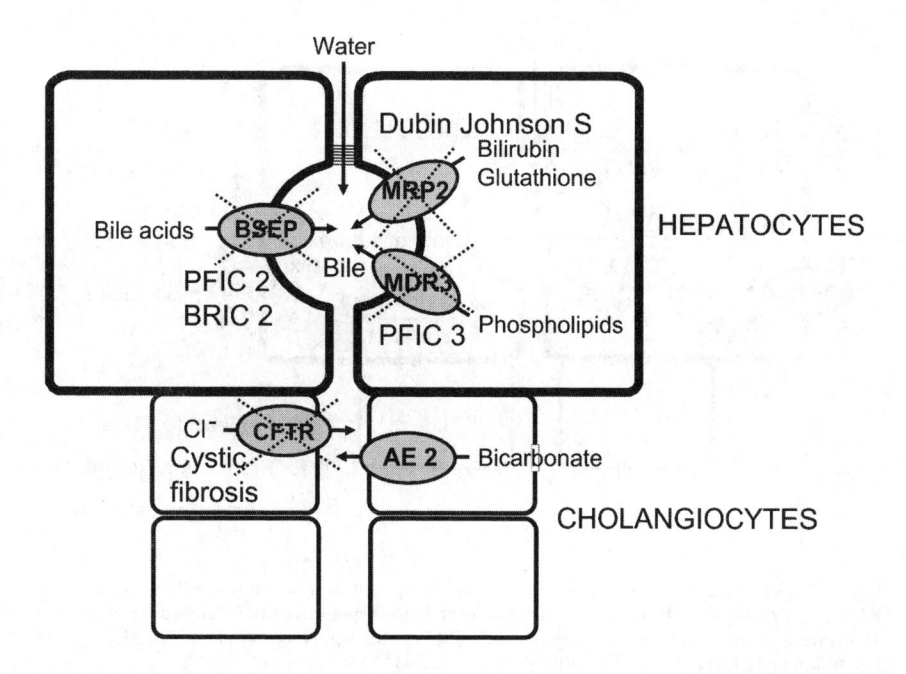

Figure 2 Inborn cholestatic disorders. AE2: anion exchanger 2; BRIC 2: benign recurrent intrahepatic cholestasis type 2; BSEP: bile salt export pump; CFTR: cystic fibrosis transmembrane regulator; MDR3: multidrug resistance P-glycoprotein 3 = phospholipid export pump; MRP2: multidrug resistance associated protein 2 = conjugate export pump; PFIC 2: progressive familial intrahepatic cholestasis type 2

Recently it has been shown that adaptive responses to cholestasis occur not only in the liver but also in the kidney and in the intestine[8–14] (Figure 3). They are mediated by nuclear receptors[12]. In the following, only the responses in the liver are briefly mentioned, since Dr Boyer in another chapter of this book will more extensively describe these adaptive changes in the kidney and in the intestine. Down-regulation of NTCP and OATP2 reduce the uptake of both bile acids and other organic anions in cholestasis, and thus protect the hepatocyte against an overload of bile aids and bilirubin[1,15,16]. At the same time there is up-regulation of MRP3 and MRP4 in the basolateral membrane[8,11,17]. These transporters pump bile acids and other organic anions from the hepatocyte into the blood and thus decrease their retention in cholestasis[9,13,18,19]. Prior to their extrusion, many xenobiotics are metabolized to more hydrophilic and less toxic compounds by cytochrome P450 (CYP) 3A enzymes, and a large fraction of bile acids is sulphated by the enzyme sulphotransferase 2A1[19] (Figure 3).

The nuclear receptor, farnesoid X receptor (FXR), which is a bile acid sensor, and the pregnane X receptor (PXR) – to which many xenobiotics bind – are among the major players in this regulation[12] (Figure 3). In humans, FXR

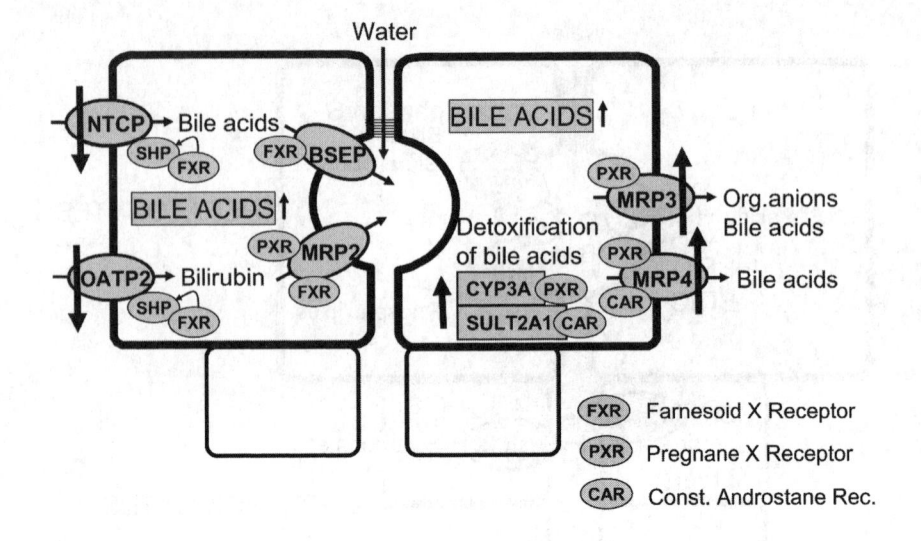

Figure 3 Adaptive responses to cholestasis. BSEP: bile salt export pump; CYP3A: cytochrome P450 enzyme 3A; OATP: organic anion transporting polypeptide; MRP: multidrug resistance associated protein; NTCP: sodium taurocholate co-transporting polypeptide; SHP: short heterodimer partner; SULT2A1: sulphotransferase 2A1

acts through SHP (short heterodimer partner), to down-regulate NTCP and OATP2[1,16]. For the up-regulation of MRP3 and MRP4, and also for the up-regulation of the bile acid metabolizing and conjugating enzymes, PXR and – as recently shown by Assem et al.[19] – the constitutive androstane receptor (CAR) play an important role. Bile acids[20] and certain synthetic bile acid derivates such as 6-ethyl chenodeoxycholic acid (6-ECDCA)[21] are agonists for FXR. Rifampicin is an example for an agonist for PXR. Bilirubin and phenobarbital are agonists for CAR.

The common consequence of all forms of cholestasis is a retention of bile acids in the hepatocytes. Elevated levels of bile acids then lead to apoptosis and necrosis of hepatocytes and, eventually, to chronic cholestatic liver disease[22]. In certain cholestatic disorders there is also leaking of bile acids into the peribiliary space causing, via induction of chemokines and cytokines, activation of hepatic stellate cells and fibrosis[13].

THERAPEUTIC TARGETS

On the basis of the above the following therapeutic targets can be identified in cholestasis (Figure 4): (a) Stimulation of secretion of bile acids and other potentially toxic cholephils into the bile and into the blood to reduce their retention in the hepatocyte; (b) stimulation of the metabolism of hydrophobic

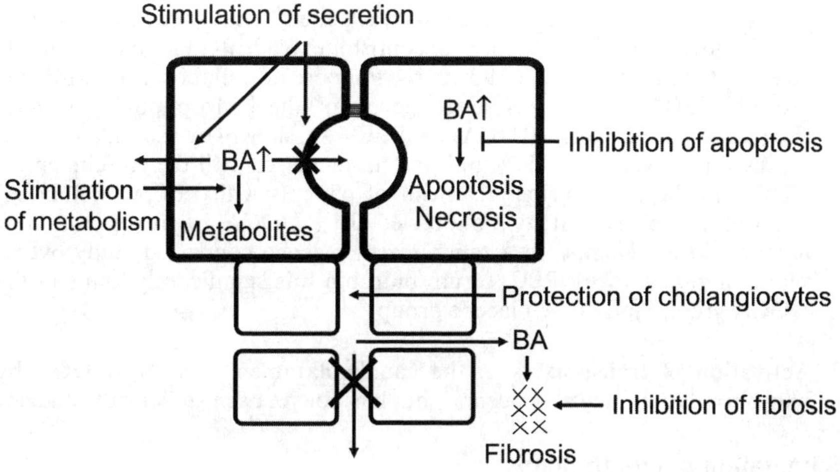

Figure 4 Targets for medical treatment in cholestasis. BA: bile acids

bile acids and other potentially toxic compounds to more hydrophilic, less toxic metabolites; (c) p-rotection of injured cholangiocytes against toxic effects of bile; (d) inhibition of apoptosis caused by elevated levels of cytotoxic bile acids; and (e) inhibition of fibrosis caused by leaking of bile acids into the peribiliary space.

Secretion of bile acids and other potentially toxic compounds

Secretion into the bile and into the blood may be stimulated by enhancing transporter expression and/or function at different levels, namely the levels of transcription, translation, targeting and protein activation:

1. Rifampicin, a ligand of PXR, stimulates transcription of the transporter, MRP2 in humans. In mice both cholic acid (CA) and ursodeoxycholic acid (UDCA) stimulate the expression of BSEP and MRP2 mRNA[23]. One must be aware that considerable species differences exist with regard to binding of bile acids to nuclear receptors and regulation of transporter expression by nuclear receptors[12].

2. UDCA stimulates targeting of the transporters BSEP and MRP2 to the canalicular membrane via at least two different signalling cascades[24–26]. Immunoelectronmicroscopy with gold particles can be employed to assess localization of BSEP in the canalicular membrane and in a subapical compartment of rat liver[24,26]. BSEP and MRP2 in the canalicular membrane were markedly reduced when taurolithocholic acid (TLCA) was administered in the perfused rat liver, but were maintained when

tauroursodeoxycholic acid (TUDCA) was added[24]. Enhanced expression of BSEP under UDCA treatment may contribute to a better elimination of bile acids from the blood. As shown by Poupon in collaboration with our group[27], UDCA decreases serum levels of the hydrophobic bile acid, chenodeoxycholic acid (CDCA) in PBC. As shown by Zollner et al.[11], expression of MRP2 mRNA and protein increases with the enrichment of UDCA in the liver during treatment of patients with PBC with UDCA. Accordingly, as shown by Poupon et al.[28], UDCA improves excretory function in PBC. Thus, in a randomized, placebo-controlled study over 2 years, in patients with PBC, serum bilirubin was significantly lower in the UDCA group than in the placebo group[28].

3. Activation of transporters in the canalicular membrane by UDCA by phosphorylation may also occur[29], but has not yet been sufficiently studied.

Stimulation of metabolism

Another therapeutic target is stimulation of the metabolism of hydrophobic bile acids to more hydrophilic, less toxic, compounds. Rifampicin, a drug used for the treatment of cholestatic pruritus, stimulates the expression of CYP3A4 mRNA in patients with gallstones[13]. In line with this, Dilger et al.[30] showed that, in patients with early-stage PBC, rifampicin stimulates CYP4A metabolic activity as assessed by urinary 6β-hydroxy cortisol, whereas UDCA has no effect.

Protection of cholangiocytes

Protection of cholangiocytes by making the bile more hydrophilic and less toxic appears to be an important therapeutic target. UDCA fulfils this requirement because it renders bile acid composition of bile more hydrophilic, and may increase biliary phospholipid secretion. As shown by Stiehl et al.[31] in patients with primary sclerosing cholangitis (PSC) and elevated serum bilirubin, UDCA stimulates not only the secretion of endogenous bile acids, but also the secretion of phospholipids.

Inhibition of apoptosis

Inhibition of apoptosis caused by elevated levels of hydrophobic bile acids may also be a therapeutic target in cholestasis. As shown by Rodrigues et al.[32,33], feeding of the hydrophobic bile acid deoxycholic acid (DCA) to rats increases hepatocyte apoptosis as assessed by the number of tunnel-positive hepatocytes. Addition of UDCA abolished this effect. Through activation of the CD95 receptor by elevated levels of hydrophobic bile acids in the hepatocyte, a death-inducing signalling complex (DISC) is formed and caspase 8 is activated. Caspase 8 then causes mitochondrial membrane permeability transition (MMPT), which leads to activation of the effector caspases and results in apoptosis. In addition, CDCA may also directly act on the mitochondrial membrane to cause MMPT with the same sequence of events. UDCA stabilizes the mitochondrial membrane and inhibits MMPT and apoptosis[32-34]. The antiapoptotic effect of UDCA has also been demonstrated in human hepatocytes[35].

Inhibition of fibrosis

An important therapeutic target in the future may become inhibition of fibrosis. Very recently, Fiorucci et al.[21] showed, in the rat with common bile duct ligation (CBDL), that fibrosis can be inhibited by 6-ethyl-CDCA (6-ECDCA). 6-ECDCA has a nearly 100–fold higher binding activity to FXR than CDCA. Hepatic stellate cells express FXR and the antifibrotic effect of 6-ECDCA appears to be mediated via FXR and SHP. It remains to be shown whether this finding is relevant for human cholestatic liver diseases, but it may indicate a promising new way for designing drugs which target nuclear receptors to inhibit cholestatic fibrosis.

CHRONIC CHOLESTATIC LIVER DISEASE

Let me now illustrate some of my points using PBC, the model disease for chronic cholestatic liver disease as an example. PBC is characterized by an inflammatory lesion of interlobular bile ducts, which results in bile duct destruction and may progress to fibrosis and cirrhosis. Since the aetiology of the disease is unknown, presently available therapies aim at inhibiting the underlying pathogenetic processes and delaying progession of the disease.

The pathogenesis of this slowly progressive disease involves: (a) a still-unknown immunological injury of small interlobular bile ducts; (b) aggravation of the bile duct lesion by cytotoxic bile acids; (c) obstruction and loss of small bile ducts followed by cholestasis and retention of bile acids; (d) hepatocyte injury, apoptosis, necrosis, fibrosis and eventually cirrhosis. If these processes progress, liver failure ensues (Figure 5).

Immunosuppressive agents – at least as monotherapies – have met with limited success. They have been found useful in combination with UDCA in selected patients. Rifampicin is used in the treatment of cholestatic pruritus when other therapies are ineffective. UDCA, at present, is the only approved drug for PBC: it appears to exert its beneficial effects by diminishing toxic effects of bile acids on the bile ducts, reducing the retention of bile acids in hepatocytes and inhibiting apoptosis. If there is insufficient response to medical therapy, liver transplantation must be considered[3,22].

In randomized, double-blind placebo-controlled trials UDCA at doses of 13–15 mg/kg per day improved serum liver tests including bilirubin and other serum markers of cholestasis[28,36-38], the Mayo risk score[38] and liver histology[28,37]. As shown by Pares et al.[36] and by Poupon et al.[39], UDCA inhibits histological progression in early-stage PBC. As shown by Corpechot et al.[40], UDCA inhibits progression to severe liver fibrosis or cirrhosis in early-stage PBC. In line with this is the observation that UDCA delays the onset of oesophageal varices[41]. Doses lower than 10 mg/kg per day of UDCA were of little benefit in PBC[42]. A combined analysis of three of the largest trials showed

Pathogenesis of PBC

```
┌─────────────────────────┐
│  Immunologic injury     │
│    of bile ducts        │
└─────────────────────────┘
            ⇓
┌─────────────────────────┐
│ Aggravation of bile duct lesion │
│    by toxic bile acids  │
└─────────────────────────┘
            ⇓
┌─────────────────────────┐
│  Cholestasis, retention │
│ of bile acids in hepatocytes │
└─────────────────────────┘
            ⇓
┌─────────────────────────┐
│ Hepatocyte injury, apoptosis, │
│ necrosis, fibrosis, cirrhosis │
└─────────────────────────┘
            ⇓
┌─────────────────────────┐
│     Liver failure       │
└─────────────────────────┘
```

Treatments of PBC

- Prednisolone*
- Budesonide (in stage I/II only)*
- Azathioprine*
- Mycophenolate* (?)

*In selected patients in combination with ursodeoxycholic acid

Ursodeoxycholic acid

Rifampicin**
**In pts. with pruritus who do not respond to other antipruritic agents

Liver transplantation

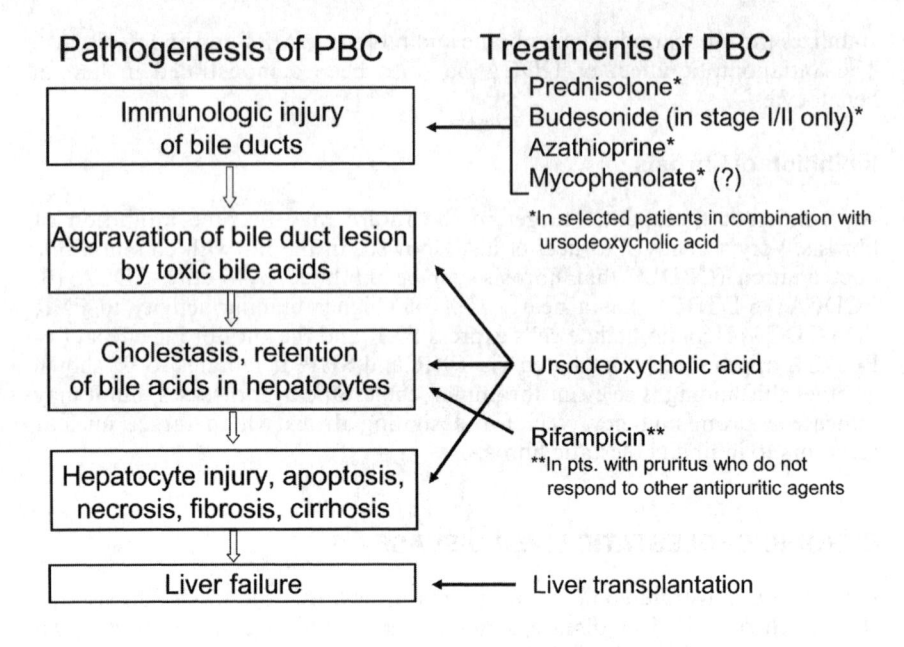

Figure 5 Pathogenetic processes and treatments in primary biliary cirrhosis (PBC)

that treatment with UDCA at doses of 13–15 mg/kg per day for up to 4 years increased the time taken to liver transplantation or death[43]. Within the first 2 years of treatment, however, a survival benefit was not seen. A meta-analysis of eight randomized trials showed no difference between UDCA and placebo in the effects on incidence of death, liver transplantation and death or liver transplantation[44]. However, it must be considered that in six of the eight studies treatment was evaluated up to 24 months only, and that the dose of UDCA was 10 mg/kg per day or lower in two of the studies. Therefore, a prolongation of transplant-free survival by UDCA therapy as shown in the combined analysis of the three largest studies with doses higher than 13 mg/kg per day and a follow-up of 4 years may have not been detectable in this meta-analysis.

UDCA therapy has been studied most extensively in PBC, and its beneficial effects in this disease have been documented by randomized controlled trials. Treatment with UDCA appears to be beneficial also in a number of other cholestatic conditions, such as primary sclerosing cholangitis (PSC), intrahepatic cholestasis of pregnancy, liver disease in cystic fibrosis, progressive familial intrahepatic cholestasis (PFIC), chronic graft-versus-host disease (GVHD) and some forms of drug-induced cholestasis[3].

SUMMARY

The major aims of medical treatment of cholestasis are reduction of the levels of bile acids and other potentially toxic compounds in the liver and diminution of bile acid-induced toxic injury of cholangiocytes and hepatocytes. Targets to reach these goals include: (a) stimulation of secretion of bile acids and other cholephils into the bile and into the blood, (b) stimulation of the metabolism of hydrophobic bile acids and other potentially toxic compounds to less toxic metabolites, (c) protection of injured cholangiocytes against the toxic effects of hydrophobic bile acids, (d) inhibition of apoptosis, and (e) inhibition of fibrosis. The clinical results of UDCA treatment of PBC may be regarded as the first success of this strategy.

References

1. Kullak-Ublick GA, Stieger B, Meier PJ. Enterohepatic bile salt transporters in normal physiology and liver disease. Gastroenterology. 2004;126:322–42.
2. van Mil SW, van der Woerd WL, van der Brugge G et al. Benign recurrent intrahepatic cholestasis type 2 is caused by mutations in ABCB11. Gastroenterology. 2004;127:379–84.
3. Paumgartner G, Beuers U. Mechanisms of action and therapeutic efficacy of ursodeoxycholic acid in cholestatic liver disease. Clin Liver Dis. 2004;8:67–81.
4. Jansen PL, Strautnieks SS, Jacquemin E et al. Hepatocanalicular bile salt export pump deficiency in patients with progressive familial intrahepatic cholestasis. Gastroenterology. 1999;117:1370–9.
5. Stieger B, Fattinger K, Madon J, Kullak-Ublick GA, Meier PJ. Drug- and estrogen-induced cholestasis through inhibition of the hepatocellular bile salt export pump (Bsep) of rat liver. Gastroenterology. 2000;118:422–30.
6. Byrne JA, Strautnieks SS, Mieli-Vergani G, Higgins CF, Linton KJ, Thompson RJ. The human bile salt export pump: characterization of substrate specificity and identification of inhibitors. Gastroenterology. 2002;123:1649–58.
7. Trauner M, Fickert P, Stauber RE. Inflammation-induced cholestasis. J Gastroenterol Hepatol. 1999;14:946–59.
8. Zollner G, Fickert P, Zenz R et al. Hepatobiliary transporter expression in percutaneous liver biopsies of patients with cholestatic liver diseases. Hepatology. 2001;33:633–46.
9. Denson LA, Bohan A, Held MA, Boyer JL. Organ-specific alterations in RAR alpha:RXR alpha abundance regulate rat Mrp2 (Abcc2) expression in obstructive cholestasis. Gastroenterology. 2002;123:599–607.
10. Bohan A, Chen WS, Denson LA, Held MA, Boyer JL. Tumor necrosis factor alpha-dependent up-regulation of Lrh-1 and Mrp3(Abcc3) reduces liver injury in obstructive cholestasis. J Biol Chem. 2003;278:36688–98.
11. Zollner G, Fickert P, Fuchsbichler A et al. Role of nuclear bile acid receptor, FXR, in adaptive ABC transporter regulation by cholic and ursodeoxycholic acid in mouse liver, kidney and intestine. J Hepatol. 2003;39:480–8.
12. Trauner M, Boyer J. Bile salt transporters: molecular characterization, function and regulation. Physiol Rev. 2003;83:633–71.
13. Fickert P, Fuchsbichler A, Wagner M et al. Regurgitation of bile acids from leaky bile ducts causes sclerosing cholangitis in Mdr2 (Abcb4) knockout mice. Gastroenterology. 2004;127: 261–74.
14. Dietrich CG, Geier A, Salein N et al. Consequences of bile duct obstruction on intestinal expression and function of multidrug resistance-associated protein 2. Gastroenterology. 2004;126:1044–53.
15. Gartung C, Ananthanarayanan M, Rahman MA et al. Down-regulation of expression and function of the rat liver Na^+/bile acid cotransporter in extrahepatic cholestasis. Gastroenterology. 1996;110:199–209.
16. Jung D, Kullak-Ublick GA. Hepatocyte nuclear factor 1 alpha: a key mediator of the effect of bile acids on gene expression. Hepatology. 2003;37:622–31.

17. Wagner M, Fickert P, Zollner G et al. Role of farnesoid X receptor in determining hepatic ABC transporter expression and liver injury in bile duct-ligated mice. Gastroenterology. 2003;125:825–38.
18. Rius M, Nies AT, Hummel-Eisenbeiss J, Jedlitschky G, Keppler D. Cotransport of reduced glutathione with bile salts by MRP4 (ABCC4) localized to the basolateral hepatocyte membrane. Hepatology. 2003;38:374–84.
19. Assem M, Schuetz EG, Leggas M et al. Interactions between hepatic Mrp4 and Sult2a as revealed by the constitutive androstane receptor and Mrp4 knockout mice. J Biol Chem. 2004;279:22250–7.
20. Trauner M. The nuclear bile acid receptor FXR as a novel therapeutic target in cholestatic liver diseases: hype or hope? Hepatology. 2004;40:260–3.
21. Fiorucci S, Antonelli E, Rizzo G, Renga B, Mencarelli A, Riccardi L, Orlandi S, et al. The nuclear receptor SHP mediates inhibition of hepatic stellate cells by FXR and protects against liver fibrosis. Gastroenterology. 2004;127:1497–512.
22. Paumgartner G, Beuers U. Ursodeoxycholic acid in cholestatic liver disease: mechanisms of action and therapeutic use revisited. Hepatology. 2002;36:525–31.
23. Fickert P, Zollner G, Fuchsbichler A et al. Effects of ursodeoxycholic and cholic acid feeding on hepatocellular transporter expression in mouse liver. Gastroenterology. 2001; 121:170–83.
24. Beuers U, Bilzer M, Chittattu A et al. Tauroursodeoxycholic acid inserts the apical conjugate export pump, Mrp2, into canalicular membranes and stimulates organic anion secretion by protein kinase C-dependent mechanisms in cholestatic rat liver. Hepatology. 2001;33:1206–16.
25. Kurz AK, Graf D, Schmitt M, Vom Dahl S, Haussinger D. Tauroursodesoxycholate-induced choleresis involves p38(MAPK) activation and translocation of the bile salt export pump in rats. Gastroenterology. 2001;121:407–19.
26. Dombrowski F, Stieger B, Beuers U. Tauroursodeoxycholic acid inserts the bile salt export pump into canalicular membranes. Hepatology. 2003;38:A688.
27. Poupon RE, Chretien Y, Poupon R, Paumgartner G. Serum bile acids in primary biliary cirrhosis: effect of ursodeoxycholic acid therapy. Hepatology. 1993;17:599–604.
28. Poupon RE, Balkau B, Eschwege E, Poupon R. A multicenter, controlled trial of ursodiol for the treatment of primary biliary cirrhosis. UDCA–PBC Study Group. N Engl J Med. 1991;324:1548–54.
29. Noe J, Hagenbuch B, Meier PJ, St-Pierre MV. Characterization of the mouse bile salt export pump overexpressed in the baculovirus system. Hepatology. 2001;33:1223–31.
30. Dilger K, Denk A, Heeg MHJ, Beuers U. No relevant effects of ursodeoxycholic acid on cytochrome P-450 3A metabolism in primary biliary cirrhosis. Hepatology. 2005;41:595–602.
31. Stiehl A, Rudolph G, Sauer P, Theilmann L. Biliary secretion of bile acids and lipids in primary sclerosing cholangitis. Influence of cholestasis and effect of ursodeoxycholic acid treatment. J Hepatol. 1995;23:283–9.
32. Rodrigues C, Fan G, Wong P, Kren B, Steer C. Ursodeoxycholic acid may inhibit deoxycholic acid-induced apoptosis by modulating mitochondrial transmembrane potential and reactive oxygen species production. Mol Med. 1998;4:165–78.
33. Rodrigues CM, Fan G, Ma X, Kren BT, Steer CJ. A novel role for ursodeoxycholic acid in inhibiting apoptosis by modulating mitochondrial membrane perturbation. J Clin Invest 1998;101:2790-2799.
34. Lazaridis KN, Gores GJ, Lindor KD. Ursodeoxycholic acid 'mechanisms of action and clinical use in hepatobiliary disorders'. J Hepatol. 2001;35:134–46.
35. Benz C, Angermuller S, Otto G, Sauer P, Stremmel W, Stiehl A. Effect of tauroursodeoxycholic acid on bile acid-induced apoptosis in primary human hepatocytes. Eur J Clin Invest. 2000;30:203–9.
36. Pares A, Caballeria L, Rodes J et al. Long-term effects of ursodeoxycholic acid in primary biliary cirrhosis: results of a double-blind controlled multicentric trial. UDCA-Cooperative Group from the Spanish Association for the Study of the Liver. J Hepatol. 2000;32:561–6.
37. Heathcote EJ, Cauch-Dudek K, Walker V et al. The Canadian Multicenter Double-blind Randomized Controlled Trial of ursodeoxycholic acid in primary biliary cirrhosis. Hepatology. 1994;19:1149–56.

38. Lindor KD, Dickson ER, Baldus WP et al. Ursodeoxycholic acid in the treatment of primary biliary cirrhosis. Gastroenterology. 1994;106:1284–90.
39. Poupon RE, Lindor K, Pares A, Chazouilleres O, Poupon R, Heathcote EJ. Combined analysis of the effects of treatment with ursodeoxycholic acid on histologic progression in primary biliary cirrhosis. J Hepatol. 2003;39:12–16.
40. Corpechot C, Carrat F, Bonnand AM, Poupon RE, Poupon R. The effect of ursodeoxycholic acid therapy on liver fibrosis progression in primary biliary cirrhosis. Hepatology. 2000;32:1196–9.
41. Lindor KD, Jorgensen RA, Therneau TM, Malinchoc M, Dickson ER. Ursodeoxycholic acid delays the onset of esophageal varices in primary biliary cirrhosis. Mayo Clin Proc. 1997;72:1137–40.
42. Eriksson LS, Olsson R, Glauman H et al. Ursodeoxycholic acid treatment in patients with primary biliary cirrhosis. Scand J Gastroenterol. 1997;32:179–86.
43. Poupon RE, Lindor KD, Cauch-Dudek K, Dickson ER, Poupon R, Heathcote EJ. Combined analysis of randomized controlled trials of ursodeoxycholic acid in primary biliary cirrhosis. Gastroenterology. 1997;113:884–90.
44. Goulis J, Leandro G, Burroughs A. Randomised controlled trials of ursodeoxycholic-acid therapy for primary biliary cirrhosis: a meta-analysis. Lancet. 1999;354:1053–60.

16
Adaptive regulation of bile salt transporters in cholestasis

J. L. BOYER, W. S. CHEN, S.-Y. CAI, G. DENK, A. BOHAN,
C. SOROKA and L. DENSON

Bile salt transporters in the liver, kidney and intestine undergo adaptive regulation in response to cholestatic liver injury. These adaptations may minimize the retention of bile salts in the liver and thus attenuate liver injury. Both transcriptional and post-transcriptional changes occur after bile duct ligation in the rat, resulting in down-regulation of the sodium taurocholate cotransporting polypeptide (Ntcp) and organic anion transporting polypeptide (Oatp2) at the sinusoidal membrane of the hepatocyte and the apical sodium-dependent bile salt transporter (Abst) in ileum and renal proximal tubule. In contrast, the canalicular bile salt export pump (Bsep), while diminished, continues to be expressed, even though there is complete bile duct obstruction. The multidrug resistance associated protein 2 (Mrp2) at the apical membrane of the hepatocyte and proximal tubule are down- and up-regulated respectively[1]. In contrast, other members of the Mrp family, Mrp3 and Mrp4, are significantly up-regulated at the sinusoidal membrane of hepatocytes but remain unchanged (Mrp3) or are post-transcriptionally down-regulated in rat kidney (Mrp4)[2].

Many of these adaptive responses are transcriptionally regulated by nuclear receptors, although the role of these nuclear receptors in cholestatic liver injury is less clear. Recent studies indicate that the Mrp2 promoter contains a retinoic acid alpha:retinoid X receptor alpha (RARα:RXRα) cis element as well as response elements for the constitutive androstane receptor (CAR), pregnane X receptor (PXR) and the farnesoid X receptor (FXR)[3]. In addition cytokines (IL-1β) can suppress Mrp2 promoter induction *in vitro*[4] and reduce RXRα nuclear protein levels[5]. Common bile duct ligation (CBDL) in the rat down-regulates liver Mrp2 RNA and protein in association with a loss of RARα and RXRα nuclear protein and diminished RNA expression. Binding of RARα:RXRα to the Mrp2 promoter is also diminished. In contrast, renal Mrp2 protein is up-regulated, RNA is unchanged and there is no change in renal RARα and RXRα nuclear protein or RNA. These studies indicate that CBDL induced cholestasis leads to differences in expression of the same ABC transporters in liver and kidney, and that these differences may relate to organ-specific effects of ligand mediated nuclear receptor regulation of gene expression. Preservation of Mrp2 expression in kidney may permit urinary excretion of toxic organic anions and xenobiotics when biliary excretion is impaired. Renal Mrp4 may also play an important role in renal excretion of cyclic nucleotides, nucleoside analogues and xenobiotics[2,6].

Recent studies also suggest that Mrp3 up-regulation can be induced by both cytokines and bile acids. CBDL in wild-type (WT) mice manifest significantly less histological necrosis, higher serum bile acids and lower hepatic bile acids than tissue necrosis factor receptor 1 (TnfrI)–/– mice in which the TNF receptor has been deleted[7]. CBDL up-regulates both Lrh-1 and Mrp3 in WT mice, a response that is blunted in TnfrI–/–, mice. Both mouse and human Mrp3/MRP3 promoters appear to be regulated by Lrh1/CPF. Thus Mrp3 expression is up-regulated by cytokines and bile acids and is hepatoprotective in obstructive cholestasis.

Other recent studies indicate that Mrp3 expression may be normally suppressed by RARα and or RXRα and that loss of these nuclear receptors during obstructive cholestasis may contribute to the up-regulation of MRP3/Mrp3 (Chen et al., submitted). This conclusion is supported by siRNA studies in which small RNA interference was used to suppress endogenous RARα in HepG2 cells. MRP3 promoter activity was significantly increased. In contrast co-transfection of RARα and RXRα and their respective ligands inhibited MRP3 promoter activity, an effect abolished by mutations in a DR2 RXRα:RARα like response element. The specificity of these effects was confirmed by electrophoretic mobility shift assays and supershift assays. Binding of these nuclear receptors to this DR2 element was significantly reduced in rat liver following common bile duct ligation.

Thus liver Mrp2 and MRP3/Mrp3 appear to be reciprocally down- and up-regulated respectively in cholestasis, in part by similar mechanisms, involving the loss of binding of RXRα:RARα nuclear receptors. Therapeutic manipulation of nuclear receptor-mediated expression of Mrps in liver and kidney could lead to new treatments for cholestatic liver disease.

References

1. Trauner M, Boyer JL. Bile salt transporters: molecular characterization, function and regulation. Physiol Rev. 2003;83:633–71.
2. Denk GU, Soroka CJ, Takeyama Y, Chen WS, Schuetz JD, Boyer JL. Multidrug resistance-associated protein 4 is up-regulated in liver but down-regulated in kidney in obstructive cholestasis in the rat. J Hepatol. 2004;40:585–91.
3. Kast HR, Goodwin B, Tarr PT et al. Regulation of multidrug resistance-associated protein 2 (ABCC2) by the nuclear receptors pregnane X receptor, farnesoid X-activated receptor, and constitutive androstane receptor. J Biol Chem. 2002;277:2908–15.
4. Denson LA, Auld KL, Schiek DS, McClure MH, Mangelsdorf DJ, Karpen SJ. Interleukin-1β suppresses retinoid transactivation of two hepatic transporter genes involved in bile formation. J Biol Chem. 2000;275:8835–43.
5. Denson LA, Bohan A, Held MA, Boyer JL. Organ-specific alterations in RARα:RXRα abundance regulate rat Mrp2 (Abcc2) expession in obstructive cholestasis. Gastroenterology. 2002;123:599–607.
6. Smeets PH, Van Aubel RA, Wouterse AC, van den Heuvel JJ, Russel FG. Contribution of multidrug resistance protein 2 (MRP2/ABCC2) to the renal excretion of p-aminohippurate

(PAH) and identification of MRP4 (ABCC4) as a novel PAH transporter. J Am Soc Nephrol. 2004;15:2828–35.
7. Bohan A, Chen WS, Denson LA, Held MA, Boyer JL. Tumor necrosis factor alpha-dependent up-regulation of Lrh-1 and Mrp3(Abcc3) reduces liver injury in obstructive cholestasis. J Biol Chem. 2003;278:36688–98.

17
Treatment of primary biliary cirrhosis: current standards

R. POUPON, C. CORPECHOT, F. CARRAT, Y. CHRÉTIEN and
R. E. POUPON

INTRODUCTION

Over the past two decades significant progress has been achieved in the management and specific treatment of primary biliary cirrhosis (PBC). The efficacy of liver transplantation was demonstrated about 15 years ago[1]. The procedure is now routinely used for end-stage disease all over the world. As far as medical therapy is concerned, two major advances have been accomplished: first ursodeoxycholic acid (UDCA) as a therapeutic agent for early-stage disease; second, the demonstration that the combination of UDCA and budesonide or prednisone is superior to UDCA alone and far better than corticosteroids alone in the short-term treatment of early-stage PBC.

This short chapter will focus on these two current aspects of the specific treatment of PBC with the aim of delineating the place and magnitude of the effects of these therapeutic options in PBC.

BACKGROUND

Controlled trials of sufficient size, duration and power to detect an effect on histological progression or survival must be carried out to demonstrate unequivocally the impact of a therapeutic strategy. In PBC there is great difficulty in following this rule, for at least the following reasons. PBC is a rare disease, the prevalence being 0.4–0.8/1000 women aged over 45 years. In the vast majority of the patients its natural course is very long, from 10 to 20 years. Recently we became aware of the heterogeneity of PBC in terms of clinical expression, severity, pathophysiology, and response to drugs; 10–15% of patients either simultaneously or successively present typical features of both PBC and autoimmune hepatitis with flares of transaminases, 'hepatic episodes' which may suddenly precipitate the patient towards end-stage disease. Severity is equally highly variable. Some patients remains asymptomatic for up to 20 years while others present with subacute disease characterized by rapid disappearance of intrahepatic bile duct, severe pruritus and frank cholestasis[2,3]. The pathophysiology of cholestasis differs in early stages compared to late stages. In early stages, cholestasis is assumed to be mainly mediated by cytokines, while in late stages, cholestasis is thought to be mainly mediated by loss of the interlobular bile ducts. Statistically, there is a significant and inverse relationship between the number of intact interlobular bile ducts and the importance of fibrosis and degree of parenchyma remodelling[4]. In some cases this is not true. Severe bile duct paucity characterized the so-called preductopenic variant of PBC, while vascular changes and portal hypertension predominate in another subset of patients[1,2]. The variability of response to drugs is illustrated in numerous past reports. Experience with methotrexate is typically representative of this paradigm[5]. Kaplan and Knox showed that low-dose weekly methotrexate in selected patients could induce marked improvement in liver biochemistries as well as in liver histology which translated into long-term stabilization of the disease[6]. However, when this drug was assessed in patients enrolled in controlled trials no such benefit could be demonstrated[6–9]. Eventually, long-term trials need important financial effort from pharmaceutical companies, which so far remain reluctant to commit in the way of a tiny market. The case of UDCA trials may serve to illustrate all these obstacles. Having defined the key question, the power of a trial depends on the number of patients required as a function of the expected magnitude of the effect, the α and β risks. In our combined analysis the individual data of the French, Mayo and Canadian trials were pooled[10–12]. The estimated survival of these patients was 95% after 2 years and 85% after 4 years of follow-up. Assuming an expected reduced risk of dying or of being transplanted of 50%, an α risk $<5\%$ and a β risk of 20%, 2500 patients should have been included to achieve such an effect in a trial of 2 years duration. Further, approximately 500 patients should have been required in a 4-year trial. In the three above-mentioned trials the planned follow-up was 2 years. However, after a 2-year double-blind period, patients having received placebo were offered UDCA for an additional 2-year period, thus allowing a comparison of survival free of liver transplantation of two arms, UDCA vs placebo + UDCA for 4 years in a total of 548 patients. Plausible statistical conditions allowing detection of a possible effect on survival were thus achieved. It should be noted that meta-analyses which fuelled the controversy regarding UDCA and PBC were carried out on less than 1300 patients followed in very short-term trials[13,14].

In the combined analysis[10] survival free of liver transplantation was significantly improved in patients treated with UDCA compared with patients originally assigned to placebo ($p<0.001$; relative risk 1.9; 95% confidence interval 1.3–2.8). Subgroup analysis showed that this results from the beneficial effect of UDCA in medium- and high-risk groups (bilirubin level >1.4 mg/dl) and histological stage IV subgroup. The approval of UDCA for PBC by the FDA is based on the results of this study.

Two other drugs, namely azathioprine and cyclosporin[15,16], have been shown to have some efficacy in PBC. In the European azathioprine trial 248 patients were enrolled and followed for up to 12 years; the 5-year mortality was about

55%. In the European cyclosporin trial 349 patients were enrolled and followed for up to 6 years; the 5-year mortality was about 30%. Assuming a decreased risk of mortality or transplantation of 50%, an α risk < 5% and a β risk of 20% these two trials met the conditions required to detect a possible effect of the drugs. The two drugs were shown to have a marginal but significant effect on survival after correcting for imbalance at entry into the trials for prognostic variables.

In short, among all the drugs assessed, only UDCA, azathioprine and cyclosporin have been shown to be effective; the great advantage of UDCA being not only its better effacy but also its lack of toxicity.

LONG-TERM STUDIES OF UDCA FOR PBC

Because UDCA trials were of very short duration, further complementary long-term observational studies were desirable to better define the role of UDCA in the management of PBC. In a cohort of 225 patients treated with UDCA (13–15 mg/kg per day) monitored from the beginning of treatment until time of last follow-up, survival without orthotopic liver transplantation (OLT) was compared with survival predicted by the Mayo model (first 7 years), and observed 10-year survival of a standardized control cohort of the French population[17]. The observed survival without OLT of UDCA-treated patients was significantly higher ($p < 0.04$) than survival predicted by the Mayo model. The observed survival was significantly lower ($p < 0.01$) than survival predicted from the French population. The observed survival of non-cirrhotic patients was not different ($p > 0.9$) from that of the French control population, but survival of cirrhotic patients was significantly lower ($p < 0.001$). Further, the study showed that the most powerful and independent predictors of death or OLT were the presence of cirrhosis and the serum bilirubin level at the onset of treatment, suggesting that UDCA is far more effective if given in early stages of PBC.

PBC AS A MULTISTATE DISEASE

To overcome the obstacle raised by the long natural course of PBC, the multistate Markov modelling method[18] could be applied to PBC. In short, this approach consists in dissecting the course of a disease into several successive pieces or states, to compute the transition rates between them, and to model the overall progression. After checking the validation of the model by comparing observed and predicted transitions, it becomes possible to identify and quantify the impact of prognostic variables or treatment on progression. PBC represents an attractive application of this approach, since the different states of the disease (histological stage 1–4); terminal phase (defined by a serum bilirubin level > 105 μmol, ±ascites ±bleeding; death or OLT) are well defined.

UDCA impact of histological progression

This approach was used to determine the influence of UDCA treatment on histological progression by using 162 pairs of liver biopsies obtained during a 4-year period in patients enrolled in our controlled trial[19]. UDCA therapy was associated with a 500% reduction of the progression rate from early-stage disease to extensive fibrosis or cirrhosis (7% per year under UDCA vs 34% per year under placebo, $p<0.002$), but was not associated with a significant difference in regression rates (3% per year under both UDCA and placebo). At 4 years the probability of UDCA-treated patients of remaining in early stage was 76% as compared to 29% in placebo-treated patients. A controlled trial and the combined analysis of individual data from four randomized studies provided confirmatory and consistent data[20,21].

Multistate modelling for long-term survival

The multistate Markov modelling was then applied to further define the impact of UDCA on progression towards cirrhosis, death and transplantation[22]. The patient population included 262 patients who had received 13–15 mg/kg UDCA daily for a mean 8-year period (range 1–22 years). Forty-five patients developed cirrhosis, 20 underwent OLT and 16 died by censor date. The overall survival rates were 92% at 10 years and 82% at 20 years. Survival rates without OLT were 84% and 66% at 10 and 20 years respectively, which was not significantly lower than the survival rate of an age- and sex-matched control population ($p = 0.1$), but better than the survival rate predicted by the updated Mayo model ($p<0.01$, RR = 0.5). The survival rate of stage 1 and 2 patients was similar to that in the control population (RR = 8.8, $p = 5$) whereas the probability of death and OLT remained significantly increased in treated patients in late histological stages (RR = 2.2; $p<0.05$). All these date show that UDCA alone normalizes the survival rate of patients with PBC when given at early stages. However, there is a continued need for new therapeutic options in patients with advanced disease.

MARKERS OF LONG-TERM UDCA FAILURE[23]

An important issue in the management of UDCA-treated PBC patients is to find early predictors of UDCA 'suboptimal response' in order to identify patients who have progressive disease and who may need adjuvant therapies. By univariate analysis the following variables were identified as associated with both histological progression and incidence of OLT; serum bilirubin level, albumin level, alkaline phosphatase activity, alanine aminotransferase activity, platelet count, interlobular bile duct paucity, lymphocytic piecemeal necrosis severity and Mayo risk score. However, multivariate analysis indicates that serum bilirubin levels (cut-off 1 mg/dl) and lymphocytic piecemeal necrosis grade for a given histological stage predict independently both the histological progression and the incidence of OLT.

COMBINATION THERAPIES FOR PBC

There is thus a need for combination therapies in patients with early predictors of long-term progression of the disease. The combination of colchicine with UDCA failed to show major additional benefits over colchicine[24]. The combination of methotrexate with UDCA, tested in two controlled studies, detected no additional benefit from the combination therapies[6,9]. In contrast, the combination of corticosteroids (either prednisone or budesonide) and UDCA in controlled studies enrolling non-cirrhotic patients with normal bilirubin levels demonstrated that the combination is superior to UDCA alone[25–27]. In particular, the study from the Leuschner group – using budesonide 9 mg/day – showed that the combination of budesonide and UDCA provides better results not only in terms of biochemistry (enzymes) but also in terms of histology. Both liver inflammation and fibrosis improved by 25% and 57% respectively in patients receiving the combination therapy. Preliminary results from Rautiainen et al.[28] are consistent with these findings. Unfortunately, these two studies did not provide quantitative date regarding the transition rates between stages. For this reason it remains unknown whether budesonide in addition to UDCA is capable of preventing the progression of PBC from early stage to cirrhosis, particularly in patients with early predictors of long-term suboptimal response to UDCA alone.

CONCLUSION AND THERAPEUTIC PROSPECT

Significant achievements have been reached. First, UDCA when given in early stages normalizes the survival rate of patients[22]. This finding observed in French patients needs to be confirmed in other centres. If we assume the result correct, there is no need to treat early-stage patients by the combination of UDCA and corticosteroids. Second, there is sufficient evidence to accept the view that corticosteroids, especially budesonide + UDCA, are superior to UDCA alone in early-stage disease. This finding should now be confirmed in PBC patients presenting with early predictors of incomplete response to UDCA in an appropriate controlled trial.

Because of their numerous side-effects, corticosteroids are not well tolerated in the long term. Moreover budesonide is a potent corticosteroid with high first-pass hepatic extraction ratio. For this reason it may be harmful in patients with cirrhosis or compromised liver function, and thus should not be prescribed in these patients[29]. Accordingly the ability of new anti-inflammatory or immunosuppressive drugs should be assessed in these settings to allow corticosteroid sparing. A good candidate is mycophenolate; this induces a selective decrease in the number and function of T and B lymphocytes; it is more effective and less toxic than azathioprine and has a corticosteroid-sparing effect in post-transplant settings. Patients with extensive fibrosis and cirrhosis should be specifically targeted with UDCA and new adjuvant therapies, since this subset of patients still has a lower survival that an age-matched control population.

References

1. Markus BH, Dickson ER, Grambsch PM et al. Efficacy of liver transplantation in patients with primary biliary cirrhosis. N Engl J Med. 1989;320:1709-13.
2. Vleggaar FP, van Buuren HR, Zondervan PE, ten Kate FJ, Hop WC. Jaundice in noncirrhotic primary biliary cirrhosis: the premature ductopenic variant. Gut. 2001;49:276-81.
3. Poupon R. Autoimmune ovelapping syndromes. Clin Liver Dis. 2003;7:865-78.
4. Poupon R, Chazouilleres O, Balkau B, Poupon RE. Clinical and biochemical expression of the histopathological lesions of primary biliary cirrhosis. UDCA-PBC Group. J Hepatol. 1999;30:408-12.
5. Kaplan MM, Knox TA. Treatment of primary biliary cirrhosis with low-dose weekly methotrexate. Gastroenterology. 1991;101:1332-8.
6. Kaplan MM, Cheng S, Lyn Price L, Bonis PAL. A randomized controlled trial of colchicine plus ursodiol versus methotrexate plus ursodiol in primary biliary cirrhosis: ten-year results. Hepatology. 2004;39:915-23.
7. Poupon R. Trials in primary biliary cirrhosis: need for the right drugs at the right time. Hepatology. 2004;39:900-2.
8. Hendrickse MT, Rigney E, Giaffer MH et al. Low-dose methotrexate is ineffective in primary biliary cirrhosis: long-term results of a placebo-controlled trial. Gastroenterology. 1999;117:400-7.
9. Combes B, Emerson SS, Flye NL. The primary biliary cirrhosis (PBC) ursodiol (UDCA) plus methotrexate (MTX) or its placebo study (PUMPS): a multicenter randomized trial. Hepatology. 2003;38(Suppl.1):210 (abstract).
10. Poupon RE, Lindor KD, Cauch-Dudek K, Dickson ER, Poupon R, Heathcote EJ. Combined analysis of randomized controlled trials of ursodeoxycholic acid in primary biliary cirrhosis. Gastroenterology. 1997;113:884-90.
11. Heathcote EJ, Cauch-Dudek K, Walker V et al. The Canadian multicenter double-blind randomized controlled trial of ursodeoxycholic acid in primary biliary cirrhosis. Hepatology. 1994;19:1149-56.
12. Lindor KD, Dickson ER, Baldus WP et al. Ursodeoxycholic acid in the treatment of primary biliary cirrhosis. Gastroenterology. 1994;106:1284-90.
13. Goulis J, Leandro G, Burroughs AK. Randomised controlled trials of ursodeoxycholic-acid therapy for primary bilairy cirrhosis: a meta-analysis. Lancet. 1999;354:1053-60.
14. Gluud C, Christensen E. Ursodeoxycholic acid (UDCA) in primary biliary cirrhosis (PBC) – a Cochrane hepato-biliary systemic review. J Hepatol. 1999;30(Suppl. 1):83.
15. Christensen E, Neuberger J, Crowe JP et al. Beneficial effect of azathioprine and prediction of prognosis in primary biliary cirrhosis. Final results of an international trial. Gastroenterology. 1985;89:1084-91.
16. Lombard M, Portmann B, Neuberger J et al. Cyclosporin A treatment in primary biliary cirrhosis: results of a long-term placebo controlled trial. Gastroenterology. 1993;104:519-26.
17. Poupon RE, Bonnand A-M, Chrétien Y, Poupon R and the UDCA-PBC Study Group. Ten-year survival in ursodeoxycholic acid-treated patients with primary biliary cirrhosis. Hepatology. 1999;29:1668-71.
18. Gentleman RC, Lawless JF, Lindsey JC, Yan P. Multi-state Markov models for analysing incomplete disease history data with illustrations for HIV disease. Stat Med. 1994;13:805-21.
19. Corpechot C, Carrat F, Bonnand A-M, Poupon RE, Poupon R. The effect of ursodeoxycholic acid therapy on liver fibrosis progression in primary biliary cirrhosis. Hepatology. 2000;32:1196-9.
20. Parés A, Caballeria L, Rodés J et al. Long-term effects of ursodeoxycholic acid in primary biliary cirrhosis: results of a double-blind controlled multicentric trial. J Hepatol. 2000;32:561-6.
21. Poupon RE, Lindor KD, Parès A, Chazouilleres O, Poupon R, Heathcote EJ. Combined analysis of the effect of treatment with ursodeoxycholic acidon histologic progression in primary biliary cirrhosis. J Hepatol. 2003;39:12-16.
22. Corpechot C, Carrat F, Bahr A, Chrétien Y, Poupon RE, Poupon R. The effect of ursodeoxycholic acid therapy on the natural course of primary biliary cirrhosis. Gastroenterology. 2005;128:297-303.

23. Corpechot C, Carrat F, Poupon R, Poupon RE. Primary biliary cirrhosis: incidence and predictive factors of cirrhosis development in ursodiol-treated patients. Gastroenterology. 2002;122:652–8.
24. Poupon R, Poupon RE. Treatment of primary biliary cirrhosis. Baillières Clin Gastroenterol. 2000;14:615–27.
25. Leuschner M, Gültdütuna S, You T, Hübner K, Bhatti S, Leuschner U. Ursodeoxycholic acid and prednisolone versus ursodeoxycholic acid and placebo in the treatment of early stages of primary biliary cirrhosis. J Hepatol. 1996;25:49–57.
26. Leuschner M, Maier K-M, Schlichting J et al. Oral budesonide and ursodeoxycholic acid for treatment of primary biliary cirrhosis: results of a prospective double-blind trial. Gastroenterology. 1999;117:918–25.
27. Wolfhagen FHJ, van Hoogstraten HJF, van Buuren HR et al. Triple therapy with ursodeoxycholic acid, prednisone, and aziathioprine in primry biliary cirrhosis: a 1-year randomized, placebo-controlled study. J Hepatol. 1998;29:736–42.
28. Rautiainen H, Karkkainen P, Karvonen AL et al. Budesonide combined with UDCA to improve liver histology in primary biliary cirrhosis: a three-year randomized trial. Hepatology. 2005;41:747–52.
29. Hempfling W, Grunhage F, Dilger K, Reichel C, Beuers U, Sauerbruch T. Pharmacokinetics and pharmacodynamic action of budesonide in early- and late-stage primary biliary cirrhosis. Hepatology. 2003;38:196–202.

18
Primary sclerosing cholangitis: neoplastic potential and chemopreventive effect of ursodeoxycholic acid

A. STIEHL and D. ROST

CLINICS

Primary sclerosing cholangitis (PSC) is chraracterized by progressive fibrosing inflammation of the bile ducts leading to cholestasis and finally to cirrhosis of the liver[1-3]. The disease is diagnosed by endoscopic retrograde cholangiography which shows the typical pearl-like picture with multiple bile duct stenoses. Alternatively, MRC (magnetic resonance cholangiography) detects PSC with a specificity and sensitivity of approximately 90%. Unspecific symptoms are fatigue and pruritus[1-3]. The disease is frequently associated with ulcerative colitis[1-4]. Of the laboratory tests alkaline phosphatase (AP) and gamma-glutamyltransferase (γ-GT) are more markedly elevated than serum transaminases. Serum bilirubin increases only in advanced stages of the disease. A problem represents the increased incidence of cholangiocarcinoma and colonic carcinomas and, according to a recent study, also pancreatic carcinomas[5].

TREATMENT

In all studies with sufficient dose, ursodeoxycholic acid (UDCA) led to significant improvement of AP, γ-GT, alanine aminotransferase (ALT), aspartate aminotransferase (AST) and in part also of serum bilirubin[6-10]. Recent data indicate that high doses of UDCA (20 mg/kg) lead to significant improvement of liver histology, whereas lower doses are less effective[9]. The efficacy of high-dose UDCA has recently been confirmed[10]. Such high doses may be needed, since in patients with cholestasis the absorption of UDCA may be reduced[11]. In the majority of patients the optimal dose[12] is between 22 and 25 mg/kg. Treatment of PSC patients with immunosuppressive, anti-inflammatory or antifibrotic agents was not very successful. Patients with an overlap syndrome with autoimmune hepatitis need additional immunosuppressive treatment with corticosteroids and/or azathioprine.

A problem in the treatment of patients with PSC is the development of dominant stenoses which occlude the major bile ducts, which cannot be expected to be treated efficiently by medical treatment[13] and which need endoscopic intervention[13–20]. When dominant stenoses of the larger bile ducts are detected by endoscopic retrograde cholangiopancreatography (ERCP) early endoscopic intervention with dilation of the duct is mandatory. In most cases a single dilation is not sufficient, and repeated dilations are necessary until the duct remains open[13,20]. Intermittent stenting also has been used[13–20] but the stents tend to occlude early due to the inflammatory material shed from the bile ducts. Moreover, in a controlled study, additional stenting was of no benefit in patients undergoing balloon dilation[18]. Since occlusion of the stent leads to bacterial infection of the proximal biliary tree stents in general should be removed or replaced early, i.e. within 2 weeks. In our hands dilation is by far the more effective form of endoscopic treatment.

It seems very important that all endoscopic procedures are performed under antibiotic prophylaxis, since bacterial cholangitis is a frequent complication of endoscopic procedures[21]. It is obvious that UDCA will have little or no effect on liver histology when dominant stenoses are present and are not treated by endoscopic means.

BILE DUCT CARCINOMA

An unresolved problem in the treatment of patients with PSC is the development of bile duct carcinomas[1–3,5]. Until now it is been very difficult to detect cholangiocarcinomas at an early stage. Brush-border cytology of dominant strictures is not sufficiently sensitive[22]. Tumour markers CEA and CA 19-9 are neither sensitive nor specific[23]. The imaging methods (computed tomography and nuclear magnetic resonance) do not allow the detection of early carcinomas, and the results with positron emission tomography[24] need further confirmation in larger trials. When the carcinoma has developed the prognosis in general is very poor.

In a large multicentre study from Sweden, in which 305 PSC patients were followed over a median follow-up time of 63 months, a bile duct carcinoma was observed in 8% of patients and 44% of these were asymptomatic at the time of diagnosis of PSC[3]. In 37% of the patients with bile duct carcinoma this diagnosis was made within 1 year after detection of PSC and, as a consequence, it seems possible that the patients already had a bile duct carcinoma when the PSC was recognized. No factors were found which would allow the identification of patients who will later develop a bile duct carcinoma.

A bile duct carcinoma rate of 8%[3] appears much lower than that observed by others[25]. Of interest is the fact that in the Swedish study overall only 8% of patients developed a cholangiocarcinoma, and in patients with endstage disease who were considered for transplantation, 30% had bile duct carcinomas[3]. These data explain why the figures on the incidence supplied by transplantation centres are always much higher than the corresponding figures from prospective studies of gastroenterology units. Very high rates of bile duct carcinomas have repeatedly been reported in studies in transplantation centres[3,25], and it appears that they reflect very select patient groups.

In a controlled study 0/52 of the patients with PSC on UDCA developed a bile duct carcinoma in comparison to 3/53 patients in the placebo group[8]. In a prospective study over 15 years, of 106 patients treated with UDCA only three developed a bile duct carcinoma[20]. In a recent study of 225 patients listed for liver transplantation hepatobiliary malignancies developed in 20% of patients, and UDCA treatment was associated with a significantly decreased incidence of hepatobiliary cancer[26]. It seems possible that the reduced inflammation around the bile ducts observed after UDCA treatment[6,7,9] may reduce the incidence of bile duct carcinomas

COLONIC CARCINOMA

Colorectal carcinoma occurs more frequently in patients with chronic inflammatory bowel disease than in the normal population. Risk factors are involvement of the whole colon and long duration of the disease. Recently it has been shown that PSC represents an independent risk factor for the development of colonic carcinoma[27]. In a study in which 40 patients with PSC and colitis were matched with 40 patients of the same age, with comparable colitis and comparable duration of the disease, the absolute cumulative risk of developing colorectal dysplasia or carcinoma in the patients with PSC was almost five times higher than in the patients without PSC. The study also indicates that patients with PSC and colitis who develop colonic dysplasia or carcinoma are at a high risk of developing cholangiocarcinoma. It is evident that patients with PSC and colitis need colonoscopic surveillance at short intervals.

In animal experiment bile acids have cocarcinogenic effects in the development of colonic adenocarcinomas. UDCA has been shown to prevent this cocarcinogenic effect[28] and as a consequence the effect of UDCA on the incidence of colonic dysplasias, adenomatous polyps and carcinomas is if great interest. After oral administration of UDCA to patients with ileostomy at the end of the ileum, of a single oral dose of 500 mg UDCA, 59% was excreted from the ileostomy (Figure 1)[29]. Thus, due to its poor absorption in the upper small intestine, substantial amounts of UDCA enter the colon where it is bacterially degraded.

In two placebo-controlled trials on the effect of UDCA on liver disease in PSC the incidence of dysplasias and carcinomas has been evaluated (Figure 2). In the first study, comprising 59 patients, the incidence of dysplasias and carcinomas in the UDCA group was 32% and in the control group it was 72%[30], the difference being significant. In a second placebo-controlled study with 52 patients, of 29 patients in the UDCA group only 10% had dysplasias or carcinomas whereas in the placebo group, of 23 patients 35% developed dysplasias or carcinomas[31] ($p < 0.05$). Thus, in two controlled trials in patients with ulcerative colitis and PSC, UDCA significantly reduced the incidence of colonic dysplasias and carcinomas.

Ileal bile acids, %

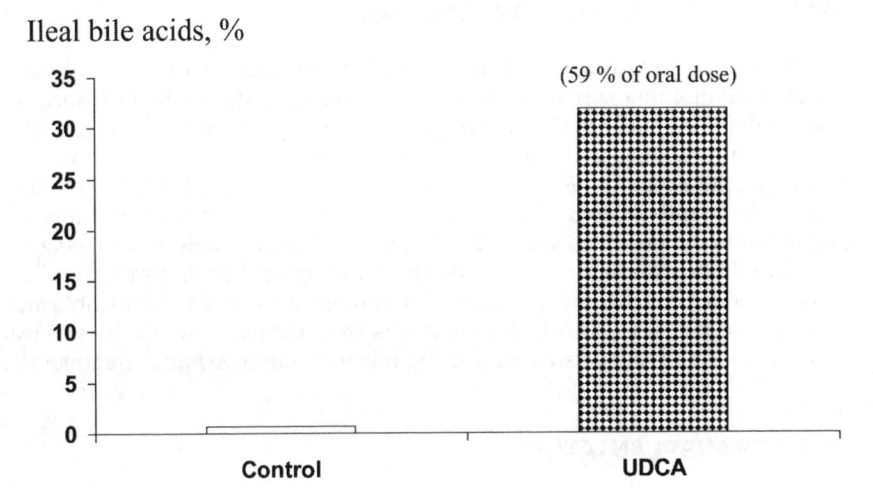

Figure 1 Ileal excretion of bile acids in patients with ileostomy. Effect of ursodeoxycholic acid administration on ileal bile acid composition and excretion. The data indicate that after a single oral dose of 500 mg of ursodeoxycholic acid, ursodeoxycholic acid represents 31.8% of ileal bile acids and 59% of the oral dose is excreted from the end of the ileum and will enter the colon (from ref. 29)

Colonic dysplasias and carcinomas, %

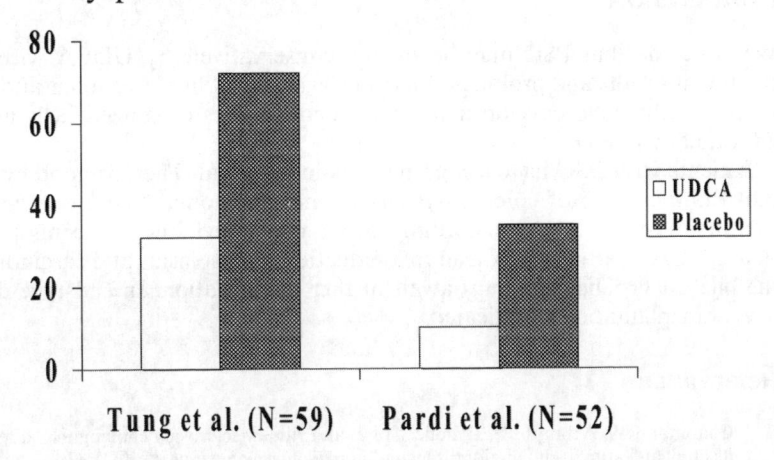

Figure 2 Effect of ursodeoxycholic acid treatment on dysplasias and carcinomas in patients with PSC and colitis (from refs 30 and 31). Ursodeoxycholic acid treatment significantly reduced the frequency of colonic dysplasias and carcinomas

EFFECT OF TREATMENT ON SURVIVAL

PSC is a progressive disease and survival of such patients is reduced. Survival is better in asymptomatic patients than in symptomatic patients. In a prospective non-randomized study performed in our institution, in which 65 patients were treated with UDCA and, whenever necessary, by additional endoscopic dilations, the actuarial Kaplan–Meier estimate of survival after treatment with UDCA and dilation of major duct stenoses was significantly improved compared to the predicted survival ($p < 0.001$)[13]. The data were confirmed after extension of this study to 106 patients and prolongation for up to 13 years[20].

The need for endoscopic treatment of dominant stenoses has been confirmed in a multicentre study in which 63 patients were included. Actuarial survival compared with predicted survival was significantly improved after treatment[19].

LIVER TRANSPLANTATION

In endstage disease liver transplantation represents the treatment of choice. The 5-year survival rate after liver transplantation for PSC is approximately 72% (European Transplant Registry). In view of the fact that the incidence of bile duct carcinomas is much lower than the lethality after transplantation it does not appear justified to recommend prophylactic liver transplantation in precirrhotic stages of the disease in order to prevent the development of bile duct carcinomas.

CONCLUSION

We conclude that PSC may be treated conservatively by UDCA with good treatment results and prolongation of survival free of liver transplantation only when patients who develop major duct stenoses are recognized early and are additionally treated by endoscopic means.

Patients with PSC have a high neoplastic potential. There is good evidence that the incidence of colonic dysplasias and carcinomas may be reduced by treatment with UDCA. According to one controlled study it seems possible that UDCA treatment may lead to a reduction of dysplasias and carcinomas of the bile ducts. These findings await further confirmation. In endstage disease liver transplantation is indicated.

References

1. Chapman RW, Arborgh BA, Rhodes JM et al. Primary sclerosing cholangitis – a review of its clinical features, cholangiography and hepatic histology. Gut. 1980;21:870–7.
2. Wiesner RH, Grambsch PM, Dickson ER et al. Natural history, prognostic factors, and survival analysis. Hepatology. 1989;10:430–6.
3. Broome U, Olson R, Lööf L et al. Natural history and prognostic factors in 305 Swedish patients with primary sclerosing cholangitis. Gut. 1996;38:610–15.
4. Olsson R, Danielsson A, Järnebrot G et al. Prevalence of primary sclerosing cholangitis in patients with ulcerative colitis. Gastroenterology. 1991;100:1319–23.

5. Bergquist A, Ekbom A, Olsson R et al. Hepatic and extrahepatic malignancies in primary sclerosing cholangitis. J Hepatol. 2002;36:321–7.
6. Stiehl A, Walker S, Stiehl L et al. Effects of ursodeoxycholic acid on liver and bile duct disease in primary sclerosing cholangitis. A 3 year pilot study with a placebo-controlled study period. J Hepatol. 1994;20:57–64.
7. Beuers U, Spengler U, Kruis W et al. Ursodeoxycholic acid for treatment of primary sclerosing cholangitis: a placebo controlled trial. Hepatology. 1992;16:707–14.
8. Lindor KD and the Mayo PSC/UDCA Study Group. Ursodiol for the treatment of primary sclerosing cholangitis. N Engl J Med. 1997; 336:691–5.
9. Mitchell SA, Bansi D, Hunt N et al. A preliminary trial of high dose ursodeoxycholic acid in primary sclerosing cholangitis. Gastroenterology. 2001;121:900–7.
10. Harnois DM, Angulo P, Jorgensen RA, LaRusso NF, Lindor KD. High-dose ursodeoxycholic acid as therapy for patients with primary sclerosing cholangitis. Am J Gastroenterol. 2001;96:1558–62.
11. Sauer P, Benz C, Rudolph G et al. Influence of cholestasis on absorption of ursodeoxycholic acid. Dig Dis Sci. 1999;44:817–22.
12. Rost D, Rudolph G, Kloeters-Plachky P, Stiehl A. Effect of high-dose ursodeoxycholic acid on its biliary enrichment in primary sclerosing cholangitis. Hepatology. 2004;40:693–8.
13. Stiehl A, Rudolph G, Sauer P et al. Efficacy of ursodeoxycholic acid and endoscopic dilation of major duct stenoses in primary sclerosing cholangitis. An 8-year prospective study. J Hepatol. 1997;26:560–6.
14. Grijm R, Huibregtse K, Bartelsman J et al. Therapeutic investigations in primary sclerosing cholangitis. Dig Dis Sci. 1986;31:792–8.
15. Johnson GK, Geenen JE, Venu RP, Hogan WJ. Endoscopic treatment of biliary duct strictures in sclerosing cholangitis: follow-up assessment of a new therapeutic approach. Gastrointest Endosc. 1987;33:9–12.
16. Lee JG, Schutz SM, England RE, Leung JW, Cotton PB. Endoscopic therapy of sclerosing cholangitis. Hepatology. 1995;21:661–7.
17. van Milligen AWM, van Bracht J, Rauws EAJ et al. Endoscopic stent therapy for dominant extrahepatic bile duct strictures in primary sclerosing cholangitis. Gastrointest Endosc. 1006;44:293–9.
18. Kaya M, Petersen BT, Angulo P et al. Balloon dilatation compared to stenting of dominant strictures in primary sclerosing cholangitis. Am J Gastroenterol. 2001;96:1059–66.
19. Baluyut AR, Sherman S, Lehman GA, Hoen H, Chalasani N. Impact of endoscopic therapy on the survival of patients with primary sclerosing cholangitis. Gastrointest Endosc. 2001;53:308–12.
20. Stiehl A, Rudolph G, Klöters-Plachky P et al. Development of bile duct stenoses in patients with primary sclerosing cholangitis treated with ursodeoxycholic acid. Outcome after endoscopic treatment. J Hepatol. 2002;36:151–6.
21. Olsson R, Björnsson E, Bäckman L et al. Bile duct bacterial isolates in primary sclerosing cholangitis: a study of explanted livers. J Hepatol. 1998;28:426–32.
22. Ponsioen C IJ, Vrouenraets SME, van Milligen AWM et al. Value of brush border cytology for dominant strictures in primary sclerosing cholangitis. Endoscopy. 1999;31:305–9.
23. Hultcrantz R, Olsson R, Danielsson A et al. A three year prospective study on serum tumor markers used for detecting cholangiocarcinoma in patients with primary sclerosing cholangitis. J Hepatol. 1999;30:669–73.
24. Keiding S, Rasmussen HH, Gee A et al. Detection of cholangiocarcinoma in primary sclerosing cholangitis by positron emission tomography. Hepatology. 1998;28:700–6.
25. Nashan B, Schlitt HJ, Tusch G et al. Biliary malignancies in primary sclerosing cholangitis: timing of liver transplantation. Hepatology. 1996;23:1105–11.
26. Brandsaeter B, Isoniemi H, Broome U et al. Liver transplantation for primary sclerosing cholangitis ; predictors and consequences of hepatobiliary malignancy. J Hepatol. 2004;40: 815–22.
27. Broome U, Löfberg R, Veress B, Erikson LS: Primary sclerosing cholangitis and ulcerative colitis: evidence for increased neoplastic potential. Hepatology. 1995;22:1404–8.
28. Earnest DL, Holubec H, Wali RK et al. Chemoprevention of azomethane-induced colonic carcinogenesis by supplemental dietary ursodeoxycholic acid. Cancer Res. 1994;54:5071–4.

29. Stiehl A, Raedsch R, Rudolph G. Ileal excretion of bile acids: comparison with biliary bile composition and effect of ursodeoxycholic acid treatment. Gastroenterology. 1988;94:1201–6.
30. Tung BY, Emond MJ, Haggitt RC et al. Ursodiol use is associated with lower prevalence of colonic neoplasia in patients with ulcerative colitis and primary sclerosing cholangitis. Ann Intern Med. 2001;134:89–95.
31. Pardi DS, Loftus EV, Kremers WK et al. Ursodeoxycholic acid as a chemoprotective agent in patients with ulcerative colitis and primary sclerosing cholangitis. Gastroenterology. 2003;124:889–93.

19
The pruritus of cholestasis: treatment options

N. V. BERGASA

INTRODUCTION

One of the most common manifestations of cholestasis is pruritus. The aetiology of the pruritus of cholestasis is unknown[1]. It is inferred that the pruritus results from the accumulation in plasma of substances that are excreted in bile normally and, as a result of cholestasis, accumulate in plasma; however, the nature of the substances, referred to as pruritogen(s), is unknown. The reason not all patients with cholestasis report pruritus is unknown but it tends to suggest that there is a subject-dependent mechanism (i.e. ability to perceive pruritus).

The idea that the pruritus of cholestasis arises from the stimulation of 'itch fibres' at the level of the skin by 'toxic compounds' that accumulate in tissues as a result of cholestasis is seductive and plausible; at present, however, there are no scientific data to demonstrate that this occurs. It is also possible that continuous pruritogenic stimuli exert changes in human perception resulting in the perception of non-pruritogenic stimuli as pruritogenic. In this context there is some experimental evidence to suggest that this change occurs in patients with chronic pruritus[2].

Bile acids have been considered to be pruritogenic substances in cholestasis, as they accumulate in plasma and tissues in cholestasis and can result in pruritus when injected into the skin of normal volunteers[3]. This experimental design, however, does not mimic the conditions of a cholestatic milieu in human beings; accordingly, the results of those studies are difficult to interpret in the context of the aetiology of the pruritus of cholestasis.

There is evidence to suggest that in cholestasis there is increased opioidergic neurotransmission, summarized as follows: (a) patients with cholestasis can experience symptoms and signs suggestive of an opiate withdrawal-like reaction when administered opiate antagonists[4], (b) a stereospecific naloxone reversible state of antinociception (analgesic) can be displayed by rats with cholestasis secondary to bile duct resection[5], and (c) there is down-regulation of mu opioid receptors in rats with cholestasis secondary to bile duct resection[6]. Increased opioidergic neurotransmission results in pruritus, considered to be pruritus of central origin. The best example of this occurrence is the pruritus that results from the intrathecal administration of morphine[7-9], an alkaloid that exerts its effect by binding to mu opioid receptors. This type of pruritus can be effectively treated by opiate antagonists[9], supporting the idea that it is opioid receptor-mediated. Patients with cholestasis can experience an amelioration of their pruritus by the administration of opiate antagonists[4,10-13]. Accordingly, the increased opioidergic tone of cholestasis may contribute to the pruritus[14]. A central mechanism has been proposed[14]; however, a peripheral component has not been excluded. The reasons for increased opioidergic neurotransmission in cholestasis are unknown, but data from an animal model[15] and from patients with cholestasis[4,16] suggest that there may be increased availability of opioid peptides (e.g. met-enkephalin and leu-enkephalin) in cholestasis; however, these two peptides have not been directly implicated in the generation of pruritus. At present it can be safely stated that, although an opioid-mediated mechanism appears to be involved in the pruritus of cholestasis, the details that lead to the perception of pruritus in liver disease are unknown but could include the formation of complex substances with affinity for opioid receptors and neurophysiological changes that result from chronic pruritus[2].

One of the obstacles in the study of pruritus is the fact that it is a sensation; accordingly, it cannot be directly quantitated. Scratching, however, is the behaviour that results from pruritus, and it can be directly quantitated. A system that records scratching activity was developed to incorporate objective methodology in studies of the pruritus of cholestasis, allowing for the collection of objective data[17].

The traditional management of the pruritus of cholestasis has been to remove the pruritogenic substance(s) from the circulation; however, this has been a difficult task as the substance(s) is unknown. Over the past 15 years the use of opiate antagonists to treat the pruritus of cholestasis has been incorporated into clinical practice, based on data from behavioural studies (i.e. measurement of scratching activity). Recently, anecdotal reports that concern the use of drugs that may alter the perception of pruritus have been published. This review will focus on the most commonly used interventions to treat the pruritus of cholestasis. A section on evolving therapy will be provided. In Table 1 details on selected therapies are listed.

TREATMENT OF THE PRURITUS OF CHOLESTASIS

Removal of pruritogenic substances

Cholestyramine is widely used to treat the pruritus of cholestasis[18]; it is a non-absorbable resin approved for the treatment of hypercholesterolaemia. Its use to treat pruritus is based on the assumption that the drug will increase the faecal excretion of the pruritogens. Interestingly, cholestyramine intake is associated with release of cholecystokinin, an endogenous antiopiate. Patients with cholestasis and pruritus may respond to cholestyramine. Sometimes there is a transient response, followed by resistance to the drug.

Table 1 Selected treatments for the pruritus of cholestasis

Medication	Potential side-effects	Dose/mode of administration/frequency	Methodology
Cholestyramine	Bloating, constipation, malabsorption of nutrients	4 g p.o. before and after breakfast; increase by 4 g at other meal times not to exceed 16 g/day	Subjective
Rifampicin	Hepatotoxicity	150 mg p.o./b.i.d. if serum bilirubin >3 mg/dl; 150 mg p.o/t.i.d. if serum bilirubin <3	Subjective
Naloxone	Opiate withdrawal-like syndrome	0.2 µg/kg/min/intravenous continuous infusions preceded by 0.4 mg intravenous bolus	Objective (i.e. behavioural studies on scratching activity)
Naltrexone	Opiate withdrawal-like syndrome, potential hepatotoxicity	25 mg p.o./b.i.d. on day 1 followed by 50 mg p.o. daily	Objective (i.e. behavioural studies on scratching activity)

Invasive procedures including plasmapheresis[19] and more recently extracorporeal albumin dialysis, have been used[20]. A substantial placebo effect is expected to involve the response to these procedures but, by their nature, designs of properly controlled trials are difficult. Their use appears justified in some clinical situations.

Enzyme inducers

Rifampicin has been widely used since the 1980s to treat the pruritus of cholestasis[21]. The mechanism of action supporting its antipruritic effect is not known. As with other treatment, not all patients with cholestasis and pruritus respond to rifampicin. In those who do, one of the concerns is hepatotoxicity[22,23], which demands careful follow-up of liver profile in patients taking this treatment.

Opiate antagonists

Naloxone, naltrexone and nalmefene have been used in the treatment of the pruritus of cholestasis[4,10–13], based on the idea that the pruritus is mediated, at least in part, but endogenous opioids. As the administration of opiate antagonists to patients with cholestasis may be associated with an opiate withdrawal-like reaction, the initiation of therapy in low doses is preferred. One option is to admit patients to the hospital for intravenous infusions of naloxone (0.002 µg/kg body weight) to be increased gradually to reach a dose of 0.2–0.8 µg/kg body weight; at this dose pruritus tends to be relieved in many patients[24,25]. The introduction of oral naltrexone following intravenous infusions of naloxone can ameliorate the development of the opiate withdrawal-like syndrome.

EVOLVING THERAPIES FOR THE PRURITUS OF CHOLESTASIS (TABLE 2)

Changes in threshold to experience nociception

Dronabinol

Dronabinol is a sesame oil preparation of delta-9-tetrahydrocannabinol, the psychoactive compound extracted from *Cannabis sative* L. (marijuana). The administration of dronabinol (Marinol) at a dose of 5 mg at bedtime to three patients with cholestasis and intractable pruritus was reported to be associated with amelioration of that symptom[26]. One consideration in interpreting the original report[27] was an increased threshold to noxious stimuli, i.e. pruritus, due to enhanced cannabinoid neurotransmission by the drug.

Table 2 Evolving therapies for the pruritus of cholestasis

Medication	Dose/mode of administration/frequency	Type of study	Methodology
Dronabinol	5 mg p.o. at bedtime	Case report	Subjective
Gabapentin	100 mg p.o. daily for first 3 days, to be increased by 300 mg every 3 days. Maximun dose used was 2400 mg per day	Double-blind, randomized, placebo controlled	Objective (i.e. behavioural study)
Sertraline	75 mg per day	Retrospective review	Subjective

Gabapentin

Gabapentin is a drug reported to change the perception of pain in animals[28,29]. In addition it is used in the treatment of neuropathy secondary to diabetes mellitus[30]; furthermore, it was reported to be effective in the treatment of radiobrachial pruritus[31]. A randomized controlled study of gabapentin for the pruritus of cholestasis that included behavioural methodology revealed that gabapentin was as good as placebo in the treatment of the pruritus of cholestasis; some patients, however, preferred gabapentin to placebo in the open phase of the trial[32].

Antidepressants

Sertraline

A small group of patients with primary biliary cirrhosis followed in a clinical trial for their disease reported improvement of the pruritus with the ingestion of sertraline[33]. Any relationship between the reported effect of sertraline on pruritus and on mood is unknown at present.

Bright-light therapy directed towards the eyes

Based on the observation that scratching behaviour can have a 24-h rhythm and that 24-h rhythms are considered to be centrally regulated by light via retinothalamic pathways[34], the effect of light therapy, as used in the treatment of seasonal affective disorder, was studied. Light, at a dose of 10 000 lux, indirectly reflected towards the eyes, at exposures of up to 60 min in the morning and in the evening, were associated with a decrease in the sensation of pruritus, a modest decrease in scratching behaviour and a significant decrease in the variability of scratching at 8 weeks of treatment[35]. The decrease in the variability of scratching is a reflection of outbursts of 'pruritus' and may suggest that light therapy may be useful in conjunction with other medications. Bright-light therapy can be associated with side-effects including episodes of mania.

Lessons from behavioural studies in primates

The administration of morphine intrathecally to monkeys is associated with scratching behaviour[36]. It is inferred that the animal scratches in response to the itch sensation. This behaviour can be effectively prevented and treated by/with opiate antagonists, suggesting it is opioid-receptor-mediated. Human experience supports that interpretation. The scratching produced by the central administration of morphine to monkeys was prevented by U-50488H, a compound that stimulates kappa receptors[37]. Butorphanol is a mixed mu/kappa agonist[38]. Butorphanol in inhaler form was used to treat a patient with chronic pruritus secondary to chronic hepatitis C. The patient associated the use of intranasal butorphanol (1 mg per sniff) with amelioration of pruritus. Her excoriations healed. The dose used was 1 mg twice a day (N.V. Bergasa, unpublished). This preliminary observation goes along with the behavioural studies done in monkeys and indeed, support the idea that the stimulation of kappa receptor may be an approach to the treatment of the pruritus of cholestasis. Butorphanol treatment can be associated with sedation, and although the addiction potential is reported as low, the use of this drug to treat pruritus cannot be recommended widely until properly designed studies are conducted.

In summary, the scientific study of pruritus is a recognized need. Behavioural studies, including those conducted in animals, can provide insight into the pathogenesis of pruritus.

References

1. Bergasa NV, Jones EA. The pruritus of cholestasis: potential pathogenic and therapeutic implications of opioids. Gastroenterology. 1995;108:1582–8.
2. Schmelz M. Itch: mediators and mechanisms. J Dermatol Sci. 2002;28:91–6.
3. Kirby J, Heaton KW, Burton JL. Pruritic effect of bile salts. Br Med J. 1974;4:693–5.
4. Thornton JR, Losowsky MS. Opioid peptides and primary biliary cirrhosis. Br Med J. 1988;297:1501–4.
5. Bergasa NV, Alling DW, Vergalla J, Jones EA. Cholestasis in the male rat is associated with naloxone-reversible antinociception. J Hepatol. 1994;20:85–90.

6. Bergasa NV, Rothman RB, Vergalla J, Xu H, Swain MG, Jones EA. Central mu-opioid receptors are down-regulated in a rat model of cholestasis. J Hepatol. 1992;15:220–4.
7. Ballantyne JC, Loach AB, Carr DB. Itching after epidural and spinal opiates. Pain. 1988;33:149–60.
8. Ballantyne JC, Loach AB, Carr DB. The incidence of pruritus after epidural morphine. Anaesthesia. 1989;44:863.
9. Slappendel R, Weber EW, Benraad B, van Limbeek J, Dirksen R. Itching after intrathecal morphine. Incidence and treatment. Eur J Anaesthesiol. 2000;17:616–21.
10. Bergasa NV, Talbot TL, Alling DW et al. A controlled trial of naloxone infusions for the pruritus of chronic cholestasis. Gastroenterology. 1992;102:544–9.
11. Wolfhagen FHJ, Sternieri E, Hop WCJ, Vitale G, Bertolotti M, van Buuren HR. Oral naltrexone treatment for cholestatic pruritus: a double-blind, placebo-controlled study. Gastroenterology. 1997;113:1264–9.
12. Bergasa NV, Alling DW, Talbot TL et al. Naloxone ameliorates the pruritus of cholestasis: results of a double-blind randomized placebo-controlled trial. Ann Intern Med. 1995;123:161–7.
13. Bergasa NV, Alling DW, Talbot TL, Wells M, Jones EA. Oral nalmefene therapy reduces scratching activity due to the pruritus of cholestasis: a controlled study. J Am Acad Dermatol. 1999;41:431–4.
14. Jones EA, Bergasa NV. The pruritus of cholestasis: from bile acids to opiate agonists. Hepatology. 1990;11:884–7.
15. Swain MG, Rothman RB, Xu H, Vergalla J, Bergasa NV, Jones EA. Endogenous opioids accumulate in plasma in a rat model of acute cholestasis. Gastroenterology. 1992;103:630–5.
16. Spivey J, Jorgensen R, Gores G, Lindor K. Methionine-enkephalin concentrations correlate with stage of disease but not pruritus in patients with primary biliary cirrhosis. Am J Gastroenterol. 1994;89:2018–32.
17. Talbot TL, Schmitt JM, Bergasa NV, Jones EA, Walker EC. Application of piezo film technology for the quantitative assessment of pruritus. Biomed Instrum Technol. 1991;25:400–3.
18. Datta DV, Sherlock S. Cholestyramine for long term relief of the pruritus complicating intrahepatic cholestasis. Gastroenterology. 1966;50:323–32.
19. Ambinder EP, Cohen LB, Wolke AM et al. The clinical effectiveness and safety of chronic plasmapheresis in patients with primary biliary cirrhosis. J Clin Apher. 1985;2:219–23.
20. Schachschal G, Morgera S, Kupferling S, Neumayer HH, Lochs H, Schmidt HH. Emerging indications for MARS dialysis. Liver. 2002;22(Suppl. 2):63–8.
21. Galeazzi R. Rifampicin-induced elevation of serum bile acids in man. Dig Dis Sci. 1980;25:108–12.
22. Prince MI, Burt AD, Jones DE. Hepatitis and liver dysfunction with rifampicin therapy for pruritus in primary biliary cirrhosis. Gut. 2002;50:436–9.
23. Ghent CN, Carruthers SG. Treatment of pruritus in primary biliary cirrhosis with rifampin. Results of a double-blind, crossover, randomized trial. Gastroenterology. 1988;94:488–93.
24. Jones EA, Dekker LR. Florid opioid withdrawal-like reaction precipitated by naltrexone in a patient with chronic cholestasis. Gastroenterology. 2000;118:431–2.
25. Neuberger J, Jones EA. Liver transplantation for intractable pruritus is contraindicated before an adequate trial of opiate antagonist therapy. Eur J Gastroenterol Hepatol. 2001;13:1393–4.
26. Neff GW, O'Brien CB, Reddy KR et al. Preliminary observation with dronabinol in patients with intractable pruritus secondary to cholestatic liver disease. Am J Gastroenterol. 2002;97:2117–9.
27. Neff GW, O'Brien CB, Regev A et al. The remedy for intractable cholestatic related pruritus (ICRP): delta-9-tetrahydrocannabinol (Marinol). Hepatology. 1999;30:328A.
28. Yoon MH, Yaksh TL. The effect of intrathecal gabapentin on pain behavior and hemodynamics on the formalin test in the rat. Anesth Analg. 1999;89:434–9.
29. Gustafsson H, Flood K, Berge OG, Brodin E, Olgart L, Stiller CO. Gabapentin reverses mechanical allodynia induced by sciatic nerve ischemia and formalin-induced nociception in mice. Exp Neurol. 2003;182:427–34.
30. Backonja M, Glanzman RL. Gabapentin dosing for neuropathic pain: evidence from randomized, placebo-controlled clinical trials. Clin Ther. 2003;25:81–104.

31. Bueller HA, Bernhard JD, Dubroff LM. Gabapentin treatment for brachioradial pruritus. J Eur Acad Dermatol Venereol. 1999;13:227–8.
32. Bergasa NV, McGee M, Ginsburg I, Engler D. Gabapentin therapy for pruritus in patients with chronic liver disease (CLD): a double-blind, randomized, placebo-controlled study. Hepatology. 2004;38(Suppl. 2):296A.
33. Browning J, Combes B, Mayo MJ. Long-term efficacy of sertraline as a treatment for cholestatic pruritus in patients with primary biliary cirrhosis. Am J Gastroenterol. 2003; 98:2736–41.
34. Moore RY. Organization of mammalian circadian system. In: Chardwick DJ, Ackrill K, editors. Circadian Clocks and their Adjustments. London, Wiley, 1993:88–106.
35. Bergasa NV, Link MJ, Keogh M, Yaroslavsky G, Rosenthal RN, McGee M. Pilot study of bright-light therapy reflected toward the eyes for the pruritus of chronic liver disease. Am J Gastroenterol. 2001;96:1563–70.
36. Ko MC, Naughton NN. An experimental itch model in monkeys: characterization of intrathecal morphine-induced scratching and antinociception. Anesthesiology. 2000;92: 795–805.
37. Ko M, Lee H, Song M et al. Activation of kappa-opioid receptors inhibits pruritus evoked by subcutaneous or intrathecal administration of morphine in monkeys. J Pharmacol Exp Ther. 2003;305:173–9.
38. Walsh S, Strain E, Abreu M, Bigelow G. Enadoline, a selective kappa opioid agonist: comparison with butorphanol and hydromorphone in humans. Psychopharmacology. 2001; 157:151–62.

Section VI
Pancreas

Chair: G. ADLER and R.W. AMMANN

20
Stages and course of chronic pancreatitis

R. W. AMMANN

INTRODUCTION

Chronic pancreatitis (CP) is a chronic inflammatory disease of the pancreas that progresses eventually over several years to pancreatic 'cirrhosis' and the typical functional consequences.

The estimated incidence of CP in industrialized countries ranges between 3.5 and 10 patients per 100 000 population per year[1], compared to acute pancreatitis[2] or pancreas cancer that is ≥2 fold higher[3].

A vast and controversial literature exists on the diagnosis and management of CP. The lack of a consensus is due to several facts; in particular (a) clinical symptoms of CP are varied and non-specific, (b) early-stage CP can be suspected but definite diagnosis relies on histology; (c) no routine biopsy method such as liver biopsy is available, (d) diagnosis of late-stage CP is reliable and easy, and (e) the natural history of CP from onset to late-stage CP is poorly defined[1,4,5].

Unfortunately, in most published series no accurate data on diagnosis, classification or staging of CP are provided. Therefore, a comparison of data from different series is not really possible. A reassessment of the current approach to diagnosis and classification of CP is particularly appropriate in view of progress in imaging technology and the recent discovery of gene mutations in CP. These issues have been discussed recently in a comprehensive review[1].

This chapter is focused on: (a) course and stages of CP, (b) mechanism(s) of pain, (c) impact of aetiology on the course of CP.

COURSE AND STAGES OF CP

Chronologically, two main stages in the evolution of CP from onset of disease may be distinguished[4,5]:

1. Early-stage CP that is dominated typically by recurrent acute pancreatitis. Diagnosis and management of acute pancreatitis (±complications) are largely standardized; however, the broad clinical overlap between acute reversible (e.g. biliary) and progressive pancreatitis (e.g. alcoholic) hinders an accurate classification in the initial phase of disease. Histology, the gold standard of early-stage CP, is rarely available.

2. Late-stage CP is dominated morphologically by fibrosis, acinar atrophy, typical ductal alterations and pancreatic calcification, and clinically by steatorrhoea and/or diabetes. Diagnosis of late-stage CP is reliable, and medical (substitutional) therapy of steatorrhoea and/or diabetes is largely standardized.

Classification and staging of CP rely primarily on four major variables (Figure 1): (a) clinical profile; (b) function tests; (c) morphology (i.e. calcification, computed tomography (CT)/sonography, ERCP/MRCP, histology, if available); (d) aetiology (see below).

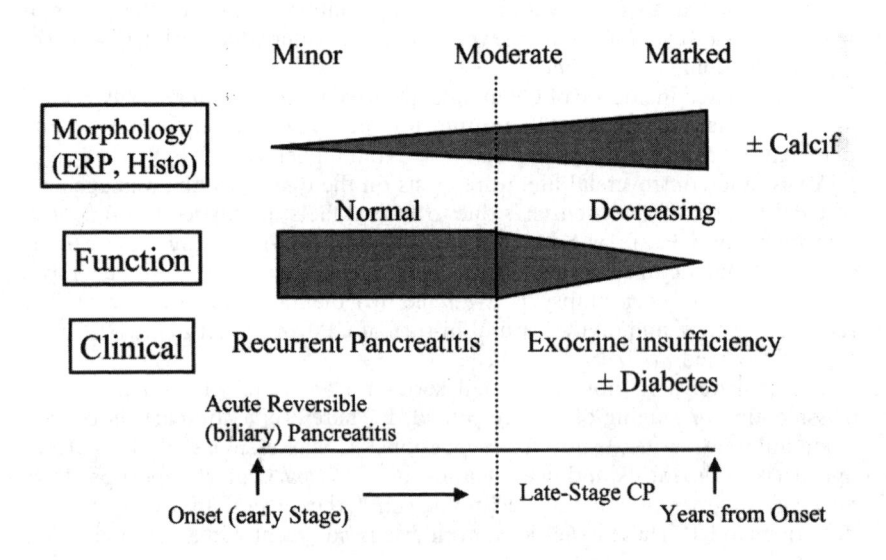

Figure 1 Scheme of the correlation of the three major variables from early- to late-stage chronic pancreatitis (CP). During evolution 2 major stages may be distinguished, namely: (a) Early-stage CP, dominated by recurrent pancreatitis and lack of exocrine insufficiency or marked morphological alteration such as calcification or major ductal alterations. The diagnostic gold standard of this stage is histology that is, however, rarely available. (b) Late-stage CP, dominated by increasing exocrine insufficiency (±diabetes) and pancreatic calcification. Diagnosis is easy and reliable by any of the clinically available methods including CT, MRCP, endoscopic ultrasound or function tests, e.g. faecal elastase 1. Of note: pancreatitis- related pain is rare or lacking in uncomplicated advanced CP (spontaneous 'burnout' !; see text)

STAGES AND COURSE OF CHRONIC PANCREATITIS

Information on the correlation of these variables from early- to late-stage CP is scarce. Especially function tests have been abandoned in many centres within the past decade. Tests of exocrine function are, however, the only reliable criterion of the acinar cell mass, and this variable is relevant both (a) for monitoring the progression of the disease process (+ diagnosis of CP) and (b) for analysing the pathomechanism(s) of pain in CP in the absence of histology[5]. Limitations of the indirect function tests such as faecal chymotrypsin or elastase in diagnosis of 'early CP' are well known, but the sensitivity of the latter tests is high in moderate/severe exocrine insufficiency that is a typical feature of advanced stages of CP[6,7].

The relation between function and histology (+calcification) has been analysed in a personal prospective series of 73 patients with alcoholic CP who had either a surgical biopsy or autopsy. Two experienced pathologists examined the series based on a defined score system. The series was subdivided into four subgroups in relation to years from onset. From early- to late-stage CP the fibrosis score (0–12) almost doubled and calcification increased about 3-fold (Figure 2)[8].

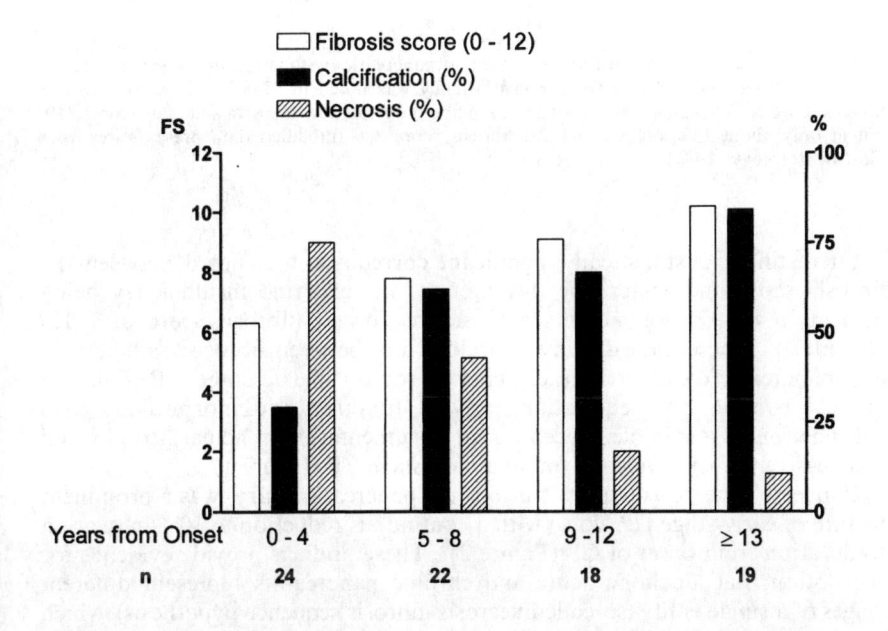

Figure 2 Correlation (histologically) of fibrosis, calcification and necrosis in relation to duration of CP in a series of 73 consecutive patients with alcoholic CP. Large pancreatic specimens (biopsy or autopsy, at different time intervals from onset) were assessed by two experienced pathologists according to a score system. The median fibrosis score (FS, 0–12) increased from 6.2 (first 4 years from onset, 24 specimens) to 10.2 (≥13 years from onset). Calcification (%) increased almost 3-fold from 30% to 84% in close correlation with the fibrosis score. In contrast, the percentage of necrosis diminished from 75% to 10% during this period (modified data presentation from Gastroenterology, 1996)

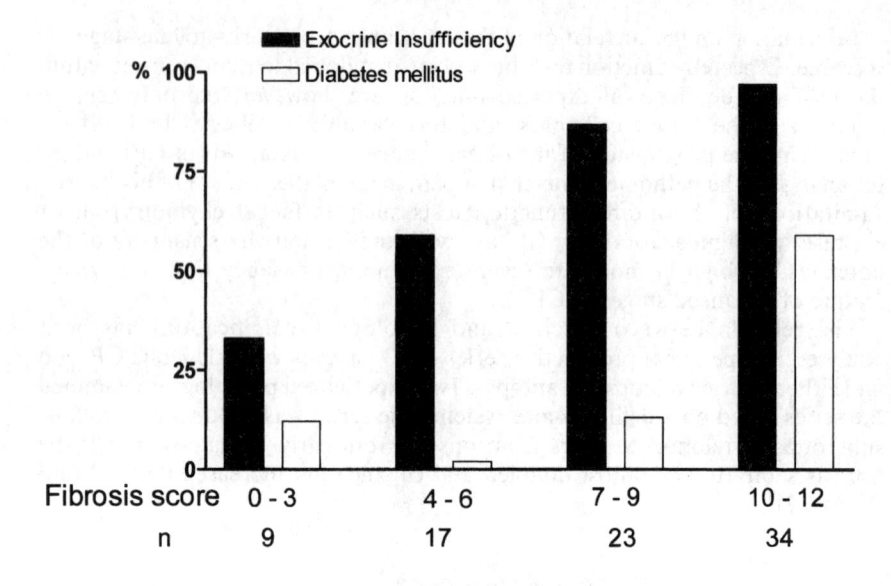

Figure 3 Correlation between fibrosis score and pancreatic dysfunction in the same series of alcoholic CP (see Figure 2). Exocrine insufficiency was noted in 87–97% of patients with a fibrosis score of 7–12. Diabetes was observed in about 60% of patients with a fibrosis score ⩾ 10, but in only about 13% of cases with a fibrosis score ⩽ 9 (modified data presentation from Gastroenterology, 1996)

Interestingly, a statistically significant correlation was noted between the fibrosis score and pancreatic dysfunction, i.e. exocrine insufficiency being present in 87–97% of patients with severe fibrosis (fibrosis score of 7–12) (Figure 3)[8]. These data document a close link between fibrosis, calcification and pancreatic dysfunction (i.e. acinar atrophy) in late-stage CP. Thus, in clinical routine, the sequential study of function and morphology (e.g. calcification) is a suitable procedure for documentation of acinar atrophy and progressive fibrosis, typically found in late-stage CP (Figure 1).

Conversely, necrosis (equivalent to acute pancreatic injury) was a prominent feature of early-stage CP (75%) with a continuous reduction to 10% in relation to duration from onset of CP (Figure 2)[8]. These findings provide evidence for the notion that alcoholic acute and chronic pancreatitis represent different stages of a single entity (so-called necrosis–fibrosis sequence hypothesis), which is in contrast to the hypothesis of the Marseille experts postulating that acute and chronic pancreatitis are two separate nosological entities which rarely merge (see refs 4, 5 and 8–15).

Unfortunately, the diagnostic accuracy of the new indirect morphological methods such as ERCP, endoscopic ultrasonography, CT or MRCP for early-stage CP is undefined[1]. Sensitivity and specificity of these new morphological methods in comparison with histology as gold standard of early-stage CP require further investigations[1]. In late-stage CP every method will be abnormal, even plain abdominal radiography for calcification.

A major clinical challenge is to diagnose CP in early-stage CP when abdominal pain is the only symptom and the imaging and function tests are not diagnostic (Figure 1). The time interval between first-onset alcoholic pancreatitis and the clinical diagnosis of definite CP averages 4.5–5.5 years[4,5,10,11]. In clinical practice (and in the absence of histology), early-stage CP is at present a diagnostic 'black box' period. Thus, the clinical long-term surveillance of suspected early-stage CP applying a 'wait-and-watch strategy' before CP can be diagnosed (or excluded) definitively represents the only rational approach, according to current knowledge[12].

Of note, the 'wait-and-watch strategy' has no direct impact on therapy (except for surgical strategy) since all therapeutic options for acute and chronic pancreatitis are palliative only, and not curative. Surgery for relief of severe pain is required primarily in early-stage alcoholic CP. For instance, in our series of alcoholic CP, 116 out of 207 patients required surgery for severe pain, but surgery had to be performed in almost 50% of patients in early-stage CP, mainly for pseudocysts, i.e. before definite CP was confirmed clinically[5]. Treating patients with suspected early-stage CP according to a strategy reserved for definite CP, i.e. pancreatic head resection, carries the risk of 'overtreament'. Therefore, we agree with the recent statement of DiMagno: 'To falsely label a person as having CP is a significant concern. A misdiagnosis of CP is difficult to correct and may harm patients, particularly if potentially injurious treatments are undertaken'[13].

In our experience CP is a benign disease which, in contrast to acute pancreatitis (and pancreatic cancer), carries a low immediate mortality. Severe pain requiring a surgical (or endoscopic) intervention occurs in about 50% of patients (primarily due to local complications) and can be relieved promptly by a drainage procedure (see below). The 50% survival of alcoholic CP is about 20 years, but death is mainly due to causes unrelated to CP (i.e. >80% severe infections, cardiovascular disease or extrapancreatic neoplasia)[4,5,14–17]. Surprisingly, less than 10% of alcoholic CP patients develop liver cirrhosis.

MECHANISM(S) OF PAIN

There is increasing evidence that pain in CP is multifactorial and may be due to more than one mechanism[13]. Several current concepts of pain mechanism(s) in CP exist[18], primarily (a) acute inflammation/necrosis as in acute pancreatitis, (b) pseudocyst formation (most often postnecrotic), (c) ductal hypertension ('obstructive' CP due to ductal strictures and/or calculi), (d) 'neuroimmune' mechanisms, (e) extrapancreatic causes, e.g. common bile duct stenosis.

CP typically starts with recurrent clinical acute pancreatitis, separated by long pain-free periods (i.e. months or years)[4,5,8–15]. Over 90% of alcoholic CP in our series presented such episodes of pancreatitis of varied severity, some of them requiring hospital admission for severe pain[5]. The management of acute (uncomplicated) pancreatitis is standardized and primarily medical. Alcohol abstinence prevents further episodes of pancreatitis in early-stage CP[19]. In addition, abstinence may delay the progression of acute to chronic pancreatitis[20].

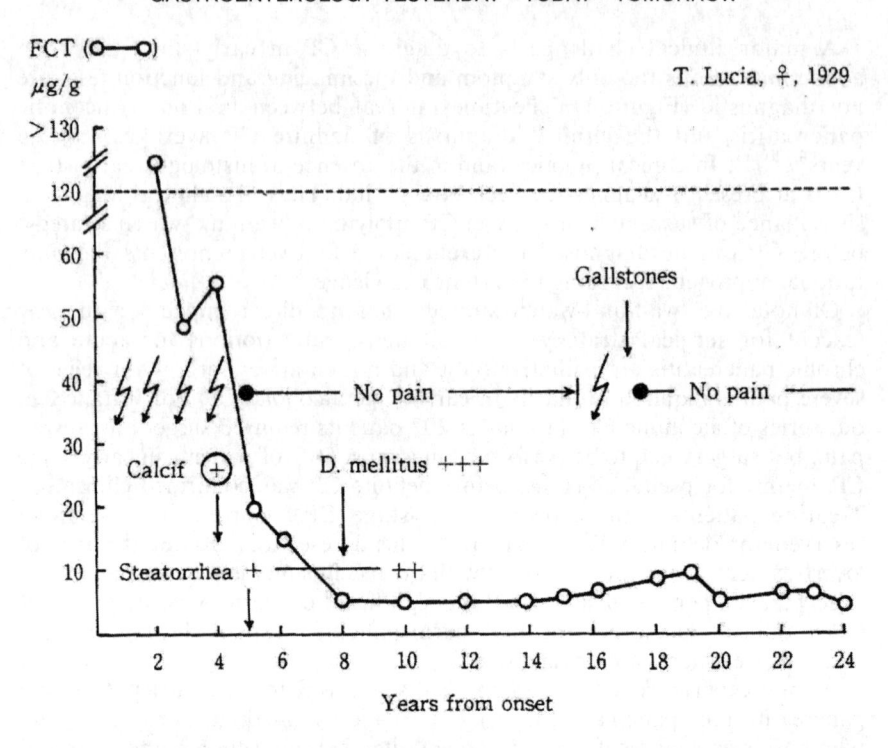

Figure 4 Typical long-term course of alcoholic CP in a 38-year-old chronic alcoholic female patient over 24 years from onset. The patient was repeatedly hospitalized for recurrent pancreatitis during the first 4 years from onset, i.e. early-stage CP. With onset of exocrine insufficiency (FCT, faecal chymotrypsin, normal >120 μm/g) and calcification at 4 years from onset, i.e. late-stage CP, the patient became spontaneously pain-free despite continued alcohol abuse. Diabetes started at 8 years from onset. At 16 years from onset the patient suffered from recurrent biliary colics that were relieved by cholecystectomy. The patient finally died at 30 years from onset of oropharyngeal cancer following 25 years without any pancreatitis-related pain

According to current opinion in most series focused on interventional procedures (i.e. surgery or endoscopy), 'severe chronic intractable pain' is the cardinal feature of CP[21–24]. In endoscopy series 'stenting' of strictures, sphincterotomy, stone extraction and/or extracorporeal lithotripsy are recommended, assuming that severe pain in CP is primarily due to ductal hypertension secondary to calculi or stricture of the main pancreatic duct, i.e. 'obstructive CP'. To our knowledge only one randomized study of endoscopic vs surgical therapy has been performed in CP[24]. The initial success rate was similar by both methods but, at the 5-year follow-up, complete absence of pain was more frequent after surgery (37% vs 14% in the endoscopy series). The very low rate of postoperative pain relief compared to the current surgical literature[21] is unexplained. Additional controlled studies on this issue are mandatory.

Surgical/endoscopic series of CP evaluating the pain mechanism(s) are biased because they focus on CP patients who needed surgery or endoscopy for severe pain[20-24]. Conversely, in mixed medical/surgical series only 27-67% of CP patients experience chronic pain severe enough to warrant a surgical intervention[5,13,15]. In a personal series of alcoholic CP, severe persistent pain (>2 months) requiring surgery occurred in 116 out of 207 patients (56%). Severe pain was predominantly caused by local complications such as pseudocysts (66%), obstructive cholestasis (16%) and probable high ductal pressure (13%). Prompt pain relief was typically achieved by a drainage procedure tailored to the local complication (endoscopy was not performed in this series) and only few patients underwent a pancreatic head resection; $n = 4$)[5].

Painful CP without need of surgery (or endoscopy) was noted in 91 of 207 patients with alcoholic CP (44%)[5]. This group of CP without surgical intervention is best suited for evaluating the natural course of pain. Interestingly, alcoholic CP becomes painless in up to 90% within 10 years from disease onset, i.e. in late-stage CP, and irrespective of surgery according to the literature[4,5,13-15]. The association of pain relief with exocrine insufficiency ('burnout-hypothesis' of CP) is debated and requires further investigation[5,13-15,25]. A typical course of CP over 24 years from onset in a chronic alcoholic patient is shown in Figure 4. The CP started with recurrent acute pancreatitis for the first 3 years associated with normal exocrine function and lack of calcification (i.e. early-stage CP). With onset of calcification and exocrine insufficiency 4 years from onset (i.e. late-stage CP), the CP became painless despite continued alcohol abuse, except at 16 years from onset when the patient developed biliary colics relieved by cholecystectomy. The patient died of oropharyngeal cancer 30 years from onset (following a painless CP course over the last 26 years).

Taken together, different major pain mechanisms are likely to exist in CP in the same patient during evolution of CP and/or in CP series, i.e. surgical/endoscopic vs. medical-surgical series, namely: (a) recurrent pancreatitis (acute inflammation/necrosis) primarily in early-stage CP; (b) pseudocysts (mainly postnecrotic, predominately in early-stage CP); (c) ductal hypertension (symptomatic large-duct CP, often associated with calculi); (d) symptomatic cholestatic obstruction, predominantly in late-stage CP; (e) 'neuroimmune mechanism' (based on surgical series[18]); (f) extrapancreatic pain causes such as peptic ulcer, gallstones, dyspepsia (maldigestion) and especially opiate addiction; (g) pancreatic cancer – increased risk in late-stage CP (e.g. cumulative risk in a large series of hereditary CP of 3.4% at 50 years and 8.6% at 70 years[26].

IMPACT OF AETIOLOGY ON THE COURSE OF CP

CP may be classified aetiologically according to the TIGAR-0 system[1]:

Toxic-metabolic, e.g. alcohol, hypercalcaemia, hyperlipaemia.
Idiopathic, e.g. idiopathic juvenile, idiopathic senile CP, tropical CP.
Genetic, e.g. autosomal dominant i.e. trypsin gene mutation or autosomal recessive/modifier genes, i.e. CFTR, SPINK 1 mutations.
Autoimmune pancreatitis.
Recurrent severe acute pancreatitis.
Obstructive.

In industrialized countries the prominent risk factors of CP are alcohol (~70%), idiopathic (~25%) or rare causes (~5%). Of major importance is the recent discovery of trypsinogen gene mutations (PRSS-1) in hereditary pancreatitis[1]. In addition, an increase of mutations of the trypsin secretory inhibitor gene (SPINK 1) and/or the cystic fibrosis genes (CFTR) have been reported primarily in idiopathic CP which seem to reflect an increased susceptibility to pancreatitis in association with other (undefined) factors[1]. These studies of molecular genetics open new perspectives in our understanding of the pathophysiology of pancreatitis and regarding an improved classification of CP, which require further investigation – a topic beyond the scope of this chapter (for recent reviews see refs 1, 9, 26–29).

Of special note is the fact that, in contrast to acute pancreatitis that is caused in 60–80% either by gallstones or alcohol, biliary pancreatitis virtually never progresses to CP[12]. On the other hand, the majority of alcoholic (acute) pancreatitis seems to progress to CP, but probably a small (undefined) percentage of patients have reversible pancreatitis similar to biliary pancreatitis[11,12]. This special, clinically relevant aspect, requires additional investigations.

Table 1 Clinical characteristics of etiology-classified CP (n = 343)

	ACP*	IJCP*	ISCP*	HP*
No. of patients	265	21	46	11
% Male	90	71	87	46
Age at onset; median, years	36	23	62	10
Follow-up from onset; median, years	16	22	14	36
% with pain	95	100	48	91
% pancreatic surgery for severe pain	57	62	27	20
Late-stage CP documented by:				
% Calcification	86	86	80	91
% Exocrine insufficiency	96	86	91	100
% Diabetes	66	33	41	73

*ACP, alcoholic CP; IJCP, idiopathic 'juvenile' CP[27]; ISCP, idiopathic 'senile' CP[27]; HP, hereditary CP.

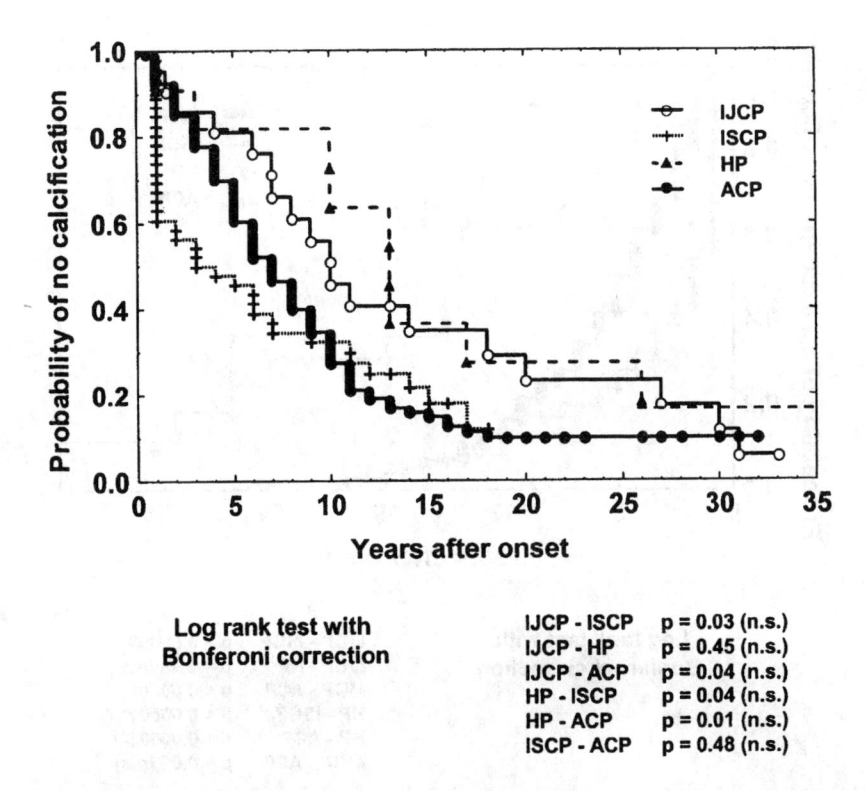

Log rank test with	IJCP - ISCP	p = 0.03 (n.s.)
Bonferoni correction	IJCP - HP	p = 0.45 (n.s.)
	IJCP - ACP	p = 0.04 (n.s.)
	HP - ISCP	p = 0.04 (n.s.)
	HP - ACP	p = 0.01 (n.s.)
	ISCP - ACP	p = 0.48 (n.s.)

Figure 5 Cumulative rate of calcification in relation to duration of CP from onset in three subgroups of non-alcoholic (IJCP, idiopathic 'juvenile'; ISCP, idiopathic 'senile' CP, and HP, hereditary CP) compared to ACP (alcoholic CP (Kaplan–Meier method). Onset of calcification was markedly delayed in IJCP and HP compared to ACP and ISCP, e.g. calcification in ACP and ISCP occurred in 50% at 4–7 years from onset, in contrast to HP and IJCP with a 50% rate of calcification at 12–15 years from onset of disease

Aetiology has a major impact on course and outcome of CP, particularly in the painful, precalcific early-stage CP, according to the literature[1,8,9,15,26,27]. Some new (unpublished) data from a prospective long-term study of three aetiological subgroups of non-alcoholic compared to alcoholic CP may be summarized as shown in Table 1.

The features of late-stage CP are comparable, supporting the notion that the long-term evolution of CP is identical irrespective of aetiology[30].

However, a marked delay in the progression rate to late-stage CP (onset of calcification (Figure 5) and exocrine insufficiency (Figure 6) was noted in HP and IJCP compared to alcoholic CP. Thus, the painful early-stage CP lasts significantly longer in HP and IJCP than in ACP. These findings confirm and extend the results of a former comparable series in which HP was not considered[15].

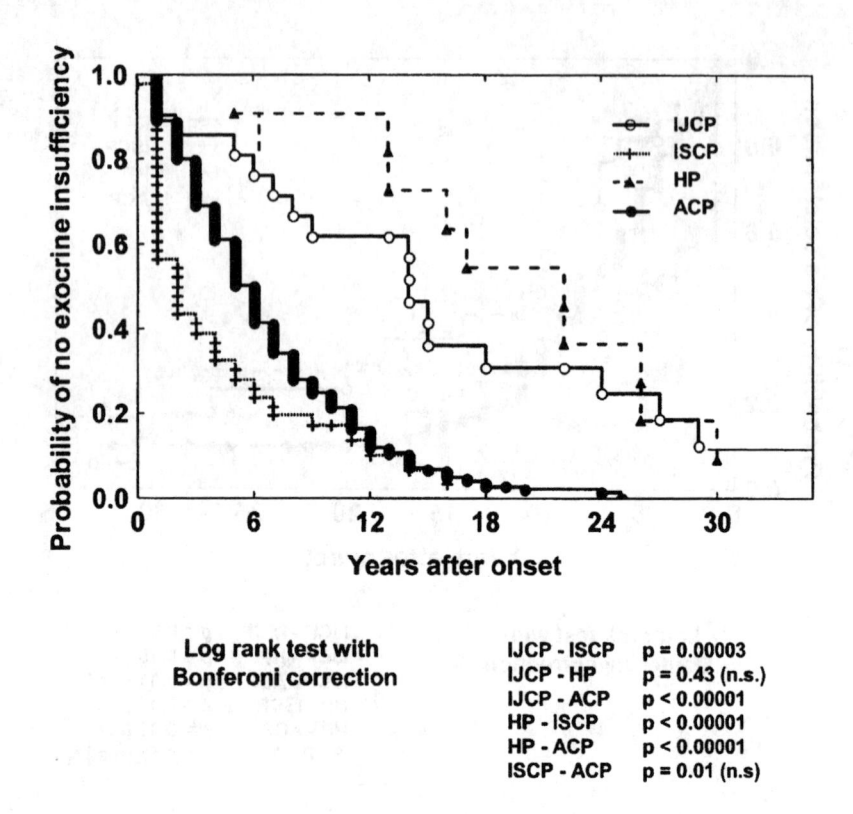

Figure 6 A significant delay in onset of exocrine insufficiency from onset (i.e. late-stage CP) in the same series (see Figure 5) was noted in HP and IJCP compared to ACP and ISCP, indicating a delayed progression rate of pancreatic damage in HP and IJCP, or in other words, a prolongation of early-stage CP in HP and IJCP compared to ACP and ISCP

Interestingly, pain relief coincided closely with calcification and exocrine insufficiency in all four aetiological subgroups (irrespective of surgery) (Figure 7) and despite the differences in the progression rate of HP/IJCP vs ACP. Thus, it appears that the 'burnout' hypothesis of painful CP is valid for uncomplicated CP regardless of surgery and aetiology.

The 50% survival in ACP and ISCP is 15–20 years, which is in contrast to a survival of about 80% at 25–35 years from onset in HP and IJCP (Figure 8).

Obviously, these data are based on a relatively small series of patients (except ACP) which have to be validated by further prospective long-term investigations of mixed medical–surgical series, especially multicentre studies utilizing standardized definitions with regard to diagnosis, staging, pain profile and classification, i.e. aetiology of CP.

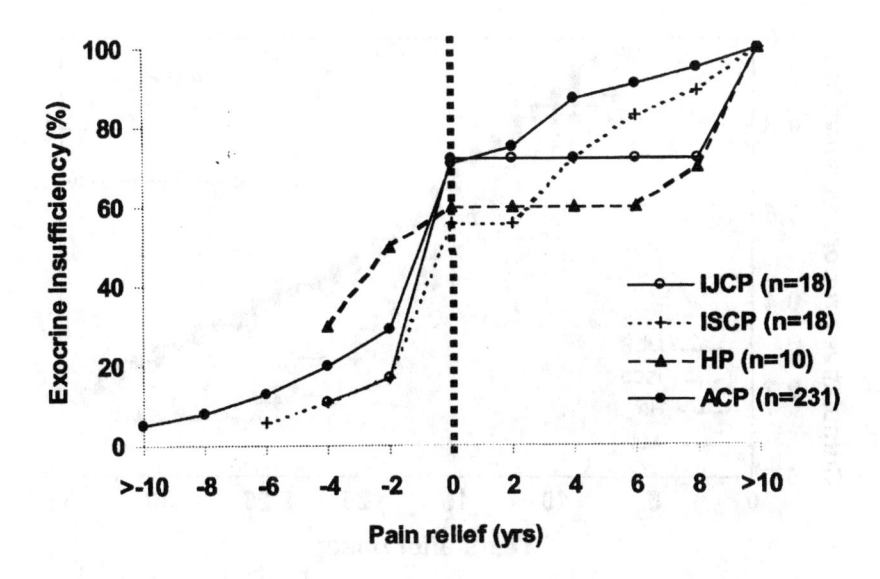

Figure 7 Close coincidence of pain relief (time 0) with exocrine insufficiency was observed in 60–80% of patients irrespective of aetiology, and despite the delayed onset of exocrine insuffiency in HP and IJCP compared to ACP and ISCP (see Figure 6). This observation supports the notion that the 'burnout' hypothesis is valid for uncomplicated CP in late-stage CP irrespective of aetiology (and surgery) (see text)

PERSPECTIVES FOR THE FUTURE

Much progress in know-how, primarily based on improved technology and molecular genetic studies, has been achieved within the past decade. The ultimate goal should be, however, to improve our knowledge of the pathophysiology of CP. Thereby, strategies of prevention of the progression from acute to chronic pancreatitis are likely to be developed, i.e. a rational basis for a curative therapy in contrast to the current palliative therapeutic approach.

References

1. Etemad B, Whitcomb DC. Chronic pancreatitis: diagnosis, classification, and new genetic developments. Gastroenterology. 2001;120:682–707.
2. Lindkvlst B, Appelros St, Manjer J, Borgström A. Trends in incidence of acute pancreatitis in a Swedish population: is there really an increase? Clin Gastroenterol Hepatol. 2004;2: 831–7.
3. Andren-Sandberg A, Bäckmann PL. Demographics of pancreatic cancer. In: Beger HG, Büchler MW, Schönberg MH, editors. Cancer of the Pancreas. Ulm: Universitätsverlag, 1996:3–7.

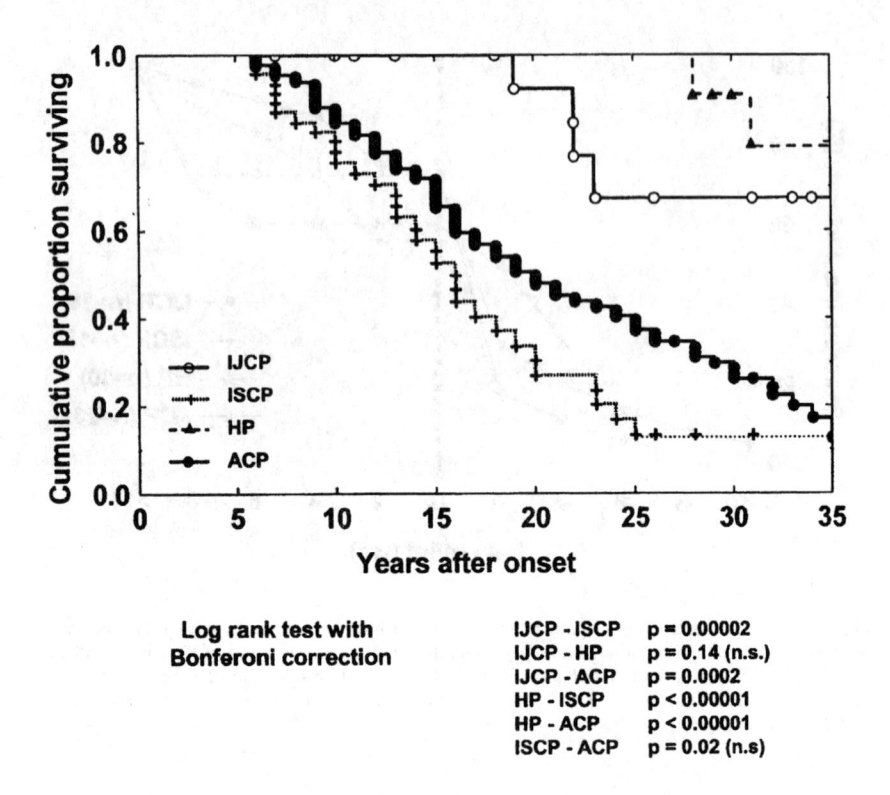

Log rank test with	IJCP - ISCP	p = 0.00002
Bonferoni correction	IJCP - HP	p = 0.14 (n.s.)
	IJCP - ACP	p = 0.0002
	HP - ISCP	p < 0.00001
	HP - ACP	p < 0.00001
	ISCP - ACP	p = 0.02 (n.s)

Figure 8 Survival in relation to aetiology (see Figure 5). The 50% survival in ACP and ISCP was 15–20 years from onset of CP. In contrast, the survival in HP and IJCP was around 70% at 25–35 years from onset of CP

4. Comfort MW, Gambill EE, Baggenstoss AH. Chronic relapsing pancreatitis: a study of 29 cases without associated disease of the biliary or gastrointestinal tract. Gastroenterology. 1946;6:239–85, 376–408.
5. Ammann RW, Mullhaupt B, Zürich Pancreatitis Study Group. The natural history of pain in alcoholic chronic pancreatitis. Gastroenterology. 1999;116:1132–40.
6. Loser C, Mollgard A, Foelsch UR. Fecal elastase 1: a novel, highly sensitive and specific tubeless pancreatic function test. Gut. 1996;39:580–6.
7. Gullo L, Ventrucci M, Tomassetti P, Migliori M, Pezzilli R. Fecal elastase 1 determination in chronic pancreatitis. Dig Dis Sci. 1999;44:210–13.
8. Ammann RW, Heitz Ph U, Klöppel G. Course of alcoholic chronic pancreatitis: a prospective clinicomorphological long-term study. Gastroenterology. 1996;111:224–31.
9. Whitcomb DC. Hereditary pancreatitis: new insights into acute and chronic pancreatitis. Gut. 1999;45:317–22.
10. Gullo L, Labo G. Natural history of acute pancreatitis and its relationship to chronic pancreatitis. In: Banks P, Porro GB, editors. Acute Pancreatitis. Milan: Masson Italia Editori, 1984:87–93.

11. Ammann RW, Mullhaupt B. Progression of alcoholic acute to chronic pancreatitis. Gut. 1994;35:552-6.
12. Ammann RW. A clinically based classification system for alcoholic chronic pancreatitis: summary of an international workshop on chronic pancreatitis in Zürich. Pancreas. 1997; 14:215-21.
13. DiMagno EP. Toward understanding (and management) of painful chronic pancreatitis. Gastroenterology. 1999;116:1252-7.
14. Ammann RW, Akovbiantz A, Largiadör F, Schüler G. Course and outcome of chronic pancreatitis. Longitudinal study of a mixed medical-surgical series of 245 patients. Gastroenterology. 1984;82:820-8.
15. Layer P, Yamamoto H, Kalthoff L, Ciain JE, Bakken L, DiMagno EP. The different courses of early- and late-onset idiopathic and alcoholic chronic pancreatitis. Gastroenterology. 1994;107:1481-7.
16. Lowenfels AB, Maisonneuve P, Cavallini G et al. Prognosis of chronic pancreatitis: an international multicenter study. Am J Gastroenterol. 1994;89:1467-71.
17. Levy P, Milan C, Pignon JP et al. Mortality factors associated with chronic pancreatitis. Unidimensional and multidimensional analysis of a medical- surgical series of 240 patients. Gastroenterology. 1989;96:1165-72.
18. Di Sebestiano P, di Mola FF, Bookman DE, Friess H, Büchler MW. Chronic pancreatitis: the perspective of pain generation by neuroimmune interaction. Gut. 2003;52:907-11.
19. Strum WB. Abstinence in alcoholic chronic pancreatitis. Effect on pain and outcome. J Clin Gastroenterol. 1995;20:37-41.
20. Gullo L, Barbara L, Labo G. Effect of cessation of alcohol use on the course of pancreatic dysfunction in alcoholic pancreatitis. Gastroenterology. 1998;95:1063-8.
21. Warshaw AL, Banks PA, Fernandez-Del Castillo C. AGA technical review: treatment of pain in chronic pancreatitis. Gastroenterology. 1998;115:765-76.
22. Rösch T, Daniel P, Scholz M et al. Endoscopic treatment of chronic pancreatitis: multicenter study of 1000 patients with long-term follow-up. Endoscopy 2002;34:765-71.
23. Cohen S, Bacon BR, Berlin JA et al. NIH state-of-the-science Conference Statement: ERCP for diagnosis and therapy. Gastrointest Endosc. 2002;56:803-9.
24. Dite P, Ruzicka M, Zboril V, Novotny I. A prospective, randomized trial comparing endoscopic and surgical therapy for chronic pancreatitis. Endoscopy. 2003;35:553-8.
25. Girdwood AH, Marks IN, Bornman PC et al. Does progressive pancreatic insufficiency limit pain in calcific pancreatitis with duct stricture or continued alcohol insult? J Clin Gastroenterol. 1981;3:241-5.
26. Howes N, Lerch MM, Greenhalf W et al. Clinical and genetic characteristics of hereditary pancreatitis in Europe. Clin Gastroenterol Hepatol. 2004;2:252-61.
27. DiMagno EP. Gene mutations and idiopathic chronic pancreatitis: clinical implications and testing. Gastroenterology. 2001;121:1508-12.
28. Truninger K, Ammann RW, Blum HE, Witt H. Genetic aspects of chronic pancreatitis: insights into aetiopathogenesis and clinical implications. Swiss Med Weekly. 2001;131:565-74.
29. DiMagno MJ, DiMagno EP. Chronic pancreatitis. Curr Opin Gastroenterol. 2004;20:444-51.
30. Lankisch PG. Natural course of chronic pancreatitis. Pancreatology. 2001;1:3-14.

21
Basis and future of enzyme replacement therapy

P. LAYER, H. PANTER and J. KELLER

INTRODUCTION

Current management of pancreatic exocrine insufficiency, one of the typical complications of chronic pancreatitis, has been based on improved understanding of its pathophysiology. Thus, in most patients steatorrhoea and malnutrition as a consequence of global nutrient malabsorption can be corrected or prevented.

Hydrolysis and breakdown of macronutrients into smaller, absorbable metabolites is crucially dependent on the action of pancreatic enzymes in the intestinal lumen. Although brush-border enzymes and several extrapancreatic enzymes participate in the digestion, they cannot prevent detrimental malabsorption as a result of untreated pancreatic exocrine insufficiency[1,2]. Knowledge of secretion and luminal fate of pancreatic enzymes and their effects on nutrient digestion under physiological and pathophysiological conditions has increased, and enabled rational treatment recommendations[3].

BASIS OF TREATMENT

Physiology

Postprandial cumulative enzyme outputs exceed more than tenfold the quantity required for digestion, physiological conditions provided. In exocrine pancreatic insufficiency less than 10% of normal prandial secretory rates may be enough to prevent steatorrhoea[4,5]. Experiments using specific enzyme inhibitors provided similar results[6]. Exposure of nutrients to the duodenal mucosa is by far the most powerful stimulus of human pancreatic exocrine secretion. As it was shown, digestive products (such as free fatty acids) rather than intact macromolecules (such as triglycerides) induce neurohormonal stimulation of the prandial enzyme response[7,8]. Even under physiological conditions the healthy human intestine is unable to digest and absorb all nutrients contained in chyme delivered from the stomach postprandially following a normal meal; by contrast, considerable nutrient quantities regularly escape intestinal absorption, pass the ileocaecal junction and contribute to upper gastrointestinal secretory and motor inhibitory regulation[9-13].

In addition, pancreatic exocrine function is coupled with gastrointestinal motility both in the fasting (interdigestive) state and following a meal, i.e. in response to endogenous stimulation[14,15]. Intraluminal pancreatic enzyme activities decrease during transit along the small intestine, but because of different stability against degradation, rate of inactivation differs between different enzymes[16,17]. Pancreatic amylase, for example, is fairly stable and not easily proteolysed, and a large amount survives duodeno-ileal transit. About two-thirds of duodenal protease activities reach the jejunum, and about one-quarter reach the ileum[17-21]. We have found that trypsin's hydrolytic activity survives better than its immunoreactivity, which suggests that its structural integrity may not be required for its enzymatic action[17,18].

By contrast, lipase is inactivated very rapidly in the absence of triglycerides, and only a small proportion reaches the distal small bowel[17,18]. More lipase activity survives in the presence of its substrate[18-22]. Chymotrypsin has been shown to be of particular importance for decreasing lipase activity and incomplete fat digestion[19,21,23,24].

Exocrine insufficiency

Exocrine insufficiency of pancreatic function occurs late in the course in the vast majority of cases of chronic pancreatitis, due to the large functional reserve of the gland[1,9,25].

Its manifestation in patients with alcoholic pancreatitis usually develops within the second decade of clinical disease, but may also appear more rapidly[2,9,26]. During the course of chronic pancreatitis exocrine secretions, including enzyme output, decrease. The clinically overt malabsorption usually develops years after onset of symptomatic disease[27].

Increasing malabsorption is associated with a shift of the site of maximal digestion and absorption from the duodenum to more distal regions of small intestine, and increased amounts of nutrients may be delivered to the distal ileum, where they influence regulation of motor and secretory function of upper gastrointestinal organs[9-13,28]. Moreover, gastroduodenal and small intestinal transit is significantly accelerated, and the available time for digestion and absorption is markedly decreased in patients with pancreatic insufficiency[28], which may further contribute to nutrient malabsorption.

This mechanism may also explain the decrease in pain in response to pancreatic enzyme supplementation in a subgroup of patients[28,29]. Steatorrhoea is the most important digestive malfunction in pancreatic exocrine insufficiency, and may be associated with malabsorption of the lipid-soluble vitamins A, D, E, and K.

Steatorrhoea develops prior to manifest malabsorption of other nutrients[26], because pancreatic lipase is crucially important for digestion of lipids. By contrast, protein digestion is induced by gastric proteolytic activity and intestinal brush-border peptidases, and is maintained even in the absence of pancreatic proteolytic activity[20]. Similarly, with lacking pancreatic amylase, starch digestion reaches about 80% due to salivary amylase and brush-border oligosaccharidases[6]. The coefficient of fat absorption indicates the efficacy of luminal fat digestion in different populations, because quantitative faecal fat excretion also depends on dietary lipid intake[30]. In contrast to steatorrhoea and creatorrhoea that can be measured in faeces as diagnostic markers of malabsorption of lipids and protein, respectively, fecal carbohydrate measurements do not represent the extent of starch malabsorption[31–34] because carbohydrates are metabolized by the intracolonic flora. On the other hand, this can be used as a measure of starch malabsorption by determining hydrogen breath concentrations[8,35–37].

Fat malabsorption occurs earlier than malabsorption of protein and carbohydrate due to an interaction of mechanisms. On the one hand acinar production and secretion of lipase decreases more rapidly compared with proteases[1,9,26]. Impaired pancreatic bicarbonate secretion characteristic for pancreatic insufficiency may be unable to maintain an intraduodenal pH >4, and may thus be insufficient to protect intraduodenal enzymes, in particular lipase, from acidic denaturation[9,38]. Lipase is also a substrate greatly susceptible to the action of proteases, and is hydrolysed more rapidly than other enzymes during small intestinal transit[17,19,21,27]. Compensatory mechanisms, in particular extrapancreatic lipolysis (e.g. lingual and gastric lipase) contribute only marginally to cumulative fat digestion[39].

Treatment modalities

For an effective treatment of exocrine pancreatic insufficiency supplemented enzymes must be delivered into the duodenal lumen simultaneously with the meal. A minimal lipase activity of 40–60 IU/ml is necessary in postprandial chyme, i.e. cumulative amounts of 25 000–40 000 IU of lipase for digestion of a regular meal[1,27].

Because ingestion of unprotected enzyme preparations is associated with rapid lipase inactivation due to acid and proteolytic destruction[19,27,38,40], it is necessary to administer up to tenfold more lipase orally to correct steatorrhoea[14]. Enteric coating of entire pancreatin tablets or capsules, which prevents acidic destruction of lipase, does not result in superior preparations compared with unprotected pancreatin.

Indeed, resistant enzyme particles of >2 mm are not delivered by the stomach with the meal (their substrate)[41–43], and the duodenal passages of nutrients and enzymes are dissociated. Modern preparations contain pancreatin protected within acid-resistant, pH-sensitive microspheres mixing intragastrically with the meal, and being emptied into, and dissolved within, the duodenum simultaneously with chyme. These preparations have superior efficacy compared with unprotected pancreatin extracts[44,45]. A further decrease in sphere size may not be associated with greater clinical benefit[46].

After reaching the duodenum enzymes are released within a few minutes; yet transit of nutrients along the small intestine may occur within this lag time, and maximal digestion and absorption may be shifted to distal segments of intestine. Thus some digestive efficacy may be lost[26,47,48]. Because in patients with pancreatic exocrine insufficiency gastrointestinal transit is significantly faster compared to healthy subjects, this shift may gain practical importance[28].

Most patients with pancreatic exocrine insufficiency are treated with pH-sensitive microsphere enzyme preparations. In many patients 25 000–50 000 IU lipase with each meal can reduce severe steatorrhoea to less than 15 g fat per day. Clinical signs such as increasing body weight and normalization of stool consistency suggest therapeutic success. In unresponsive patients, dosages should increase and nutrient intake should be distributed across 5–6 smaller meals[9]. If lack of patient compliance is suspected, faecal chymotrypsin should be measured; inadequate intake of enzymes is associated with low activities of chymotrypsin.

Ultrahigh dosages of pancreatic enzymes have been suspected to induce stenotic fibrosing colonopathy in patients with cystic fibrosis, and its risk correlates with the amount of substituted enzymes[49,50]. However, no comparable complications have been observed in patients with enzyme-treated chronic pancreatitis.

Nevertheless doses more than 75 000 IU of lipase per meal are generally not recommended. In compliant patients without satisfactory benefit the combination of unprotected enzyme preparations with proton pump inhibitor treatment often improves maldigestion[1,51–53]. Other causes of refractory steatorrhoea, such as intestinal infections with *Giardia lamblia*, bacterial overgrowth[55], villous atrophic conditions, or other associated intestinal absorption disorders, as well as previous gastric and/or intestinal resections, may require specific diagnostic efforts and medical or surgical intervention.

After gastric resection or gastroenterostomies gastric emptying is accelerated. These patients should be treated with pancreatic enzyme granulate or powder. Achlorhydric patients, and patients under therapy with acid blockers, show most benefit under conventional, i.e. unprotected, enzyme preparations. Medium-chain triglycerides do not improve lipid absorption in supplemented patients[54].

FUTURE TREATMENT

The mechanisms outlined above, which all contribute to the pivotal importance of lipase deficiency in pancreatic exocrine insufficiency, form the pathophysiological background before which future developments evolve. Consequently, these focus mostly on substitution of lipolytic activity. It should be kept in mind, however, that malabsorption of carbohydrates is probably of minor importance for overall caloric losses, but may induce abdominal symptoms due to osmotic effects and bacterial metabolism.

However, alternative lipase preparations appear on the horizon as potential future therapeutic perspectives Several microorganisms produce lipase activity, and several of these possess potentially attractive properties. Fungal lipase preparations have been available for many years, but combine several biochemical disadvantages and have not been shown to be superior to porcine preparations[56–59].

By contrast, bacterial lipase has shown encouraging results. Notably the *Burkholderia plantarii* species synthesizes and secretes a lipase that has been shown to be stable in acid and neutral pH settings and also against destruction by proteolytic hydrolysis or inactivation by bile acids[60]. Bacterial lipase has remarkable effects on lipid digestion under experimental conditions in dogs, and has been found to be superior to porcine enzymes even at milligram quantities. According to these results the amount of enzyme supplementation might be reduced by more than 90% and still improve total fat digestion[61,62]. Bacterial lipase appears to possess the potential to markedly improve maldigestion because of its stability against denaturation and hydrolysis on the one hand, and high digestive effectiveness on the other hand. However, so far there are only reports obtained from animal studies, and no human data have been published.

Another source for pancreatic enzymes may be found in genetically generated lipase. Thus, pancreatic enzymes were produced successfully after transferring human lipase genes via a recombinant adenovirus into specific cell lines such as human gallbladder cells or sheep gallbladder *ex vivo*, or even rodine bile ducts *in vivo*[63,64].

Hence it appears conceivable that future therapeutic strategies may evolve and be based on, or at least include, novel treatments involving genetic engineering for production of pancreatic lipase within the human biliary system, or possibly bioengineered human lipase preparations.

Acknowledgements

Own studies cited in this chapter were supported by the German Research Foundation (DFG, grants La 483/5), the Anna-Lorz-Foundation, and the Esther-Christiansen Foundation.

References

1. Di Magno EP, Clain JE, Layer P. Chronic pancreatitis. In: Go VLW, Dimagno EP, Gardner JD et al., editors. The Pancreas: Biology, Pathobiology, and Diseases, 2nd edn. New York: Raven Press, 1993:665–706.
2. Layer P, DiMagno EP. Natural histories of alcoholic and idiopathic chronic pancreatitis. Pancreas. 1996;12:318–19
3. Layer P, Keller J. Pancreatic enzymes: secretion and luminal nutrient digestion in health and disease. J Clin Gastroenterol. 1999;28:3–10.
4. DiMagno EP, Go VLW, Summerskill WHJ. Relations between pancreatic enzyme outputs and malabsorption in severe pancreatic insufficiency. N Engl J Med. 1973;288:813–15.
5. Hiele M, Ghoos Y, Rutgeerts P, Vantrappen G. Starch digestion in normal subjects and patients with pancreatic diseases, using a $^{13}CO_2$ breath test. Gastroenterology. 1989;96:503.
6. Layer P, Zinsmeister AR, DiMagno EP. Effects of decreasing intraluminal amylase activity on starch digestion and postprandial gastrointestinal function in humans. Gastroenterology. 1986;91:41–8.
7. Guimbaud R, Moreau JA, Bouisson M et al. Intraduodenal free fatty acids rather than triglycerides are responsible for the release of CCK in humans. Pancreas. 1997;14:76–82.
8. Layer P, Holtmann G. Pancreatic enzymes in chronic pancreatitis (state-of-the-art). Int J Pancreatol. 1994;15:1–11.
9. Read NW, McFarlane A, Kinsman RJ et al. Effect of infusion of nutrient solutions into the ileum on gastrointestinal transit and plasma levels of neurotensin and enteroglucagon. Gastroenterology. 1984;86:274–80.
10. Spiller RC, Trotman IF, Higgins BE et al. The ileal brake-inhibition of jejunal motility after ileal fat perfusion in man. Gut. 1984;25:365–74.

11. Layer P, Peschel S, Schlesinger T, Goebell H. Human pancreatic secretion and intestinal motility: effects of ileal nutrient perfusion. Am J Physiol. 1990;258:G196–201.
12. Layer P, Schlesinger T, Goebell H. Modulation of periodic interdigestive gastrointestinal motor and pancreatic function by the ileum. Pancreas. 1993;8:426–32.
13. Keller J, Rünzi M, Goebell H, Layer P. Duodenal and ileal nutrient deliveries regulate human intestinal motor and pancreatic responses to a meal. Am J Physiol. 1997;272:G632–7.
14. DiMagno EP, Layer P. Human exocrine pancreatic enzyme secretion. In: Go VLW, Di Magno EP, Gardner JD et al., editors. The Pancreas: Biology, Pathobiology, and Diseases, 2nd edn, New York, Raven Press, 1993;275–300.
15. Layer P, Chan ATH, Go VLW, DiMagno EP. Human pancreatic secretion during phase II antral motility of the interdigestive cycle. Am J Physiol. 1988;254:G249–53.
16. Borgström B, Dahlqvist A, Lundh G, Sjövall J. Studies of intestinal digestion and aborption in the human. J Clin Invest 1957;36:1521–36.
17. Layer P, Go VLW, DiMagno EP. Fate of pancreatic enzymes during aboral small intestinal transit in humans. Am J Physiol. 1986;251:G475–80.
18. Granger M, Abadie B, Marchis-Mouren G. Limited action of trypsin on porcine pancreatic amylase: characterization of the fragments. FEBS Lett. 1975;56:189–93.
19. Layer P, Jansen JBMJ, Cherian L, Lamers CBHW, Goebell H. Feedback regulation of human pancreatic secretion: effects of protease inhibition on duodenal delivery and small intestinal transit of pancreatic enzymes. Gastroenterology. 1990;98:1311–19.
20. Layer P, Baumann J, Hellmann C, vd Ohe M, Gröger G, Goebell H. Effect of luminal protease inhibition on prandial nutrient digestion during small intestinal chyme transit. Pancreas. 1990;5:718.
21. Holtmann G, Kelly DG, Sternby B, DiMagno EP. Survival of human pancreatic enzymes during small bowel transit: effect of nutrients, bile acids, and enzymes. Am J Physiol. 1997;273:G553–8.
22. Kelly DG, Sternby B, DiMagno EP. How to protect human pancreatic enzyme activities in frozen duodenal juice. Gastroenterology. 1991;100:189–95.
23. Thiruvengadam R, DiMagno EP. Inactivation of human lipase by proteases. Am J Physiol. 1988;255:G476–81.
24. Layer P, Hellmann C, Baumann J, vd Ohe M, Gröger G, Goebell H. Modulation of physiologic fat malabsorption in humans. Digestion. 1990; 46:153.
25. DiMagno EP, Go VLW, Summerskill WHJ. Relations between pancreatic enzyme outputs and malabsorption in severe pancreatic insufficiency. N Engl J Med. 1973;288:813–15.
26. DiMagno EP, Malagelada JR, Go VLW. Relationship between alcoholism and pancreatic insufficiency. NY Acad Sci. 1975;252:200–7.
27. Layer P, Yamamoto H, Kalthoff L, Clain JE, Bakken LJ, DiMagno EP. The different courses of early- and late-onset idiopathic and alcoholic chronic pancreatitis. Gastroenterology. 1994;107:1481–7.
28. Layer P, von der Ohe MR, Holst JJ et al. Altered postprandial motility in chronic pancreatitis: role of malabsorption. Gastroenterology. 1997;112:1624–34.
29. Slaff J, Jacobson D, Tillmann CR, Curington C, Toskes PP. Protease-specific suppression of pancreatic exocrine secretion. Gastroenterology. 1984;87:44–52.
30. Nakamura T, Takeuchi T. Pancreatic steatorrhea, malabsorption, and nutrition biochemistry: a comparison of japanese, european and american patients with chronic pancreatitis. Pancreas. 1997;14:323–33.
31. Bond JH. Fate of soluble carbohydrate in the colon of rats and man. J Clin Invest. 1976;57:1158–64.
32. Bond JH, Currier BE, Buchwald H, Levitt MD. Colonic conservation of malabsorbed carbohydrate. Gastroenterology. 1980;78:444–7.
33. Stephen AM, Haddad AC, Phillips SF. Passage of carbohydrate into the colon. Gastroenterology. 1983;85:589–95.
34. Flourie B, Florent C, Jouany JP et al. Colonic breakdown of 50 g wheat starch in healthy man: effect on symptoms and fecal outputs. Gastroenterology. 1986;90:111–19.
35. Mackie RD, Levine AS, Levitt MD. Malabsorption of starch in pancreatic insufficiency. Gastroenterology. 1981;80:1220.

36. Patel VP, Jain NK, Agarwal N, GeeVarghese PJ, Pitchumoni CS. Comparisons of bentiromide test and rice flour breath hydrogen test in the detection of exocrine pancreatic insufficiency. Pancreas. 1986;1:172.
37. Kerlin P, Wong L, Harris B, Capra S. Rice flour, breath hydrogen, and malabsorption. Gastroenterology. 1984;87:578.
38. DiMagno EP, Malagelada JR, Go VLW, Moertel CG. Fate of orally ingested enzymes in pancreatic insufficiency: comparison of two dosage schedules. N Engl J Med. 1977;296: 1318–22.
39. Sternby B, Holtmann G, Kelly DG, DiMagno EP. Effect of gastric or duodenal nutrient infusion on gastric and pancreatic lipase secretion. Gastroenterology. 1992:102:A292.
40. Heizer WD, Cleaveland CR, Iber FL. Gastric inactivation of pancreatic supplements. Bull Johns Hopkins Hosp. 1965;116:261–70.
41. Goebell H, Klotz U, Nehlsen B, Layer P. Oroileal transit of slow release 5-ASA. Gut. 1993; 34:669–75.
42. Code CF, Schlegel JF. The gastrointestinal interdigestive housekeeper: motor correlates of the interdigestive myoelectric complex of the dog. In: Daniel EE, editor. Proceedings of the 4th International Symposium on Gastrointestinal Motility. Vancouver: Mitchell Press, 1973:631–4.
43. Schlegel JF, Code CF. The gastric peristalsis of the interdigestive housekeeper. In: Vantrappen G, editor. Proceedings of the 5th International Symposium on Gastrointestinal Motility. Leuven: Typoff-Press, 1975:321.
44. Kölbel C, Layer P, Hotz J, Goebell H. Der Einfluß eines säuregeschützten, mikroverkapselten Pankreatinpräparats auf die pankreatogene Steatorrhö. Med Klin. 1986;81:85–6.
45. Lankisch PG, Lembcke B, Göke B, Creutzfeldt W. Therapie der pankreatogenen Steatorrhoe: Bietet der Säureschutz für Pankreasenzyme Vorteile? Verh Dtsch Ges Inn Med. 1983; 89:864–7.
46. Meyer JH, Lake R. Mismatch of duodenal deliveries of dietary fat and pancreatin from enterically coated microspheres. Pancreas. 1997;15:226–35.
47. Dutta SK, Rubin J, Harvey J. Comparative evaluation of the therapeutic efficacy of a pH-sensitive enteric-coated pancreatic enzyme preparation with conventional pancreatic enzyme therapy in the treatment of exocrine pancreatic insufficiency. Gastroenterology. 1983;84:476–82.
48. Hendeles L, Dorf A, Stecenko A, Weinberger M. Treatment failure after substitution of generic pancrelipase capsules. Correlation with *in vitro* lipase activity. J Am Med Assoc. 1990;263:2459–61.
49. FitzSimmons SC, Burkhart GA, Borowitz D et al. High-dose pancreatic enzyme supplements and fibrosing colonopathy in children with cystic fibrosis. N Engl J Med. 1997;336: 1283–9.
50. MacSweeney EJ, Oades PJ, Buchdahl R, Rosenthal M, Bush A. Relation of thickening of colon wall to pancreatic-enzyme treatment in cystic fibrosis. Lancet. 1995;345:752–6.
51. Regan PT, Malagelada JR, DiMagno EP, Glanzman SL, Go VLW. Comparative effects of antacids, cimetidine, and enteric coating on the therapeutic response to oral enzymes in severe pancreatic insufficiency. N Engl J Med. 1977;297:854–8.
52. Carroccio A, Pardo F, Montalto G et al. Use of famotidine in severe exocrine pancreatic insufficiency with persistent maldigestion on enzymatic replacement therapy. Dig Dis Sci. 1992;37:1441–6.
53. Heijerman HG, Lamers CB, Bakker W. Omeprazole enhances the efficacy of pancreatin (Pancrease) in cystic fibrosis. Ann Intern Med. 1991;114:200–10.
54. Caliari S, Benini L, Sembenini C, Gregori B, Carnielli V, Vantini I. Medium-chain triglyceride absorption in patients with pancreatic insufficiency. Scand J Gastroenterol. 1996;31:90–4.
55. Casellas F, Guarner L, Vaquero E, Antolin M, de Gracia X, Malagelada JR. Hydrogen breath test with glucose in exocrine pancreatic insufficiency. Pancreas. 1998;16:481–6.
56. Zentler Munro PL, Assoufi BA, Balasubramanian K et al. Therapeutic potential and clinical efficacy of acid-resistant fungal lipase in the treatment of pancreatic steatorrhoea due to cystic fibrosis. Pancreas. 1992;7:311–19.
57. Schneider MU, Knoll-Ruzicka ML, Domschke S, Heptner G, Domschke W. Pancreatic enzyme replacement therapy: comparative effects of conventional and enteric-coated

microspheric pancreatin and acid-stable fungal enzyme preparations on steatorrhea in chronic pancreatitis. Hepatogastroenterology. 1985;32:97–102.
58. Griffin SM, Alderson D, Farndon JR. Acid resistant lipse as replacement therapy in chronic pancreatic exocrine insufficiency: a study in dogs. Gut. 1989;30:1012–15.
59. Moreau J, Bousson M, Saint Marc Girardin MF, Pignal F, Bommelaer G, Ribet A. Comparison of fungal lipase and pancreatic lipase in exocrine pancreatic insufficiency in man. Study of their *in vitro* properties and intraduodenal bioavailability. Gastroenterol Clin Biol. 1988;12:787–92.
60. Raimondo M, DiMagno EP. Lipolytic activity of bacterial lipase survives better than that of porcine lipase in human gastric and duodenal content. Gastroenterology. 1994;107:231–5.
61. Suzuki A, Mizumoto A, Sarr MG, DiMagno EP. Bacterial lipase and high-fat diets in canine exocrine pancreatic insufficiency: a new therapy of steatorrhea? Gastroenterology. 1997;112:2048–55.
62. Suzuki A, Mizumoto A, Rerknimitr R, Sarr MG, DiMango EP. Effect of bacterial or porcine lipase with low- or high-fat diets on nutrient absorption in pancreatic-insufficient dogs. Gastroenterology. 1999;116:431–7.
63. Kuhel DG, Zheng S, Tso P, Hui DY. Adenovirus-mediated human pancreatic lipase gene transfer to rat bile: gene therapy of fat malabsorption. Am J Physiol Gastrointest Liver Physiol. 2000;279:G1031–6.
64. Maeda H, Danel C, Crystal RG. Adenovirus-mediated transfer of human lipase complementary DNA to the gallbladder. Gastroenterology. 1994;106:1638–44.

22
Hedgehog signalling in pancreatic cancer

M. HEBROK

PANCREATIC ADENOCARCINOMA

Pancreatic adenocarcinoma, the fourth leading cause of cancer death in the United States, constitutes a devastating disease that carries a dismal prognosis. Due to the absence of early markers diagnosis frequently occurs at a time when the primary tumour has metastasized into adjacent tissues. Chemotherapeutic treatment of this aggressive tumour has proven ineffective, leaving surgery as the main treatment option. However, even after removal of the primary tumour, the mean 5-year survival rate is low and decreases substantially over the following years. The progression of pancreatic cancer from normal pancreatic exocrine cells to malignant carcinoma has been classified into different stages, known as pancreatic intraepithelial lesions (PanIN)[1]. While mutations in tumour-suppressor genes and other genes linked to the cell cycle are characteristic markers of later PanIN stages, the molecular changes causing the initiation of tumour formation are still unknown (reviewed in ref. 2). Discovery of these genes in conjunction with the development of potential antagonists blocking their activities would be highly desirable. Here, we discuss the role of the Hedgehog signalling pathway during the formation and growth of pancreatic adenocarcinoma.

HEDGEHOG SIGNALLING

Embryonic signalling pathways, including the Hedgehog and Wnt signalling pathways, are known to regulate cell–cell interactions during tissue and organ formation[3,4]. In addition to these early functions, embryonic signalling pathways also play important roles in maintenance of adult organ function; however, increasing evidence suggests that deregulation of pathway activities in adult tissues can also result in tumour formation. The Hedgehog (Hh) signalling pathway was first identified in a large mutant screen in *Drosophila melanogaster*[5]. Flies mutant for the *hedgehog* gene displayed epidermal spikes in larval segments that are normally devoid of these extensions. Gene

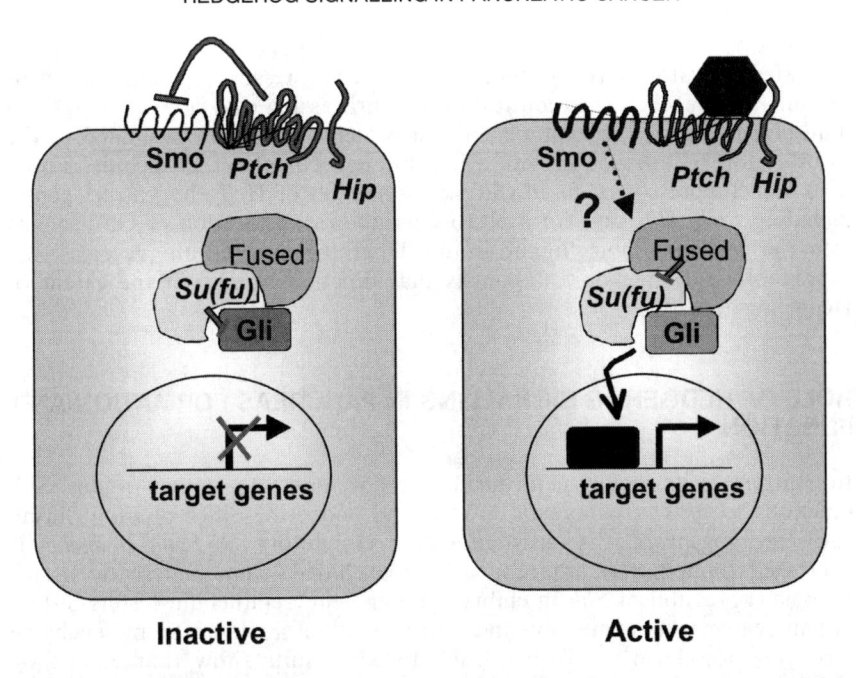

Figure 1 Hedgehog signalling pathway. In its inactive state, Patched (Ptch) mediated suppression of Smoothened (Smo) function prevents translocation of cytoplasmic Gli transcription factors into the nucleus. In the presence of Hedgehog ligands, Ptch inhibition of Smo is alleviated and Gli proteins dislocate from a multiprotein complex that includes Fused and Suppressor of Fused (Su(fu)). Within the nucleus, Gli proteins activate transcription of Hedgehog target genes, including Gli1, Ptch and Hip, another Hedgehog binding protein that restricts the diffusion of Hedgehog ligands

duplication events resulted in three distinct *Hedgehog* family members in mammals, *Sonic (Shh), Desert (Dhh)* and *Indian Hedgehog (Ihh)*, all of which code for secreted proteins.

Hedgehog signalling is mediated via a series of inhibitory steps (Figure 1). All three Hedgehog ligands have been shown to bind to transmembrane receptors, Patched 1 (Ptch1) and Patched 2 (Ptch2), present in cells with active Hedgehog signalling. Similarly, Hedgehog ligands also bind to Hip1, a transmembrane protein that does not share sequence homology with the Ptch proteins. The exact details of ligand–receptor signalling have not been fully explored; however, the current model proposes that, in the absence of ligands, Ptch receptors block the function of another transmembrane protein, Smoothened (Smo), and that this inhibition is relieved upon ligand binding. Once activated, Smo initiates a signalling cascade that results in the activation of Gli transcription factors (the vertebrate homologue of the *Drosophila* Cubitus interruptus, Ci) (reviewed in ref. 6). Three vertebrate Gli proteins, Gli1, Gli2, and Gli3, have been identified that regulate Hedgehog responses in a tissue-specific manner. Cleavage of the Gli proteins results in N-terminal truncated activators and C-terminally truncated repressor fragments; however, the intricate mechanisms controlling Gli processing and activation remain unresolved. Within the cyptoplasm, Gli proteins appear to be linked to the cytoskeleton by interaction with a multiprotein complex that includes Fused (Fu) and Suppressor of fused (SuFu). Activation of Hedgehog target genes, including *Ptch*, *Hip*, and *Gli* itself, occurs upon translocation of Gli proteins into the nucleus. Thus, ligand-induced pathway activation increases the expression of Hedgehog antagonists that function to restrict the extent of Hedgehog activity.

ROLE OF HEDGEHOG SIGNALLING IN PANCREAS FORMATION AND FUNCTION

In contrast to its requirement during the development of other organs, Shh functions to restrict pancreatic growth and endocrine differentiation during early embryogenesis[7-14]. Consistent with this inhibitory role *Sonic Hedgehog* is expressed immediately adjacent to, but excluded from, pancreatic tissue. Ectopic expression of *Shh* in embryonic pancreatic epithelium results in loss of pancreas marker expression and transformation of pancreatic mesenchyme into gut mesoderm[7,11]. By contrast, recent results show that Hedgehog signalling is required for insulin transcription and secretion in cultured insulinoma cells[15,16]. Furthermore, expression of Hedgehog signalling components, including the ligands *Ihh* and *Dhh*, as well as the receptor *Ptch*, are found by reverse transcriptase polymerase chain reaction (RT-PCR) in developing pancreatic tissue[17]. Thus, Hh signalling is active at low levels during pancreas organogenesis. In mice carrying the *LacZ* gene under control of the *Ptch* promoter, β-galactosidase activity is detected in mature pancreatic ducts and islets, a finding that further confirms active Hh signalling in adult pancreatic tissue. More importantly, it indicates that pancreatic duct cells, the putative progenitor cells of pancreatic adenocarcinoma, receive and respond to Hh signalling.

PATHWAY COMPONENTS THAT CAUSE CANCER

With the potential exception of colon carcinoma, ectopic activation of the Hedgehog signalling pathway has been implicated in tumour formation and progression[6,18,19]. Analysis of different tumour types has revealed mutations in several pathway components. For example, mutations in *SONIC HEDGEHOG* have been identified in basal cell carcinoma and medulloblastoma[20]. Furthermore, ectopic expression of *SHH* has been shown to result in basal cell carcinoma while mutations in *SMOOTHENED* and *GLI1* have been identified in basal cell carcinomas and gliomas, respectively[21,22]. Interestingly, ectopic expression of *Gli1* and *Gli2*, the most downstream components of the pathway, can induce tumour formation[23-25]. In addition, loss-of-function mutations have been identified in Hedgehog signalling components known to antagonize the activity of the pathway. Mutations in *PTCH1* and *SUFU* have been noted in medulloblastoma, and transgenic mice carrying the loss of one *Ptch1* allele develop defects similar to those observed in patients suffering from basal cell nevus syndrome (also known as Gorlin syndrome)[9]. These examples illustrate that ectopic activation of the Hedgehog signalling pathway can result in tumour formation in a variety of different tissues. However, increasing evidence suggests that normal levels of Hedgehog signalling are required for proper organ formation during embryogenesis and maintenance of adult tissue function, including maintenance of stem cell function[26]. Thus, it appears that the level of Hedgehog activity has to be tightly controlled to prevent unwanted effects on tissue organization and function.

HEDGEHOG SIGNALLING IN PANCREATIC CANCER

Our studies have shown that deregulation of this pathway is also implicated in the formation as well as maintenance of pancreatic adenocarcinoma[27]. Ectopic expression of *Sonic Hedgehog* under control of the *pancreatic and duodenal homeobox factor (Pdx-1)* promoter severely disrupts pancreas formation, and transgenic mice usually die within 3–4 weeks of age[7]. Within the pancreatic remnants, pancreatic lesions are found that resemble pancreatic intraepithelial neoplasia (PanIN) commonly observed in patients suffering from pancreatic adenocarcinoma[1]. In addition, signature mutations in the *K-ras* oncogene known to occur in almost all human PanIN[2] have also been found in a subset of the PanIN found in *Pdx1-Shh* transgenic mice. Thus, ectopic activation of the Hedgehog pathway during pancreas embryogenesis initiates the first steps of pancreatic cancer. However, an apparent caveat with this model is the fact that the pathway becomes activated during embryogenesis. Future studies should address whether deregulation of the pathway in mature pancreatic tissue is sufficient to induce formation of pancreatic neoplasia.

To determine whether Hedgehog signalling remains active in pancreatic tissue we performed RT-PCR experiments on a large number of human adenocarcinoma cell lines. A total of 26 lines were tested for expression of *GLI1*, *PTCH*, and *HIP1*, all of which are transcriptional target genes of Hedgehog signalling. In addition, we analysed the lines for expression of *SMOOTHENED*, a membrane protein known to be the 'bottleneck' of the signalling pathway, as all known Hedgehog signals require SMOOTHENED function. Cell lines were originally established either from primary tumours (e.g. the Panc series, Panc01.28–Panc10.05[28] or from liver, lymph node and spleen metastases (CFPAC1, Hs766T and SW1990, respectively). All lines tested expressed two or more components of Hh signalling, suggesting that the Hedgehog pathway is active in these tumour cells. Luciferase assays with reporter plasmids containing Gli-binding sites on a subset of these cell lines further confirmed the activity of the pathway[27].

Pancreatic adenocarcinomas are characterized by high metastatic potential, one of the parameters associated with the poor prognosis after diagnosis. As mentioned above, the pancreatic cells analysed also included a subset of lines that were derived from metastasis of primary pancreatic adenocarcinoma. In one set of lines the metastatic potential had been significantly increased via selection of metastatic variants from human pancreatic adenocarcinoma cells by using orthotopic implantation into immunocompromised nude mice[29]. Injection of the parental COLO 357 cells[30] resulted in the derivation of L3 cells that were subsequently used to generate the highly aggressive L3.6sl subclone. Interestingly, the expression of Hedgehog signalling components in parental and successor cells is maintained[27], suggesting that increased Hedgehog signalling might provide survival benefits to metastatic cells. Thus, active Hedgehog signalling appears to be a common feature of both primary tumours and metastasis-derived human pancreatic adenocarcinoma cell lines.

REQUIREMENT OF HEDGEHOG SIGNALLING FOR CANCER CELL SURVIVAL

While the Hedgehog signalling pathway is complex, with many distinct components, recent studies have identified a number of antagonists that specifically inhibit pathway activation[18]. The original compound identified is cyclopamine, a plant-derived steroid alkaloid that has been shown to specifically inhibit the function of SMOOTHENED through binding to the heptahelical bundle of the transmembrane protein[31]. To test the requirement of Hedgehog signalling in pancreatic cancer cells, five different cell lines were initially cultured with 10 µM cyclopamine for 7 days[27]. While control cultures grew normally, significant cell loss was observed in a subset of the cyclopamine-treated cell lines (CFPAC, L3.6sl, Panc5.04). Two cell lines (BxPC3, Panc1.28) did not show any obvious changes in cell morphology or number, further confirming previous results indicating that cyclopamine is not a general cell toxin but specifically inhibits the Hedgehog pathway. Cyclopamine inhibits SMO function and the observation that Panc1.28 cells are not affected by cyclopamine treatment further supports the specific activity of this compound.

To obtain more accurate information regarding the percentage of pancreatic cancer cell lines that rely on Hedgehog signalling for growth and survival, a total of 13 cell lines were tested for cyclopamine responsiveness[27]. Rather than relying on cell morphology to determine cell proliferation and survival, cells were incubated with CSFE, a fluorescent dye that permanently attaches to cells and their progeny. CSFE-labelled cells were treated with or without cyclopamine and analysed by fluorescent-activated cell sorting (FACS) to determine cell proliferation in individual cell lines. As expected, SMO-negative Panc1.28 cells did not show any effect upon treatment. By contrast, six of the remaining 12 cell lines showed markedly reduced proliferation in cyclopamine-treated cultures (five with strong response, one with marginal response), demonstrating that approximately 50% of pancreatic cancer cell lines are responsive to cyclopamine treatment[27]. These results are in line with the expectation that inhibition of the Hedgehog pathway at the level of SMO (early in the signalling cascade) cannot block potentially activating mutations downstream of SMO. Furthermore, mutations in *SMO* itself have been shown to cause pathway activation while being partially resistant to cyclopamine treatment[32]. Thus, future studies will address whether cyclopamine resistance observed in some cell lines is caused by mutations in *SMO* or by mutations in other Hedgehog signalling components downstream of *SMO*. Alternatively, deregulation of other signalling pathways that would not be affected by cyclopamine treatment could also substitute for loss of Hedgehog signalling.

In additional studies one control (BxPC3) and two cyclopamine-responsive cell lines (L3.6sl, Panc05.04) were injected subcutaneously into nude mice to test whether tumour growth can be blocked by cyclopamine treatment. Cyclopamine treatment resulted in a dramatic reduction in tumour mass varying from 50% to 60% reduction when cyclopamine was injected after tumours were palpable (delayed treatment) to 86% reduction compared to untreated controls when cyclopamine treatment was initiated at the same time as cells were transplanted (concurrent treatment). Thus, Hh signalling is essential for growth and survival of human pancreatic adenocarcinoma cells in cell culture and xenotransplanted tumours.

INTERACTION BETWEEN HEDGEHOG AND Wnt SIGNALLING

A particularly interesting but poorly understood aspect is the question of how the level of Hh signalling is regulated in pancreatic tissue and how interaction between independent signalling pathways controls tissue organogenesis. Studies in *Drosophila* and mouse have revealed interactions between the Wnt and Hedgehog signalling pathways in wing discs and limb buds, respectively[33–37]. Wnt ligands bind to frizzled receptors, thereby initiating a signalling cascade that results in nuclear localization of β-catenin (Figure 2A)[38]. The binding of β-catenin and TCF/LEF transcription factors induces expression of target genes, and Wnt signalling has been shown to maintain expression of Hedgehog ligands in both wing discs and limb buds. Conversely, Hedgehog activity is needed to stabilize Wnt expression in *Drosophila* wings[39,40], indicating that both pathways crossregulate each other's activity. Our preliminary results indicate that Hedgehog and Wnt signalling interact to govern pancreas formation. This raises the intriguing possibility that deregulation of Wnt signalling could also be implicated in formation and growth of pancreatic tumours.

Wnt SIGNALLING AND CANCER

Similar to Hedgehog signalling, deregulated Wnt signalling has been implicated in the formation of numerous cancers, mainly of gastrointestinal origin[38]. A number of Wnt signalling components, including the ligand *Wnt 2b, 5a, 5b, 7b, 11*, the receptors *Frizzled FZD3, FZD5, and FZD8*, the co-receptors *LRP5* and *LRP6*, as well as the transcriptional activator β-*catenin*, are expressed in pancreatic tissue[41–46]. More importantly, increasing evidence suggests that deregulation of the Wnt pathway contributes to pancreatic adenocarcinoma in humans and mice[45,47–49]. So far, the hypothesis that Wnt signalling plays a role in the formation or growth of pancreatic adenocarcinoma is mainly based on immunohistochemical staining that

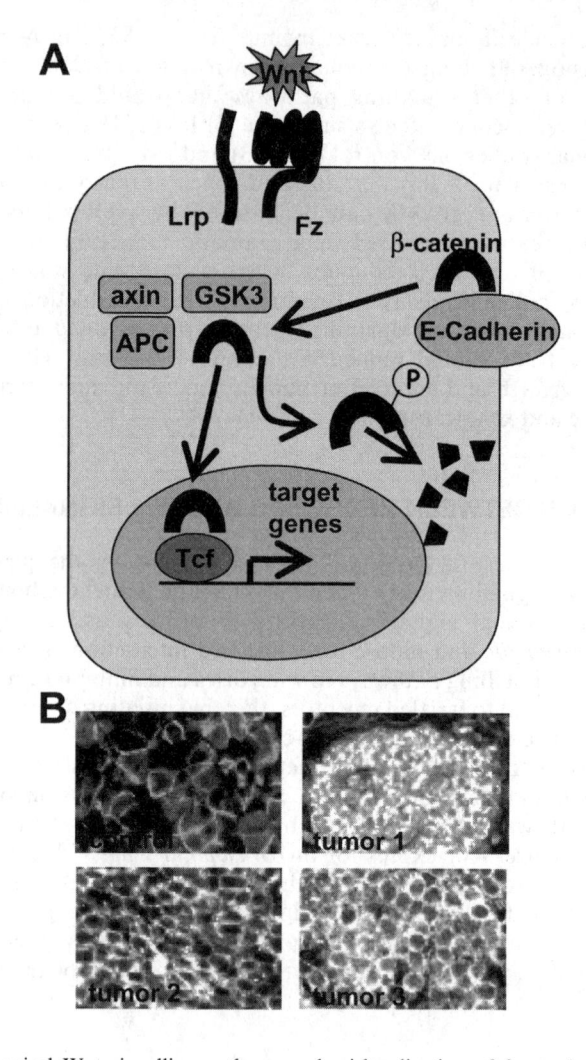

Figure 2 Canonical Wnt signalling pathway and mislocalization of β-catenin in pancreatic adenocarcinoma. **A**: Binding of Wnt ligands to the Frizzled receptor activates intracellular signals that allow β-catenin to translocate from the membrane, where it is normally bound to E-cadherin, to the cytoplasm and nucleus. Within the nucleus, β-catenin binds to TCF transcription factors to initiate transcription of Wnt target genes. In the absence of Wnt ligands, cytoplasmatic β–catenin becomes trapped in a multiprotein complex, including axin, GSK3, and APC, that results in β-catenin phosphorylation and degradation. Increasing evidence suggests that expression of cytoplasmic and nuclear β-catenin is upregulated in pancreatic adenocarcinoma. Lrp, co-receptor; Tcf/LEF, transcription factor family; Wnt, ligand. **B**: β-catenin expression pattern in normal adult pancreas and pancreatic adenocarcinoma. In untransformed tissue β-catenin is localized to the plasma membrane. In a subset of pancreatic adenocarcinoma an overall increase of β-catenin levels with cytoplasmic localization is observed. In few tumours nuclear β-catenin expression is found. Both increased cytoplasmic and nuclear β-catenin expression are indicative of increased Wnt activity

indicates pathway activation as measured by changes in protein localization of β-catenin (Figure 2B). Future studies will address whether increases in cytoplasmic and nuclear β-catenin localization that are known to occur in other gastrointestinal cancers mark a functional role for Wnt signalling in formation and maintenance of pancreatic adenocarcinoma. In addition, it will be important to test whether the activity of other embryonic signalling pathways involved in pancreatic cancer, e.g. Notch signalling[50], interacts with Hedgehog and/or Wnt pathways to regulate growth of pancreatic tumours. Unravelling these interactions is potentially important, as these studies might reveal novel targets for therapeutic intervention. Recent advances in biological chemistry have led to the identification of small chemical compounds that can be used to specifically block the function of embryonic signalling pathways[51,52]. Given the role these pathways play in other gastrointestinal tumours, future studies will address whether it is feasible to develop novel therapeutic strategies to combat pancreatic cancer that are based on the inhibition of embryonic signalling pathways.

Acknowledgements

M.H. was funded by grants from the NIH, Lustgarten Foundation, and the Juvenile Diabetes Research Foundation (JDRF).

References

1. Hruban RH, Adsay NV, Albores-Saavedra J et al. Pancreatic intraepithelial neoplasia: a new nomenclature and classification system for pancreatic duct lesions. Am J Surg Pathol. 2001;25:579–86.
2. Bardeesy N, DePinho RA. Pancreatic cancer biology and genetics. Nat Rev Cancer. 2002; 2:897–909.
3. Wang J, Wynshaw-Boris A. The canonical Wnt pathway in early mammalian embryogenesis and stem cell maintenance/differentiation. Curr Opin Genet Dev. 2004;14: 533–9.
4. Ingham PW, McMahon AP. Hedgehog signaling in animal development: paradigms and principles. Genes Dev. 2001;15:3059–87.
5. Nüsslein-Volhard C, Wieschaus E. Mutations affecting segment number and polarity in *Drosophila*. Nature. 1980;287:795–801.
6. Ruiz i Altaba A, Sanchez P, Dahmane N. Gli and hedgehog in cancer: tumours, embryos and stem cells. Nat Rev Cancer. 2002;2:361–72.
7. Apelqvist A, Ahlgren U, Edlund H. Sonic hedgehog directs specialised mesoderm differentiation in the intestine and pancreas. Curr Biol. 1997;7:801–4.
8. Chiang C, Litingtung Y, Lee E et al. Cyclopia and defective axial patterning in mice lacking sonic hedgehog function. Nature. 1996;383:407–13.
9. Goodrich LV, Milenkovic L, Higgins KM, Scott MP. Altered neural cell fates and medulloblastoma in mouse patched mutants. Science. 1997;277:1109–13.
10. Goodrich LV, Jung D, Higgins KM, Scott MP. Overexpression of ptc1 inhibits induction of Shh target genes and prevents normal patterning in the neural tube. Dev Biol. 1999;211: 323–34.
11. Hebrok M, Kim SK, Melton DA. Notochord repression of endodermal Sonic hedgehog permits pancreas development. Genes Dev. 1998;12:1705–13.
12. Motoyama J, Liu J, Mo R, Ding Q, Post M, Hui CC. Essential function of Gli2 and Gli3 in the formation of lung, trachea and oesophagus. Nat Genet. 1998;20:54–7.
13. Ramalho-Santos M, Melton DA, McMahon AP. Hedgehog signals regulate multiple aspects of gastrointestinal development. Development. 2000;127:2763–72.

14. Hebrok M. Hedgehog signaling in pancreas development. Mech Dev. 2003;20:45–57.
15. Thomas MK, Lee JH, Rastalsky N, Habener JF. Hedgehog signaling regulation of homeodomain protein islet duodenum homeobox-1 expression in pancreatic beta-cells. Endocrinology. 2001;142:1033–40.
16. Thomas MK, Rastalsky N, Lee JH, Habener JF. Hedgehog signaling regulation of insulin production by pancreatic beta-cells. Diabetes. 2000;49:2039–47.
17. Hebrok M, Kim SK, St Jacques B, McMahon AP, Melton DA. Regulation of pancreas development by Hedgehog signaling. Development. 2000;127:4905–13.
18. Pasca di Magliano M, Hebrok M. Hedgehog signaling in cancer formation and maintenance. Nature Rev Cancer. 2003;3:903–11.
19. van den Brink GR, Bleuming SA, Hardwick JC et al. Indian Hedgehog is an antagonist of Wnt signaling in colonic epithelial cell differentiation. Nat Genet. 2004;36:277–82.
20. Oro AE, Higgins KM, Hu Z, Bonifas JM, Epstein EH Jr, Scott MP. Basal cell carcinomas in mice overexpressing sonic hedgehog. Science. 1997;276:817–21.
21. Xie J, Murone M, Luoh SM et al. Activating Smoothened mutations in sporadic basal-cell carcinoma. Nature. 1998;391:90–2.
22. Kinzler KW, Bigner SH, Bigner DD et al. Identification of an amplified, highly expressed gene in a human glioma. Science. 1987;236:70–3.
23. Dahmane N, Lee J, Robins P, Heller P, Ruiz i Altaba A. Activation of the transcription factor Gli1 and the Sonic hedgehog signalling pathway in skin tumours. Nature. 1997;389:876–81.
24. Nilsson M, Unden AB, Krause D et al. Induction of basal cell carcinomas and trichoepitheliomas in mice overexpressing GLI-1. Proc Natl Acad Sci USA. 2000;97:3438–43.
25. Grachtchouk M, Mo R, Yu S et al. Basal cell carcinomas in mice overexpressing Gli2 in skin. Nat Genet. 2000;24:216–17.
26. Beachy PA, Karhadkar SS, Berman DM. Tissue repair and stem cell renewal in carcinogenesis. Nature. 2004;432:324–31.
27. Thayer SP, di Magliano MP, Heiser PW et al. Hedgehog is an early and late mediator of pancreatic cancer tumorigenesis. Nature. 2003;425:851–6.
28. Jaffee EM, Schutte M, Gossett J et al. Development and characterization of a cytokine-secreting pancreatic adenocarcinoma vaccine from primary tumors for use in clinical trials. Cancer J Sci Am. 1998;4:194–203.
29. Bruns CJ, Harbison MT, Kuniyasu H, Eue I, Fidler IJ. In vivo selection and characterization of metastatic variants from human pancreatic adenocarcinoma by using orthotopic implantation in nude mice. Neoplasia. 1999;1:50–62.
30. Morgan RT, Woods LK, Moore GE, Quinn LA, McGavran L, Gordon SG. Human cell line (COLO 357) of metastatic pancreatic adenocarcinoma. Int J Cancer. 1980;25:591–8.
31. Chen JK, Taipale J, Cooper MK, Beachy PA. Inhibition of Hedgehog signaling by direct binding of cyclopamine to Smoothened. Genes Dev. 2002;16:2743–8.
32. Taipale J, Chen JK, Cooper MK et al. Effects of oncogenic mutations in Smoothened and Patched can be reversed by cyclopamine. Nature. 2000;406:1005–9.
33. Berman DM, Karhadkar SS, Maitra A et al. Widespread requirement for Hedgehog ligand stimulation in growth of digestive tract tumours. Nature. 2003;425:846–51.
34. Tabata T, Kornberg TB. Hedgehog is a signaling protein with a key role in patterning Drosophila imaginal discs. Cell. 1994;76:89–102.
35. Yang Y, Niswander L. Interaction between the signaling molecules WNT7a and SHH during vertebrate limb development: dorsal signals regulate anteroposterior patterning. Cell. 1995;80:939–47.
36. Pinson KI, Brennan J, Monkley S, Avery BJ, Skarnes WC. An LDL-receptor-related protein mediates Wnt signalling in mice. Nature. 2000;407:535–8.
37. Parr BA, McMahon AP. Dorsalizing signal Wnt-7a required for normal polarity of D-V and A-P axes of mouse limb. Nature. 1995;374:350–3.
38. Lustig B, Behrens J. The Wnt signaling pathway and its role in tumor development. J Cancer Res Clin Oncol. 2003;129:199–221.
39. Hidalgo A. Interactions between segment polarity genes and the generation of the segmental pattern in Drosophila. Mech Dev. 1991;35:77–87.
40. Hidalgo A, Ingham P. Cell patterning in the Drosophila segment: spatial regulation of the segment polarity gene patched. Development. 1990;110:291–301.

41. Kirikoshi H, Sekihara H, Katoh M. Molecular cloning and characterization of human WNT11. Int J Mol Med. 2001;8:651–6.
42. Kirikoshi H, Koike J, Sagara N et al. Molecular cloning and genomic structure of human frizzled-3 at chromosome 8p21. Biochem Biophys Res Commun. 2000;271:8–14.
43. Saitoh T, Hirai M, Katoh M. Molecular cloning and characterization of human Frizzled-5 gene on chromosome 2q33.3-q34 region. Int J Oncol. 2001;19:105–10.
44. Saitoh T, Hirai M, Katoh M. Molecular cloning and characterization of human Frizzled-8 gene on chromosome 10p11.2. Int J Oncol. 2001;18:991–6.
45. Watanabe I, Hasebe T, Sasaki S et al. Advanced pancreatic ductal cancer: fibrotic focus and beta-catenin expression correlate with outcome. Pancreas. 2003;26:326–33.
46. Heller RS, Dichmann DS, Jensen J et al. Expression patterns of Wnts, Frizzleds, sFRPs, and misexpression in transgenic mice suggesting a role for Wnts in pancreas and foregut pattern formation. Dev Dyn. 2002;225:260–70.
47. Kongkanuntn R, Bubb VJ, Sansom OJ, Wyllie AH, Harrison DJ, Clarke AR. Dysregulated expression of beta-catenin marks early neoplastic change in Apc mutant mice, but not all lesions arising in Msh2 deficient mice. Oncogene. 1999;18:7219–25.
48. Karayiannakis AJ, Syrigos KN, Polychronidis A, Simopoulos C. Expression patterns of alpha-, beta- and gamma-catenin in pancreatic cancer: correlation with E-cadherin expression, pathological features and prognosis. Anticancer Res. 2001;21:4127–34.
49. Li YJ, Ji XR. Relationship between expression of E-cadherin-catenin complex and clinicopathologic characteristics of pancreatic cancer. World J Gastroenterol. 2003;9:368–72.
50. Miyamoto Y, Maitra A, Ghosh B et al. Notch mediates TGF alpha-induced changes in epithelial differentiation during pancreatic tumorigenesis. Cancer Cell. 2003;3:565–76.
51. Frank-Kamenetsky M, Zhang XM, Bottega S et al. Small-molecule modulators of Hedgehog signaling: identification and characterization of Smoothened agonists and antagonists. J Biol. 2002;1:10.
52. Lepourcelet M, Chen YN, France DS et al. Small-molecule antagonists of the oncogenic Tcf/beta-catenin protein complex. Cancer Cell. 2004;5:91–102.

Section VII
Intestinal disorders II

Chair: D.P. JEWELL and F. GUARNER

23
Does JC virus initiate chromosomal instability in colorectal cancer?

C. R. BOLAND, A. GOEL, L. LAGHI and L. RICCIARDIELLO

INTRODUCTION

It is currently appreciated that colorectal cancer (CRC) develops through a multistep process involving alterations at a number of critical genes that regulate growth and other cellular behaviours. In the case of CRC, the identity of many of these genes is known, at least in part. Several types of genetic alterations participate in the multistep carcinogenesis process[1]. Point mutations are typically alterations that change a single nucleotide and which lead to a structural change in the encoded protein. In some instances the point mutation leads to inappropriate activation of the gene, as in the case of Ras. In other instances the point mutation leads to loss of function of the gene, as occurs in APC or p53. However, it has been demonstrated that point mutations are not very common in CRC.

ALLELIC DELETIONS AND CHROMOSOMAL INSTABILITY (CIN)

A much more frequent genetic alteration that leads to the inactivation of a gene is its deletion from the genome. Allelic deletion has been termed loss of heterozygosity or 'LOH', based upon the techniques initially used to find this. If one hunts for LOH events in CRC, one finds a very large number of them; in fact, many more than would be needed for the generation of a tumour[2]. More than half of all CRC have widespread LOH events throughout the genome, and this has been attributed to a form of genomic instability called chromosomal instability, or CIN. CIN is the process that leads to aneuploidy, which is a ubiquitous feature of most cancers[3]. Although this phenomenon has been recognized for over a century, the mechanism responsible for it is unknown, in spite of the fact that it has been the focus of attention for a number of laboratories[4]. Many hypotheses have been proposed to account for this, including mutations in a number of genes involved in the orderly segregation of chromosomes at the time of mitosis. Unfortunately, in no instance are any of these mutations commonly found in tumours, and there is no unifying mechanism for CIN.

POLYOMAVIRUSES AND CANCER

Approximately 10 years ago our laboratory began exploring the possibility that a polyomavirus might be responsible for the process of CIN in colorectal cancer. The rationale for this hypothesis was that several members of the polyomavirus family are capable of transforming cells *in vitro* and, when they do so, aneuploidy is commonly a consequence. There is no question that SV40, the monkey virus discovered as a contaminant of the early batches of polio vaccine, has transforming ability by virtue of encoding of a T (or 'transforming') antigen. SV40 is a small (~ 5.2 kb), closed circular DNA virus that encodes for only six genes. When injected into experimental animals, tumours were a common result. Subsequently, the T antigen gene was developed for use in a variety of laboratory settings to immortalize cells. Although highly controversial, SV40 has been suggested as a possible cancer-causing human virus, particularly in the brain[5,6].

JC VIRUS (JVC)

There are two common (and a number of other less common) polyomaviruses that infect humans. JC virus (JCV) was first found in 1971 in the spinal fluid of a patient (whose initials were 'J.C.'), who had a lymphoma and was receiving immunosuppressive chemotherapy. The virus was recognized morphologically in the spinal fluid. JCV is a small (5.13 kb), closed circular DNA virus, structurally similar to the other polyomaviruses (see Figure 1). Subsequently, it has been recognized that, in patients with AIDS, JCV can become activated, which causes the demyelinating disease called progressive multifocal leucoencephalopathy (PML). A second, closely related virus is called BK virus, discovered at the same time as JCV in the urine of a renal transplant patient in Great Britain (whose initials were B.K.), and this virus also had tumorigenic properties in experimental animals[7].

However, nearly 90% of the population shows antibody titres to JCV, a phenomenon that can be seen in every part of the world. Thus, nearly all of mankind has been exposed to this virus[8]. It appears to be latent for most people for most of their lives, and may never lead to illness. In the case of PML, it can be reactivated and cause a deadly disease. Importantly, like the closely related virus SV40, injection of JCV into the central nervous systems of experimental animals (hamsters or monkeys) produces brain tumours.

In 1996, Neel et al. demonstrated a link between JCV and a type of aneuploid lymphocyte which they termed 'rogue' lymphocytes. Rogue lymphocytes appear to be harmless; however, Neel et al. suggested that this form of genomic instability might be triggered by an alteration in the virus. This group also demonstrated that inoculation of human fetal brain cells led to aneuploidy, similar to what was observed routinely with SV40[9].

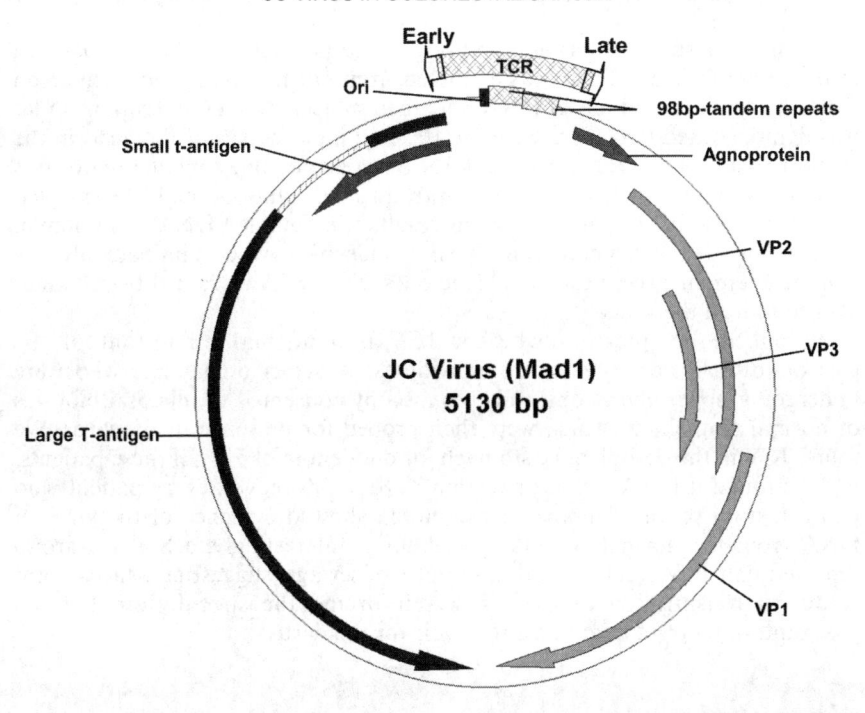

Figure 1 The JC viral genome (Mad-1 strain). JCV is a closed, circular, 5.13 kb DNA virus that encodes six genes. T antigen ('Large T') and t antigen ('small t'), are the 'early' genes, encoded counterclockwise from the bidirectional transcription control region (TCR). The late genes are the agnoprotein, and three viral capsid proteins VP1, VP2, and VP3. Ori refers to the origin of replication. The TCR contains a variable number of 98 base pair tandem repeats, two of which are seen in the Mad-1 sequence

JCV IS IN THE HUMAN COLON AND CRC

In response to Neel et al.'s provocative observation, we determined whether JCV DNA sequences might be present in specimens of CRC. We obtained a bank of DNA specimens extracted from frozen human CRC and, using the polymerase chain reaction (PCR), we were able to amplify JCV sequences from colon cancers and from the normal colon adjacent to the resected tumour specimen. The identities of the DNA sequences found by PCR were confirmed both by Southern blot and by cloning and sequencing the DNA sequences. The sequences were a match for JCV, but not for the closely related viruses BK virus and SV40. Several different genomic locations on the T antigen gene were amplified by PCR, and these results excluded the likelihood of laboratory contamination, or confusion with DNA from commonly used laboratory plasmids[10].

Because we had found the virus in both normal tissue and in cancer DNA, we proposed that it may exist in a latent form in the normal colonic epithelium but could undergo an alteration and become responsible for clonal expansion in the tumours. Thus, DNA was extracted from normal tissue and from colon cancers, identical amounts of DNA were then subjected to serial dilution, and it was demonstrated that there were 10–100-fold more copies of the virus in the tumour tissue than in the normal colon. Since one possible explanation for this observation was that lymphocytes infiltrating the tumours might be infected with the virus, and contaminating our results, we obtained DNA from human CRC xenografts, which had been grown in nude mice, which eliminates all cells from the tumour except the neoplastic ones. The DNA extracted from tissues also contained the virus[10].

We asked the question whether JCV is a normal inhabitant of the gastrointestinal tract of healthy individuals. A series of patients who were undergoing upper endoscopy and colonoscopy consented to mucosal biopsies of normal epithelium, which were then probed for presence of the virus. We found JCV in the oesophagus, stomach, or duodenum of 71% of these patients, and we found it in the colon or rectum of 81%. Moreover, every patient who had a history of an adenoma or carcinoma showed evidence of the virus in DNA from the normal colonic epithelium[11]. Interestingly, a Spanish group reported that JCV can be found in samples of sewage, suggesting a faecal–oral route of transmission of the virus, reinforcing the speculation that the gastrointestinal tract might be a reservoir for this virus[12].

THE TRANSCRIPTION CONTROL REGION (TCR) OF JCV

These findings raised the question whether some alteration in viral gene expression might be caused by a rearrangement in the promoter sequences of the virus. The JCV promoter is referred to as the transcription control region or 'TCR'. The TCR of JCV is a 350–400-nucleotide sequence immediately adjacent to the origin of replication of the virus. It is a bidirectional promoter. In the counterclockwise direction it mediates the transcription of the JCV T antigen gene, which is an 'early gene' in the life cycle of this virus. In the clockwise direction of transcription in this circular virus the TCR mediates the expression of the late genes, which include three viral capsid genes (VP1, VP2, and VP3), and a protein involved in viral assembly called the agnoprotein. Interestingly, the T antigen can be alternately spliced into two functionally different protein products referred to as large T and small t antigens. Both of these gene products have separate roles in maintaining transformation of cells. Furthermore, the early gene products (T, t) are involved in increasing expression of the late genes[13].

A very large number of rearrangements have been reported in the TCR from JCV. Many of these result in length polymorphisms, which can be readily detected by PCR. We screened approximately 250 clones of JCV from normal colons and colon cancers, and then subsequently subjected these to DNA sequence analysis. First, we found that all of the TCR from JCV found in the gut were the Mad-1 strain, representing a family of promoter sequences. Within the Mad-1 family of promoters we found additional TCR rearrangements. Interestingly, we found nearly all of the rearrangements in the specimens of cancer, and rarely found them in the normal colon. All eight of the colon cancer specimens had at least one rearranged Mad-1 TCR (and this represented 22/128 clones), whereas we found a rearranged Mad-1 TCR in only 1/156 clones from the normal colon. Thus, we have hypothesized that the rearrangements of the Mad-1 promoter may be involved in altering the transcription activity of JCV, which may play a role in carcinogenesis[14].

Having found JCV in most colon cancers we turned our attention to *in-vitro* models to determine whether JCV can infect human colonic epithelial cells. First, we obtained from Kazuo Nagashima (Hokkaido University School of Medicine, Japan) a cell line, JCI, which is productive of JCV. Three different models have been developed which indicate that this virus can induce CIN in diploid cells (unpublished).

INDUCTION OF ANEUPLOIDY BY JCV IN A DIPLOID COLON CELL LINE

The JCV genome was cloned into the pBR322 plasmid, and then transfected into the RKO colon cancer cell line. RKO is a diploid cell line with microsatellite instability secondary to hypermethylation-induced silencing of the hMLH1 promoter. This cell line has wild-type p53, APC, and β-catenin genes. After transfection of the plasmid containing the JCV genome into this cell line, integration of JCV was demonstrated, and T antigen protein expression occurred within 7 days. In addition, the capsid protein VP1 was also expressed, indicating expression of the late genes, similar to what would occur in a replicating virus, although this occurred in the early phases and at a very low level, indicating early replication[15].

Expression of T antigen induced nuclear β-catenin expression in the RKO cells, which does not occur in the uninfected cells, as the APC and β-catenin genes are not mutated in this model. Moreover, dual immunofluorescence studies demonstrated co-localization of β-catenin and T antigen when the latter gene was expressed, and this finding was confirmed by immunoprecipitation experiments. In the RKO model, p53 expression increased after JCV genome transfection, and immunostaining and immunoprecipitation experiments confirmed the interaction between T antigen and p53 in transfected cells.

Most importantly, transfection of the JCV genome into RKO cells induced CIN within seven days. Thus, introduction of the JCV genome into the diploid cell line RKO led to stabilization and nuclear localization of β-catenin, interaction between T antigen and p53, and the induction of CIN[15].

Finally, the fact that T antigen can stabilize β-catenin, and leads to its nuclear localization, would suggest that the neoplastic phenotype could occur even prior to the loss of the APC gene. In collaboration with Dennis Ahnen (University of Colorado, USA) and Michiko Iwamoto (Jichi Medical School, Japan), immunohistochemistry and loss of heterozygosity experiments were performed with a series of small adenomas. In these experiments the stabilization of β-catenin preceded the loss of heterozygosity on chromosome 5q and loss of APC staining by immunohistochemistry (unpublished results).

SUMMARY

In summary, JCV is present in the gastrointestinal tract of most healthy people. An increase in copy numbers is found in the DNA of colorectal cancers. We have evidence that JCV can induce CIN in several models and, in particular, can result in the stabilization of β-catenin, an interaction with p53, and the induction of CIN in the RKO diploid colon cancer cell line. Future studies will be directed towards determination of the mechanism by which the latent form of the virus can be converted into one that can induce CIN, and the long-term goal will be to determine whether immunization against this virus might be a reasonable strategy to prevent CRC.

Reference

1. Vogelstein B, Fearon ER, Hamilton SR et al. Genetic alterations during colorectal-tumor development. N Engl J Med. 1988;319:525–32.
2. Vogelstein B, Fearon ER, Kern SE et al. Allelotype of colorectal carcinomas. Science. 1989;244:207–11.
3. Lengauer C, Kinzler KW, Vogelstein B. Genetic instability in colorectal cancers. Nature. 1997;386:623–7.
4. Wang Z, Cummins JM, Shen D et al. Three classes of genes mutated in colorectal cancers with chromosomal instability. Cancer Res. 2004;64:2998–3001.
5. Butel JS, Jafar S, Stewart AR, Lednicky JA. Detection of authentic SV40 DNA sequences in human brain and bone tumours. Dev Biol Stand. 1998;94:23–32.
6. Carbone M, Bocchetta M, Cristaudo A et al. SV40 and human brain tumors. Int J Cancer. 2003;106:140–2.
7. Imperiale MJ. The human polyomaviruses, BKV and JCV: molecular pathogenesis of acute disease and potential role in cancer. Virology. 2000;267:1–7.
8. Brown P, Tsai T, Gajdusek DC. Seroepidemiology of human papovaviruses. Discovery of virgin populations and some unusual patterns of antibody prevalence among remote peoples of the world. Am J Epidemiol. 1975;102:331–40.
9. Neel JV, Major EO, Awa AA et al. Hypothesis: 'Rogue cell'-type chromosomal damage in lymphocytes is associated with infection with the JC human polyoma virus and has implications for oncogenesis. Proc Natl Acad Sci USA. 1996;93:2690–5.
10. Laghi L, Randolph AE, Chauhan DP et al. JC virus DNA is present in the mucosa of the human colon and in colorectal cancers. Proc Natl Acad Sci USA. 1999;96:7484–9.
11. Ricciardiello L, Laghi L, Ramamirtham P et al. JC virus DNA sequences are frequently present in the human upper and lower gastrointestinal tract. Gastroenterology. 2000;119:1228–35.
12. Bofill-Mas S, Girones R. Role of the environment in the transmission of JC virus. J Neurovirol. 2003;9(Suppl. 1):54–8.
13. Raj GV, Khalili K. Transcriptional regulation: lessons from the human neurotropic polyomavirus, JCV. Virology. 1995;213:283–91.
14. Ricciardiello L, Chang DK, Laghi L, Goel A, Chang CL, Boland CR. Mad-1 is the exclusive JC virus strain present in the human colon, and its transcriptional control region has a deleted 98-base-pair sequence in colon cancer tissues. J Virol. 2001;75:1996–2001.
15. Ricciardiello L, Baglioni M, Giovannini C et al Induction of chromosomal instability in colonic cells by the human polyomavirus JC virus. Cancer Res. 2003;63:7256–62.

24
Testing the gut and its function – faecal samples – breath tests and more?

I. BJARNASON, L. MAIDEN and K. TAKEUCHI

INTRODUCTION

The history of medicine is in many respects not too dissimilar from the trends that we see in popular culture in respect of fashion, where designer clothes come and go with old themes re-emerging when least expected. This is well illustrated in gastroenterology, whereby late nineteenth- and early twentieth-century physicians designed numerous non-invasive methods for assessing gastrointestinal function which were indicative of diseases that led to therapeutic interventions (not particularly effective by modern standards) and often surprisingly accurate predictions of prognosis. In the early part of the latter half of the twentieth century the investigation of gastrointestinal disorders was characterized by the availability of numerous absorption tests, not least gastric acid secretion tests, and faecal tests. However, practices changed dramatically with the introduction of flexible endoscopy, so much that nowadays a significant proportion of the population in developed countries have been subjected to endoscopy in one form or other, the wireless capsule enteroscope being the latest development. The functional tests then fell into disrepute, and we have grown accustomed to treating diseases according to morphology rather than by the degree of malfunction (which cannot be assessed from visualization of the bowel). Although non-invasive tests of intestinal function have been, and continue to be, developed by a handful of investigators, most gastroenterologists do not use them. There are many reasons for this; perhaps the most important one is that there is no financial remuneration for doing these tests, trainees are not taught about them and accordingly there is little pressure for clinical biochemistry laboratories to offer them as a service. However, those that are involved in developing these tests foresee a bright future as conservative self-serving interests give way to patient interest.

There is a rheumatological analogy to this way of thinking. The treatment of rheumatoid arthritis, for instance, has been transformed from simple management of symptoms (analgesic anti-inflammatory drug treatment) to therapeutic interventions with a whole variety of second-line agents (that modify the natural history of disease) that are largely used according to laboratory parameters. Some of us foresee a similar development within gastroenterology, which will benefit patients with many gastrointestinal diseases. For instance it is now possible to predict accurately which patients with clinically quiescent inflammatory bowel disease are at significant risk of clinical relapse[1-5]. This, of course, offers the opportunity to specifically treat the inflammatory component of the disease and hence potentially to alter the natural history of inflammatory bowel disease. Here we review some of the potential uses of the 'newer generation' of non-invasive functional tests.

THE OLD AND TESTED

Intestinal absorption and permeability

The small bowel has the apparent paradoxical function of simultaneously facilitating and limiting the permeation of molecules across the mucosa. The way it achieves this is not significantly different from other mammals, and these functions are, of course, the final outcome of millions of years of evolution. The main determinant of the absorptive capacity of the small bowel is its enormous effective surface area (length of small bowel 5–8 m with mucosal folds, villi and microvilli) approximating the size of a tennis court, trans-membranous brush-border carriers (that are conventionally classified as aqueous pores, active and passive carrier-mediated transporters) for hydrophilic substances and the composition of the lipophilic brush-border membrane which, along with luminal factors such as bile acids, regulate the amount of fat absorbed[6]. The size of the absorbed substrate is important, as well as its water- and lipid-solubility, and there appears to be a cut-off point whereby the permeation of hydrophilic molecules of molecular weight over 200–300 Da (equivalent to $\geqslant 0.5$ nm molecular radius) is very poor, presumably as their permeation is then confined to the paracellular route[7,8]. The permeation of lipid-soluble compounds is far less restricted (transcelluar) and even compounds of molecular weight over 1000 Da can partition across the intestinal mucosa in significant quantities.

Most of the essential nutrients, along with water and electrolytes that are required to sustain life, are absorbed as small water-soluble molecules, and are then metabolically incorporated into the macromolecular machinery of the organism, while many of the more toxic compounds (many bacterial degradation products) are large macromolecules of mixed solubility, which renders them poorly absorbed. By careful consideration of these characteristics and normal human biochemistry and physiology we are able to successfully design non-invasive tests (urinary excretion rates following oral administration) that are relevant for absorption–nutrition as well as the intestinal barrier function which requires somewhat more complicated methods[9].

The requirements of a suitable absorptive test substance are well documented[6,7]. For the non-invasive assessment of monosaccharide absorptive capacity there are three well-established probes. These are:

1. 3-O-methyl-D-glucose, which uses the intestinal glucose transporters (active carrier-mediated absorption)

2. D-xylose, which uses a passive carrier-mediated transport system (facilitated diffusion). The main drawback with this probe is that there is variable hepatic metabolism, so that urinary excretions underestimate somewhat the amount absorbed. It follows that chronic liver disease may affect the test procedure.

3. L-rhamnose or mannitol that permeate via aqueous pores in the brush-border membrane by passive diffusion.

It is problematic to assess amino-acid absorption non-invasively as there are no readily available analogues that resist metabolic activity and that are quantitatively excreted in urine after intravenous instillation. Similarly lipid-soluble probes are retained within the body following absorption, which means that investigation of lipid malabsorption requires a different approach.

Tests of intestinal permeability were introduced with a view to investigate the intestinal barrier function; indeed these terms are often regarded as synonymous. Such investigations may relate to at least three purposes. These are:

1. The detection of intestinal disease, e.g. clinical screening tests.

2. To monitor responses to therapy and confirmation of diagnosis (e.g. gluten withdrawal and challenge in coeliac disease).

3. To assess the importance of the intestinal barrier function in the aetiology, pathophysiology and pathogenesis of intestinal and systemic disease.

Unfortunately there has been a tendency to underestimate the complexity of factors affecting the outcome of these non-invasive procedures, as well as the marker analyses, but there are some excellent and detailed papers relating to this subject[6,7,9,10].

Perhaps the most important point of note concerning tests of intestinal absorption and permeability is that they use hydrophilic–lipophobic markers. This is particularly important for interpretation of increased intestinal permeability as the permeability increase may not apply to the molecules (most bacterial toxins have mixed solubility) that are mostly implicated in local and systemic problems. Nevertheless there is a remarkable correlation between increased intestinal permeability and intestinal inflammation[11]. The clinical implications of intestinal inflammation, on the other hand, relate to its intensity (inflammatory bowel disease) and complications of blood and protein loss[12].

The insurmountable problem that we face with the use of a macromolecular probe marker that is amphipathic is the variable retention within the body, variable protein binding and thus very erratic and incomplete urinary excretion. This might be overcome by integrating the amounts appearing in serum after oral ingestion with the disappearance curve following intravenous administration, but such methods[13] would be useful only in the experimental setting.

In the society of plenty, malnutrition due to dietary factors is rare, and diagnosis is straightforward. However, distinguishing between diseases presenting with maldigestion and malabsorption requires targeted investigation. Perhaps the best disease to demonstrate the use of absorption-permeability tests and other non-invasive small bowel tests is by reviewing the data from patients with HIV AIDS.

HIV AIDS

Intestinal absorption

Prior to the introduction of effective treatments for HIV, patients with advanced AIDS had a particularly miserable downhill course in their final months of life, characterized by severe diarrhoea, loss of appetite and wasting[14,15]. The question was whether the loss of weight was due to malabsorption as well as reduced food intake. Figure 1 shows a representative absorption study in HIV-infected patients at various stages of their disease[16]. There is clearly malabsorption of 3-O-methyl-D-glucose, and even more severe malabsorption of D-xylose. The malabsorption was proportional to and correlated significantly with the degree of immune suppression and not the mucosal abnormalities seen on jejunal biopsy (or the results of intestinal microbiology)[16]. The severity of the malabsorption in advanced AIDS was in many cases more severe than that seen in coeliac disease. Indeed in some patients it was so severe as to preclude any attempts at improving nutritional status by administering orally certain chemically defined liquid diets (such as elemental diet or peptide–protein-based ones). These attempts failed. An unexpected feature of pressing ahead with oral (nasogastric or through a percutaneous gastrostomy) treatment with liquid diets was that patients experienced severe nausea with projectile vomiting. This was very unlike what was seen in other diseases, such as when elemental diets are used as primary treatment for Crohn's disease[17].

There are a number of studies that show the importance of these absorption tests in clinical practice as well as in research. There are two particularly good examples of this. First Wicks et al. assessed if it was essential to administer nutrition parenterally after liver transplants, as was the routine at the time[18]. The prevalent thought was that, following major surgery, there was gastrostasis and an ileus that precluded attempts at oral intake. However, when patients were studied in the days following liver transplants it was evident (provided that the test substances were administered intrajejunally) that the surgery (or the postoperative ileus) did not interfere with absorption. Jejunal administration of elemental diets were therefore tried, and patients tolerated the feeds well. As a result of this study most patients undergoing liver

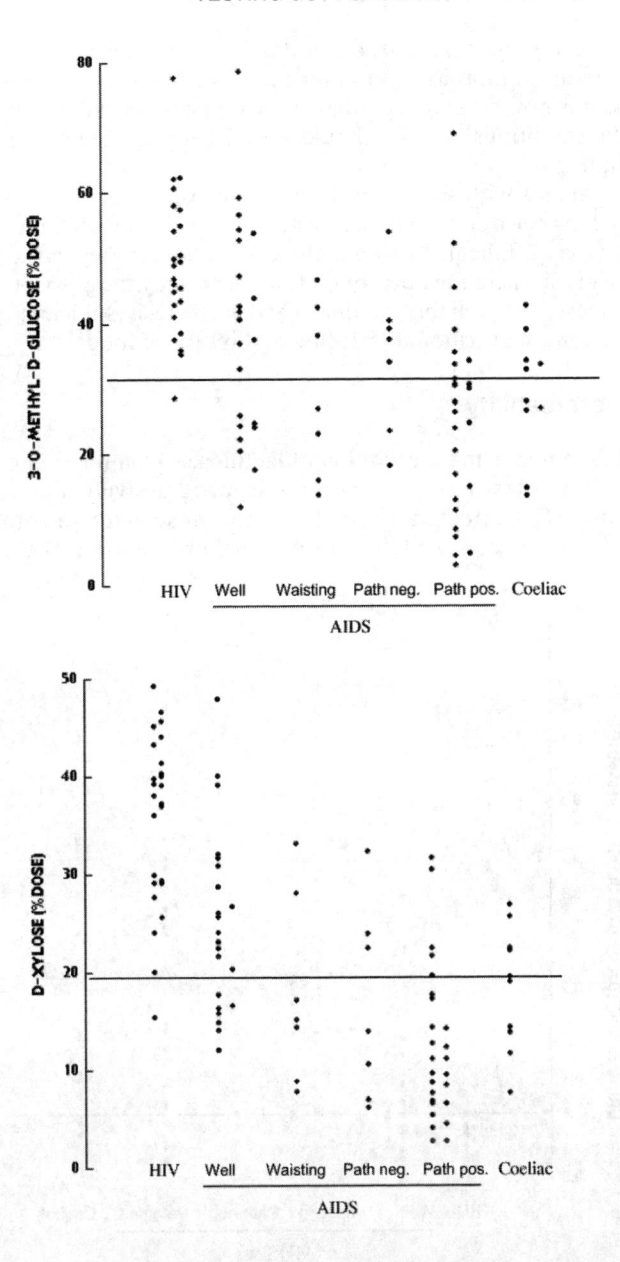

Figure 1 Five-h urinary excretion of 3-*O*-methy-D-glucose and D-xylose in patients with HIV AIDS and untreated coeliac disease. Many patients with AIDS have malabsorption of both monosaccharides, which is in many cases more severe than in patients with coeliac disease. The AIDS patients are grouped according to clinical well-being with the most immune-compromised being in the pathogen-negative and -positive group (all of whom had diarrhoea). The horizontal line indicates the lower limit of normal for the absorption of the sugars

transplants today receive enteral nutrition postoperatively. This has significantly reduced morbidity and mortality, and it comes with considerable cost savings. It is now clear that jejunal feeds are possible and effective in other postoperative conditions[19,20]. We should soon be seeing the final days of total parenteral nutrition.

Secondly, patients with short bowel syndrome, especially children, are often managed by long-term total parenteral nutrition, with predictable morbidity. However, it is very difficult to assess clinically whether they can tolerate full oral intake. This is where the absorption tests, especially the absorption of 3-O-methyl-D-glucose, can reliably predict whether there is sufficient absorptive capacity to maintain nutritional status by oral intake of food[21,22].

Intestinal permeability

Using the differential urinary excretion of lactulose/L-rhamnose it can be seen (Figure 2) that intestinal permeability is progressively impaired from asymptomatic HIV-infected individuals to those with cryptosporidial diarrhoea in advanced AIDS. Many workers related the increased

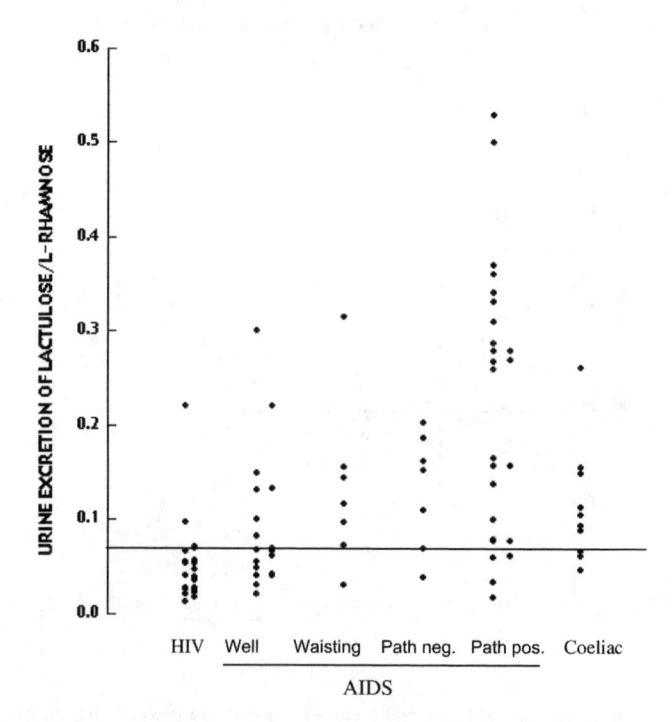

Figure 2 Intestinal permeability (differential urinary excretion of lactulose/L-rhamnose in 5-h urines). Patients with AIDS have increased intestinal permeability proportional to the degree of immune suppression. This permeability increase is in many cases greater than that seen in patients with untreated coeliac disease. The horizontal line indicates the upper limit of normal for the differential urinary excretion of lactulose/L-rhamnose

permeability to the precise infectious agent found in the stool of these patients. However, there is an interdependence between the degree of immune suppression and infection, and it now seems clear that the increased intestinal permeability relates best to the degree of immune suppression (CD4 counts)[16]. The precise clinical implications of increased intestinal permeability in HIV AIDS needs to be judged in a wider context, as discussed above, but there is no doubt that the permeability tests have identified a number of small bowel disease where none was thought to exist[11,23].

Intestinal inflammation

The gold standard for assessing intestinal inflammation is the faecal excretion of ^{111}Indium white cells (predominantly neutrophils). However, this requires specialized labelling facilities, involves radiation comparable to a barium enema and is demanding, as complete stool collections are required over 4 days.

A more convenient way of assessing intestinal inflammation is analysis of calprotectin, a neutrophil selective protein that resists bacterial degradation, in single stool samples. The method has been extensively validated[24-27] and is suitable as a screening test in children[28,29], as well as adults with abdominal symptoms. The importance of measuring calprotectin in stool rather than serum is its specificity for intestinal disorders. Other faecal markers in development, such as lactoferrin, may very well be equally suitable for assessing intestinal inflammation[30], but there has been surprisingly little validation data published with this probe[31].

Assessment of intestinal inflammation in HIV AIDS mirrors the intestinal permeability results with a moderate increase (2–3-fold) in inflammatory activity[32]. The clinical importance of this inflammation is again uncertain, and needs to be assessed in the wider context of intestinal function in HIV AIDS. The location of the inflammation in HIV AIDS appears to be in the distal ileum (from scintigraphic studies)[32]. The natural continuation of these studies was therefore to assess ileal function.

Ileal function

Ileal disease can be diagnosed during ileocolonoscopy, sonde enteroscopy and somewhat less satisfactorily by small bowel barium studies (preferably enteroclyses). However, capsule enteroscopy is poised to make a significant impact on visualizing small bowel diseases, and it seems probable that it will supersede barium studies. Unfortunately, the capsule imaging method has not been used in HIV AIDS, so that we do not know precisely the true prevalence of ileal mucosal inflammation and ulceration in these patients. However, the terminal ileum is the site of two specialized processes, namely vitamin B_{12} and bile acid absorption. When these functions are studied in patients with AIDS (Figure 3) and Crohn's ileitis it is clear that both vitamin B_{12} and SeHCAT (bile acid malabsorption) are severely impaired in both conditions[32]. This suggests that one of the mechanisms in HIV AIDS diarrhoea may involve bile acid malabsorption, and that Questran may be beneficial.

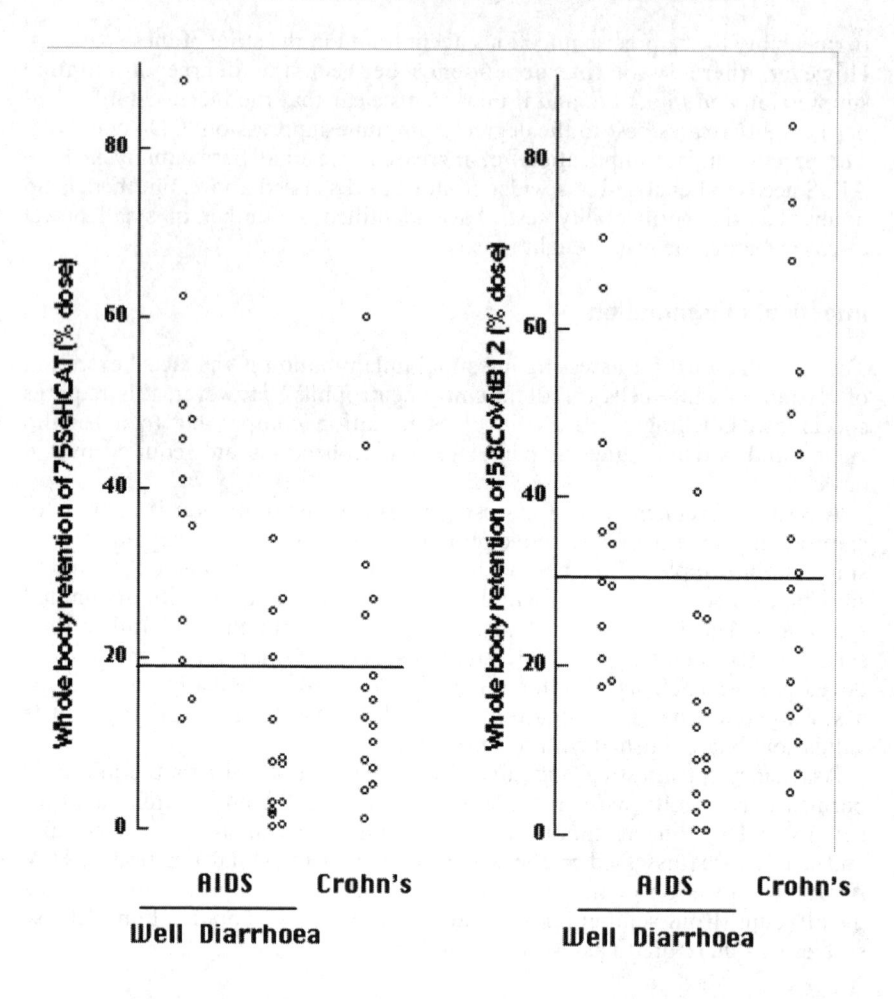

Figure 3 The whole body retention of radiolabelled SeHCAT and vitamin B_{12} following oral administration in patients with AIDS and terminal ileal Crohn's disease. The degree of malabsorption of the two markers in patients with AIDS and diarrhoea is in many cases more severe than seen in Crohn's ileitis

Transit tests

The combination of early satiety, nausea and vomiting, along with watery diarrhoea, is reminiscent of the effect of an autonomic neuropathy in diabetic patients (characterized by gastrostasis and rapid intestinal transit). Available transit tests (liquid or solid meals) assess oral to caecum transit so that any change in small bowel transit may be underestimated. In order to overcome these problems a new test was designed from a previously published blueprint[33] which involves ingestion of 3-O-methyl-D-glucose (absorbed from the duodenum; its first presence in serum gives the gastric emptying time) and sulphasalazine with measurement of the monosaccharide and sulphapyridine (sulphasalazine is degraded by colonic bacteria (azo-reductase) rendering sulphapyridine) in serum over the next few hours[34]. The time of appearance of sulphapyridine less that of 3-O-methyl-D-glucose gives the small bowel transit time. Figure 4 shows the results in a patient with AIDS where the gastric emptying time is severely prolonged while small intestinal transit is very rapid. This in turn explains why the bile acid malabsorption (above) may be so severe in HIV AIDS, as it is caused by an inflammatory process as well as rapid transit.

Small bowel bacterial overgrowth

There are virtually dozens of tests to document small bowel overgrowth. Direct intubations with culture (presence of coliform bacteria) is the most widely accepted test, but it is invasive and only samples a small part of the small bowel. Breath tests employing labelled glucose, D-xylose, lactulose and other degradable sugars have been successfully used to document non-specific small intestinal bacterial overgrowth, but a rapid intestinal transit may give false-positive results. As small intestinal transit is so rapid in HIV AIDS these non-invasive tests are unreliable. A way to overcome this is to combine the breath tests with the transit test, as the latter would overcome these shortcomings. Furthermore, if the above transit test is carried out, there is a low level of sulphapyridine in the serum (small bowel coliform bacteria have azo-reductase) before the major increase occurs on arrival at the caecum, and this is excellent evidence for coliform overgrowth in the small bowel[34].

Intestinal disaccharidase activities

Intestinal disaccharidase deficiencies can be primary (genetic) or secondary to intestinal diseases. There is no shortage of tests to diagnose intestinal disaccharidase deficiency. The crudest is simply to place patients on a low lactose-containing diet or to administer a test dose of milk (lactose) and assess symptomatic responses. Others utilize the breath test principle, but this is subject to the same problems as the small bowel bacterial overgrowth breath tests, the test results are not quantitative, and they do not discriminate between primary and secondary disaccharidase deficiencies.

Menzies and co-workers overcame most of these problems by designing a combined absorption–permeability–disaccharidase test[35]. The test exploits the so-called 'principle of differential urinary excretion' of sugars[7]. In short the test contains absorption markers (3-O-methyl-D-glucose, D-xylose and L-rhamnose), intestinal permeability markers (lactulose/L-rhamnose) and the disaccharides lactose, sucrose and palatinose, all of which are hydrolysed by different disaccharidases[36,37]. The differential urinary excretion of these sugars after ingestion (lactose/lactulose, sucrose/lactulose, palatinose/lactulose) relates inversely to the degree of disaccharidase impairment in the small bowel[37]. At the same time the test indicated if the disaccharidase deficiency is

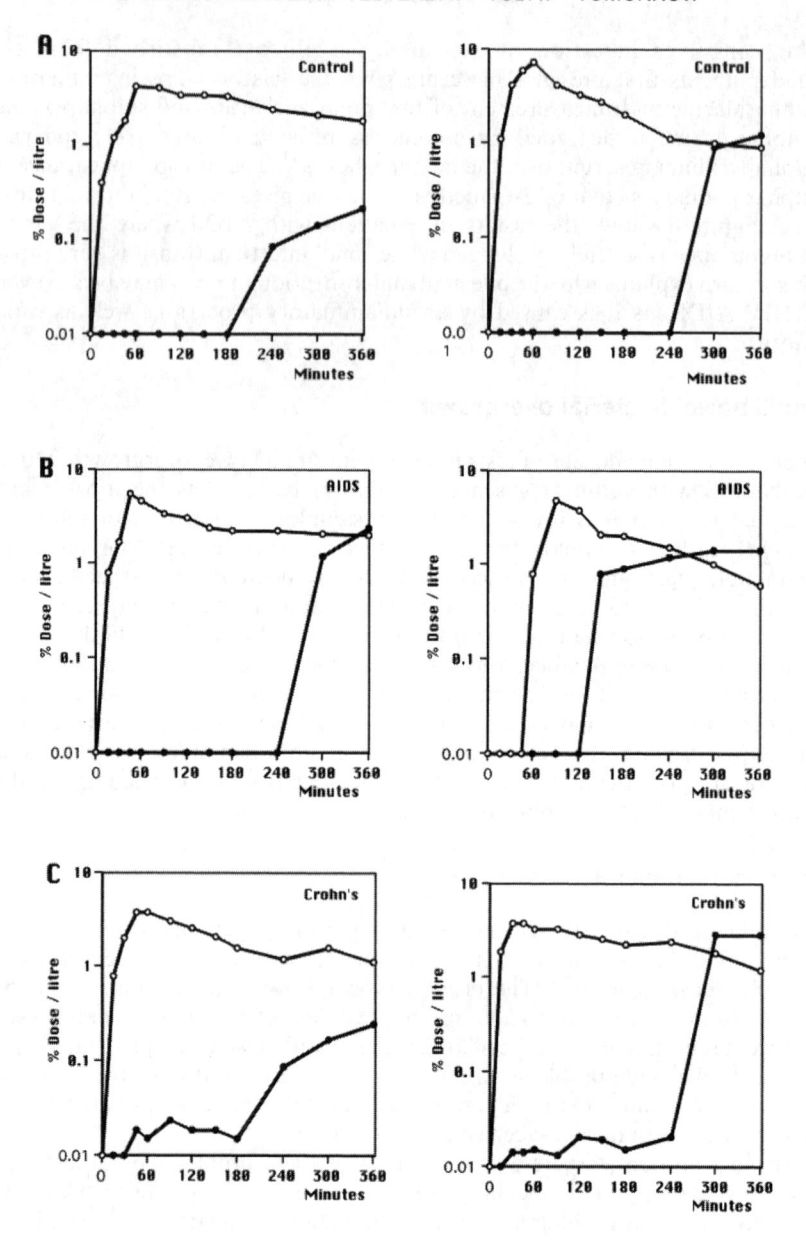

Figure 4 Serum profile of 3-*O*-methyl-D-glucose (open circle) and sulphapyridine (closed circle) after oral administration in **A**: normal subjects demonstrating a gastric emptying time of 15 min or less and a gastric to caecal transit time of 4–5 h; **B**: a well patient with AIDS on the left, demonstrating a normal profile, and on the right an AIDS patient with delayed gastric emptying (60 min) and a small intestinal transit of 2 h or less; **C**: two patients with ileal Crohn's disease, demonstrating normal profiles apart from the low levels of sulphapyridine, which suggest small bowel bacterial overgrowth

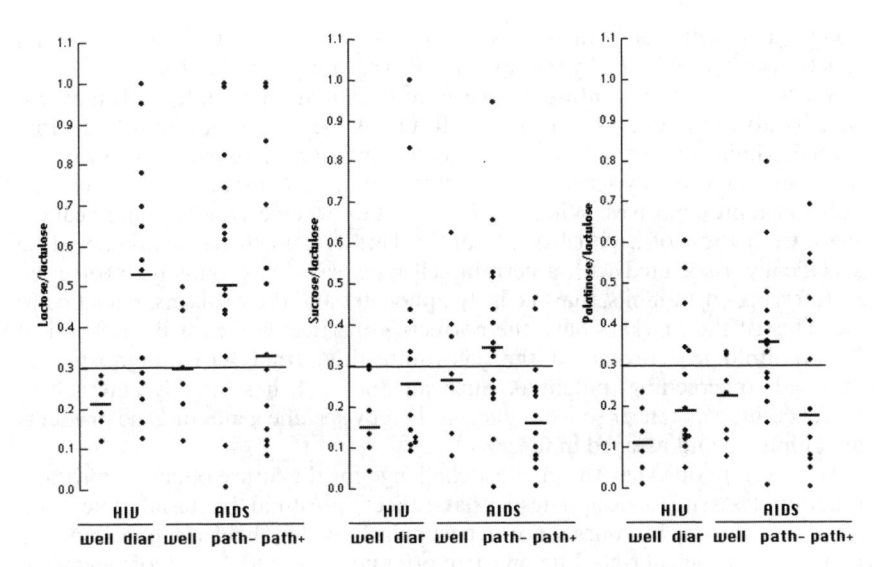

Figure 5 *In-vivo* intestinal disaccharidase activities. Each graph shows the differential urinary excretion (10 h) of a hydrolysable and non-hydrolysable (lactulose) disaccharidase after their oral administration. The upper limit of normal is represented by the horizontal line (0.3). Above this value represents increasing severity of loss of disaccharidase activities. Lactose/lactulose represents lactase activity, sucrose/lactulose sucrase activity, and palatinose/lactulose palatinase activity. Intestinal disaccharidase activities are impaired in most of the HIV AIDS groups. As there is a decline in all of the disaccharides this represents secondary damage as opposed to genetic variants. The test solution also contained absorption and permeability markers that provided further information on intestinal function

confined to a single enzyme (genetic) or more (secondary) with a concomitant change in intestinal permeability adding further weight for a secondary deficiency.

Using the combined test in patients with HIV AIDS (Figure 5) it is clear that a clinically significant secondary intestinal disaccharidase deficiency is evident. Furthermore in combination with the above findings (showing maldigestion, malabsorption and rapid intestinal transit) it suggests that the intestinal 'failure' in AIDS is so severe (and difficult to treat) because there are so many functional aspects to the symptoms.

THE FUTURE?

There are a number of intestinal tests that are difficult to better, such as the [51]chromium red blood cell test and [51]chromium labelled albumin for intestinal bleeding and protein loss, respectively, but these are no longer used except for research purposes. Similarly tests for quantitating fat maldigestion–malabsorption are now clinically obsolete, as current technology allows us to pinpoint the defects by other means. What is increasingly clear is that our ability to invent non-invasive tests that accurately reflect certain intestinal functions is limited only by the myopia of the grant-giving bodies.

Where do we see the future in respect of intestinal function tests? It may not be advisable to pierce too far into the future as the visionaries, mostly doctors turned administrators–politicians who have little or no research skills (young man/woman look at your head of institution!), are as unreliable as our elected political representatives. What is almost certain to emerge in coming years is the introduction of a panel of faecal markers[31,38]. Each test marker will be specifically associated with a certain cell type, say neutrophils (calprotectin–lactoferrin), eosinophils, mast cells, lymphocytes and their subsets, goblet cells, etc. This (if the markers have the correct properties) will provide a chemical histopathological profile of the gastrointestinal tract with diagnostic, as opposed to screening, potential. Such an approach has already emerged in faecal colorectal cancer screening tests whereby specific genes or gene products are amplified and assayed in faeces.

However, in our view the greatest challenge for the future of gastrointestinal function tests is to design tests that reflect intestinal bacterial types and function. This is, of course, not a particularly widely held opinion, but one that is worth considering. Life on earth originated around 3.5 billion years ago in the form of anaerobic prokaryotes (cells lacking a defined nucleus), subdivided into the superkingdoms of Bacteria and Archaea[39,40]. Over the next billion years developing microbes transformed earth's surface and, more importantly, photosynthetic bacteria emerged that released reactive oxygen, thereby causing an atmospheric change that has prevailed, allowing the evolution of eukaryotes (cells with a defined nucleus and membrane-bound organelles) from *circa* 1700 million years ago[39]. From the early eukaryotes came four separate groups: Animalia, Fungi, Plantae and Protista[40]. However, this evolution was allowed to occur only because there was some benefit to the prokaryotes[41]. Nowhere is this more evident than in the gastrointestinal tract of humans where the bacteria are provided with a continuous source of nutrition under optimal temperature and humidity. When, in death, we no longer provide them with the standard of living that they have become accustomed, they consume our bodies! What are the benefits to humans? Preciously few we suspect, and indeed the Grand Unified Theory (GUT) of the pathogenesis of gut diseases suggests that these bacteria play a significant part in most if not all of the intestinal diseases[11]. Some of the intestinal bacteria are clearly less bad than others. However, at present the sheer number of bacteria and their interrelations can only be at best approximated by culturing techniques with around 400 bacterial species currently identified and more yet to be discovered and absolute counts in the colon between 10^{10} and 10^{12} bacteria per gram of faeces. A simpler approach, and the one we foresee, is that it will be possible to measure a range of metabolic bacterial products in stool that might then reflect the spectrum and functional activity of the intestinal flora.

References

1. Teahon K, Smethurst P, Macpherson AJ, Levi AJ, Menzies IS, Bjarnason I. Intestinal permeability in Crohn's disease and its relation to disease activity and relapse following treatment with elemental diet. Eur J Gastroenterol Hepatol. 1993;5:79–84.

2. Wyatt J, Vogelsang H, Hubl W, Waldhoer T, Lochs H. Intestinal permeability and the predictor of relapse in Crohn's disease. Lancet. 1993;341:1437–9.
3. Arnott ID, Kingstone K, Ghosh S. Abnormal intestinal permeability predicts relapse in inactive Crohn disease. Scand J Gastroenterol. 2000;35:1163–9.
4. Hilsden RJ, Meddings JB, Hardin J, Gall DG, Sutherland LR. Intestinal permeability and postheparin plasma diamine oxidase activity in the prediction of Crohn's disease relapse. Inflamm Bowel Dis. 1999;5:85–91.
5. Tibble J, Sigthorsson G, Fagerhol M, Bjarnason I. Surrogate markers of intestinal inflammation are predictive for relapse in patients with inflammatory bowel disease. Gastroenterology. 2000;119:15–22.
6. Bjarnason I, Menzies IS. Causes and consequences of altered gut permeability. In: Brostoff J, Challacombe S, editors. Food Allergy and Intolerance, 2nd edn. London: Saunders, Elsevier, 2002:241–57.
7. Menzies IS. Transmucosal passage of inert molecules in health and disease. In: Skadhauge E, Heintze K, editors. Intestinal Absorption and Secretion. Falk Symposium 36. Lancaster: MTP Press, 1984:527–43.
8. Maxton DG, Bjarnason I, Reynolds AP, Catt SD, Peters TJ, Menzies IS. Lactulose, ^{51}CrEDTA, L-rhamnose and polyethylene glycol 400 as probe markers for '*in vivo*' assessment of human intestinal permeability. Clin Sci. 1986;71:71–80.
9. Menzies IS. Medical importance of sugars in the alimentary tract. In: Grenby TH, Parker KJ, Lindley MG, editors. Developments in Sweeteners – 2. London: Applied Science Publishers, 1983:89–117.
10. Menzies IS, Turner MW. Intestinal permeation of molecules in health and disease. In: MacDonald, T.T., editor. Immunology of Gastrointestinal Disease. Dordrecht: Kluwer Academic Publishers, 1992:173–91.
11. Bjarnason I, Takeuchi K, Bjarnason A, Adler SN, Teahon K. The G.U.T. of gut. Scand J Gastroenterol. 2004;39:807–15.
12. Bjarnason I, Hayllar J, Macpherson AJ, Russell AS. Side effects of nonsteroidal anti-inflammatory drugs on the small and large intestine. Gastroenterology. 1993;104:1832–47.
13. Love AGH, Rhode JE, Abrams ME, Veall N. The measurement of bi-directional sodium fluxes across the intestinal wall in man using whole gut perfusion. Clin Sci. 1973;44:267–78.
14. Blanshard C, Gazzard BG. Natural history and prognosis of diarrhoea of unknown cause in patients with acquired immunodeficiency syndrome (AIDS). Gut. 1995;36:283–6.
15. Sharpstone D, Ross H, Gazzard BG. The metabolic response to oppertunistic infections in AIDS. AIDS. 1996;10:1529–33.
16. Keating J, Bjarnason I, Somasundaram S et al. Intestinal absorptive capacity, intestinal permeability and jejunal histology in HIV infected patients and their relation to diarrhoea. Gut. 1995;37:623–9.
17. Teahon K, Bjarnason I, Pearson M, Levi AJ. Ten years experience with elemental diet in the management of Crohn's disease. Gut. 1990;31:1133–7.
18. Wicks C, Somasundaram S, Menzies IS, Bjarnason I, Williams R. Intestinal function and postoperative enteral nutrition following liver transplants. Gut. 1993;34(Suppl. 1):S65.
19. Mack LA, Kaklamanos IG, Livingstone AS et al. Gastric decompression and enteral feeding through a double-lumen gastrojejunostomy tube improves outcomes after pancreaticoduodenectomy. Ann Surg. 2004;240:845–51.
20. Senkal M, Haaker R, Deska T et al. Early enteral gut feeding with conditionally indispensable pharmaconutrients is metabolically safe and is well tolerated in postoperative cancer patients – a pilot study. Clin Nutr. 2004;23:1193–8.
21. D'Antiga L, Dhawan A, Davenport M, Mieli-Vergani G, Bjarnason I. Intestinal absorption and permeability in paediatric short bowel syndrome. J Paediatr Gastroenterol Nutr. 1999; 29:588–93.
22. Sigalet DL, Martin GR, Meddings JB. 3-O methylglucose uptake as a marker of nutrient absorption and bowel length in pediatric patients. J Parent Ent Nutr. 2004;28:158–62.
23. Bjarnason I, Macpherson AJM, Hollander D. Intestinal permeability: an overview. Gastroenterology. 1995;108:1566–81.
24. Roseth A, Teahon K, Rihani H et al. A new method for assessing intestinal inflammation in man. Lancet. 1997 (Submitted).

25. Roseth AG, Fagerhol MK, Aadland E, Schjonsby H. Assessment of the neutrophil dominating calprotectin in feces. A methodologic study. Scand J Gastroenterol. 1992;27: 793–8.
26. Roseth AG, Kristinsson J, Fagerhol MK et al. Faecal calprotectin: a novel test for the diagnosis of colorectal cancer? Scand J Gastroenterol. 1993;28:1073–6.
27. Roseth AG, Schmidt PN, Fagerhol MK. Correlation between faecal excretion of indium-111-labelled granulocytes and calprotectin, a granulocyte marker protein, in patients with inflammatory bowel disease. Scand J Gastroenterol. 1999;34:50–4.
28. Bunn SK, Main MJ, Grav ES, Olson S, Golden B. Fecal calprotectin as a measure of disease activity in childhood inflammatory bowel disease. J Pediatr Gastroenterol Nutr. 2001;32:171–7.
29. Carroll D, Corfield A, Spicer R, Cairns P. Faecal calprotectin concentrations and diagnosis of necrotising enterocolitis. Lancet. 2003;361:310–11.
30. Kane SV, Sandborn WJ, Rufo PA et al. Fecal lactoferrin is a sensitive and specific marker in identifying intestinal inflammation. Am J Gastroenterol. 2003;98:1309–14.
31. Tibble JA, Bjarnason I. Non-invasive investigation of inflammatory bowel disease. World J Gastroenterol. 2001;7:460–5.
32. Bjarnason I, Sharpstone D, Francis N et al. Intestinal inflammation, ileal structure and function in HIV. AIDS. 1996;10:1385–91.
33. Teahon K, Somasundaram S, Smith T, Menzies I, Bjarnason I. Assessing the site of increased intestinal permeability in coeliac and inflammatory bowel disease. Gut. 1996;38: 864–9.
34. Sharpstone D, Neild P, Crane R et al. Gastric emptying, and small bowel transit, absorption and permeability in AIDS patients with and without diarrhoea. Gut. 1999;45: 70–6.
35. Noone C, Menzies IS, Banatvala JE, Scopes JW. Intestinal permeability and lactulose hydrolysis in human rotaviral gastroenteritis assessed simultaneously by non-invasive differential sugar permeation. Eur J Clin Invest. 1986;16:217–25.
36. Bjarnason I, Batt R, Catt S, Macpherson A, Maxton D, Menzies IS. Evaluation of differential disaccharide excretion in urine for non-invasive assessment of intestinal disaccharidase activity caused by a-glucosidase inhibition, primary hypolactasia and coeliac disease. Gut. 1996;39:374–81.
37. Taylor C, Hodgson K, Sharpstone D et al. The prevalence and severity of intestinal disaccharidase deficiency in HIV-infected subjects. Scand J Gastroenterol. 2000;35:599–606.
38. Larsen A, Hovdenak N, Karlsdottir A, Wentzel-Larsen T, Dahl O, Fagerhol MK. Faecal calprotectin and lactoferrin as markers of acute radiation proctitis: a pilot study of eight stool markers. Scand J Gastroenterol. 2004;39:1113–18.
39. Campbell NA, Reece JB, Mitchell LG. Biology, 5th edn. California: Benjamin/Cummings, 1999:490–2.
40. Lawrence E. Henderson's Dictionary of Biological Terms, 12th edn. Essex: Pearson Education, 2000.
41. Alberts B. Molecular Biology of the Cell, 4th edn. New York: Garland Science, 2002:30–1

Section VIII
Intestinal disorders II

Chair: R.B. SARTOR and J. SCHÖLMERICH

25
Regulatory T cells in animal models: therapeutic potential

C. O. ELSON, Y. CONG, A. KONRAD, N. IQBAL and C. T. WEAVER

INTRODUCTION

The intestine is the major interface between the host and the external environment. In addition to food antigens the mucosal immune system must deal with a huge number of antigens and adjuvant molecules produced by the enteric microbiota.

Despite this enormous antigenic challenge, the immune response in the intestine, although substantial, remains relatively limited, indicating that the immune response there is tightly regulated. Until recent years the cellular and molecular mechanisms maintaining such immune homeostasis in the intestine have been obscure. In the past decade there has been a leap forward in our understanding of the key pathways involved in immune homeostasis, particularly from experiments involving gene-targeted mice. Hundreds of different genes encoding immune molecules have either been selectively deleted or transgenically overexpressed in mice. A small number of such 'induced mutant' mice have gone on to develop inflammatory bowel disease. A common feature in these induced mutant mice that develop colitis has been that CD4[+] T cells are the effector cell in most all of them, and secondly that the bacterial microbiota is the stimulus driving the inflammatory disease (for review see ref. 1).

It has become clear from such experiments that the immune response to the bacterial microbiota is tightly regulated and that this regulation occurs at multiple levels, including both innate and acquired immune mechanisms. Many different cell types contribute to intestinal immune regulation, including CD4[+] and CD8[+] T cells, NK-T cells, B cells, and γδ T cells. These have all been demonstrated to have some beneficial effect in different models of intestinal inflammation. However, most prominent among these regulatory cells are the CD4[+] T cell lineage which itself includes multiple subsets, including T-regulatory-1[2], T-helper-3[3], and the CD25[+]CD4[+] (refs. 4 and 5) T cell subsets. The identification of these subsets has led to reinterpretation of the current paradigm in which T-helper-1 (Th1) cells are thought to regulate T-helper-2 (Th2) cells and vice-versa. An emerging concept is that Th1 and Th2 cells both are effector subsets able to cause disease. That is certainly true in the intestine where both Th1 and Th2 cells have been shown to be able to cause colitis[6]. CD4$^+$ T regulatory cell subsets appear able to control both Th1 and Th2 responses[7,8]. Based on this new paradigm many of the experimental models of inflammatory bowel disease (IBD) can be classified as representing either impaired regulatory cell activity or as representing excessive T cell effector function which overcomes a normal level of immune regulation (Table 1).

Table 1 Mechanistic clustering of mouse models of IBD

Impaired T cell regulation	Excessive T cell effector function
CD45RB transfer model	Stat 4 transgenic
IL-2, IL-2Rα deficient	IL-7 transgenic
BM→Tgε26 transfer model	TNF-α 'knock-in'
	? TCR-α deficient
IL-10 deficient	CD40L transgenic*
CRF 2-4 deficient (IL-10Rβ)	
Mφ-PMN Stat 3 deficient	
TGF-β deficient*	
TGF-βRII deficient	
SMAD3 deficient	

Selected experimental models can be assigned to either a category of 'impaired T cell regulation' or to a category of 'excessive T cell effector function', as shown. The net effect of either is the same, i.e. chronic intestinal inflammation. Within the impaired regulation group several models can be clustered further into an IL-10 pathway, and others into a TGF-β pathway, in which deficiency of the cytokine, its receptor, or its key intracellular signalling molecule can all result in disease.

*Generalized inflammation not limited to intestine.

Among the models classified as representing impaired T cell regulation, some molecular pathways to IBD can be identified. For example, mice with induced mutations of the IL-10 gene[9], the IL-10 receptor gene (CRF2-4)[10], or the gene encoding the transcription factor STAT-3 in macrophages and neutrophils[11], all result in a similar phenotype of colitis, thus defining an IL-10 pathway. In a similar fashion mice deficient in either TGF-$β_1$ gene[12], the TGF-β receptor II gene[13], or in the transcription factor SMAD3[11] display diffuse inflammation including colitis. Thus the IL-10 pathway and the TGF-β pathway both seem to be crucial for maintenance of intestinal immune homeostasis and for the prevention of excessive responses to the antigens of the intestinal microbiota. Interestingly, these pathways appear to reflect the activity of two subsets of CD4$^+$ T regulatory subsets, namely the Tr1 subset that produces high amounts of IL-10 and the Th3 subset that produces high amounts of TGF-$β_1$. These two subsets have been implicated as mediating oral tolerance, and both have been shown able to inhibit induction of colitis in adoptive hosts. It remains unclear whether these are two separate subsets or the same subset that produces high amounts of TGF-$β_1$ under some circumstances and high amounts of IL-10 under others. It is clear that these two cytokines are interrelated, and that each is able to induce the production of the other.

WHERE ARE T REGULATORY CELLS GENERATED, PARTICULARLY THOSE THAT REGULATE IMMUNE RESPONSES TO THE ENTERIC MICROBIOTA?

This remains an open question. The $CD4^+CD25^+$ lineage is known to be generated in the thymus early in life. This subset comprises some 5–10% of both thymic and peripheral $CD4^+$ T cells in adults. This subset clearly plays an important role in maintenance of tolerance to autoantigens, such as those in the stomach, thyroid and adrenals. Indeed, depletion of this subset in mice, for example by thymectomy on day 3 of life, results in autoimmunity in these organs later in life[14]. However, such thymectomy has not been reported to induce colitis. Thus, it is unclear whether this subset, generated in a sterile thymus, induces cells that are able to regulate responses to exogenous antigens such as those of the enteric bacteria. Indeed, T regulatory cells can be generated in the periphery, in addition to in the thymus. Using transgenic technology aberrant expression of antigen on thymic stromal cells generated $CD4^+CD25^+$ T regulatory cells. However, aberrant expression of the same antigen by non-activated haematopoietic cells peripherally produced $CD4^+CD25T^-$ regulatory cells[15]. Indeed, a recent paper has described a dendritic cell subset that is able to induce Tr1 cell differentiation *in vivo*. This dendritic cell subset is normally less than 1% of the total dendritic cell population and is marked by expression of $CD11c^{lo}CD45RB^{hi}$ surface markers[16]. These cells have a plasmacytoid morphology and would be considered an immature phenotype of dendritic cell. They secrete IL-10 upon activation and are able to induce the generation of antigen-specific T regulatory-1 cells and tolerance *in vivo*[16]. Whether such dendritic cells are preferentially located in the intestine or draining lymph nodes is as yet unknown. However, intestinal $CD4^+$ T cells with Tr1-like activity, and that are reactive to enteric bacterial antigens, have been identified in both humans and mouse[17,18].

CAN T REGULATORY CELLS PREVENT COLITIS?

The answer to this question is unequivocally yes for $CD4^+$ T regulatory cells. In fact, each of the subsets mentioned above, including $CD4^+CD25^+$, $CD4^+$ Th3 cells and $CD4^+$ Tr1 cells, has been shown to prevent colitis in different model systems. One of the earliest demonstrations of this was in the $CD45RB^{hi}$ adoptive transfer model. In this model $CD4^+CD45RB^{hi}$ naive T cells are adoptively transferred into RAG-1-deficient mice or SCID mice. As these expand and develop in the new host they develop an unrestrained reactivity against antigens of the enteric microbiota and induce colitis. In the experiment in question, Tr1 cells reactive to ovalbumin were co-transferred with the potentially pathogenic $CD4^+CD45RB^{hi}$ T cells. The OVA-specific Tr1 cells were able to prevent the induction of colitis if the mice were fed low amounts of OVA antigen in order to trigger the Tr1 cells[7]. There was no effect if the animals were not fed the ovalbumin. This experiment demonstrates that T regulatory cells are specific in regard to their activation but non-specific in their inhibitory phase once activated. In this instance OVA-specific regulatory cells were suppressing the reactivity to antigens of the enteric bacteria unrelated to OVA, a phenomenon which has been called bystander suppression. A Tr1 subset reactive to the enteric bacteria has also been shown to be able to inhibit colitis induced by a memory effector T cell subset that was reactive to the enteric bacteria also in the C3H/HeJBir model[18]. Thus, Tr1 cells were able to inhibit both naive and memory T cell responses to the enteric bacteria.

CAN T REGULATORY CELLS TREAT AN ESTABLISHED COLITIS?

This is an important question in relation to the potential translation of regulatory T cell therapy for humans with inflammatory bowel disease because patients generally present at the clinic with established active disease. There is not much data on this point, but recent studies in the CD45RB^{hi} transfer model have demonstrated the ability of T regulatory cells to actively treat an ongoing colitis[19]. Much less is known about such T regulatory subsets in humans and thus it is unclear whether human T regulatory subsets would be able to treat active disease or even whether they would be able to prevent relapse in inactive disease.

WHAT IS THE MECHANISM OF T REGULATORY CELL ACTION?

This remains somewhat controversial and variable, depending on how the regulation is being measured. However, three mechanisms have been identified to date: the production of high amounts of IL-10 which is particularly evident in Tr1 cells, the production of high amounts of TGF-β_1 which is a hallmark of the Th3 subset, and a cytokine-independent cell contact mechanism. In *in-vitro* systems, particularly with CD4$^+$CD25$^+$ T cells, the cell contact mechanism appears sufficient on its own, and neither IL-10 or TGF-β are required[14]. The presence of TGF-β_1 on the surface of CD4$^+$CD25$^+$ cells has been reported as a mechanism of such cognate inhibition[20]; however, this observation has not yet been reproduced. The situation *in vivo* is obviously more complex, with the effector and regulatory cells dispersed and not in close apposition. Not surprisingly, T regulatory cell inhibition *in vivo* appears to require inhibitory cytokines such as IL-10 and/or TGF-β_1[21]. The cellular target of T regulatory activity is also a bit dependent on experimental conditions. Some T regulatory subsets appear able to directly inhibit effector cells such as Th1 cells *in vitro*. However, the Tr1 subset, particularly the one identified in C3H/HeJBir mice that is reactive to enteric bacteria, inhibit antigen presenting cells such as dendritic cells rather than having a direct effect on Th1 cells[22]. It seems likely that all three mechanisms, namely IL-10, TGF-β_1 and cell contact, operate simultaneously, and the relative predominance of any one of the mechanisms depends on the conditions and microenvironment involved.

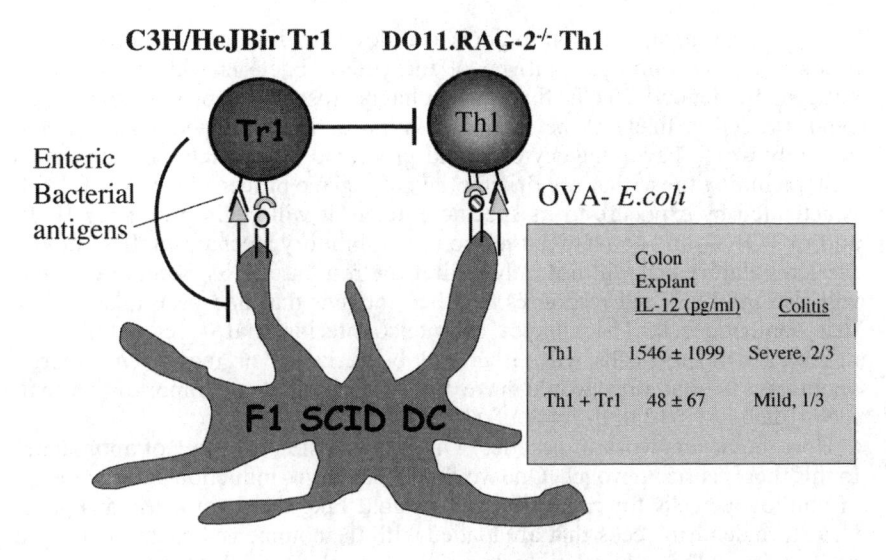

Figure 1 Bystander inhibition as a potential therapeutic approach to IBD. The T regulatory cell (Treg) interacts with a dendritic cell (DC) via TCR:MHC interactions. This results in inhibition of the DC such that it is unable to present antigen or provide cytokine costimulation to a pathogenic Th1 cell. The latter either fails to expand, or more likely undergoes apoptosis in the absence of DC stimulation. Some preliminary data are presented in the box insert using a variation of a previously described antigen-specific model of colitis[6]. In this experiment C3H/HeJBir Tr1 cells specific for enteric bacterial antigens were cotransferred with DO11.RAG-2$^{-/-}$ Th1 effector cells, specific for OVA, into a (C3H × BALB)F1 scid/scid recipient mouse. The box insert shows the results at sacrifice 8 weeks later. IL-12 production by colon explant cultures and histological colitis were both substantially reduced in the group receiving both Tr1 and Th1 cells compared to recipients of only the pathogenic Th1 cells. If this preliminary data can be reproduced it will provide proof of principle that bystander inhibition/regulation can be a therapeutic modality in IBD

CAN T REGULATORY CELLS BE USED FOR THE TREATMENT OF HUMAN IBD?

The answer to this question is unknown, and will clearly lie in future research. However, on a theoretical basis stimulation of antigen-specific T regulatory cells would represent a potentially ideal therapy, one that could suppress the pathogenic response while leaving the rest of the immune system intact. A key question yet to be answered is whether bystander inhibition by T regulatory cells is a robust phenomenon and can be demonstrated in other experimental systems and in humans. To date, bystander inhibition of experimental colitis has only been shown in a system using cells from a T cell receptor transgenic mouse[7]. It will be particularly important to determine whether bystander inhibition can be triggered by defined enteric bacterial antigens that would be present locally in the gut. This will be crucial, particularly in humans, because in most patients we will not be able to identify exactly what antigens are driving the pathogenic response.

A potential therapeutic paradigm is as follows: a T regulatory cell reactive to a common environmental antigen of the enteric bacteria will encounter its antigen on dendritic cells that have phagocytosed and processed it. This dendritic cell is likely to be in the intestine or draining nodes and almost certainly would have phagocytosed and processed other bacterial antigens as well, including those that are driving the pathogenic process. Once the Tr1 cell is activated by exposure to its specific antigen, it will begin producing IL-10 and/or TGF-β, and activate the cell contact inhibitory mechanism. In so doing, the T regulatory cell will not only inhibit the response to its own antigen, but will also inhibit T cell responses to other antigens that had been taken up by that dendritic cell. Th1 effector cells encountering that T regulatory cell-inhibited dendritic cells will either not be activated or may even undergo apoptosis, in that they would have been deprived of an important growth factor such as IL-12 in the case of Th1 cells[23].

How might this work in practice? One can envision a variety of approaches to this therapeutic approach. One would be the *ex-vivo* induction and expansion of autologous cells for reinfusion. This might take the form of expansion of immature dendritic cells that are loaded with the commensal bacterial antigen and reinfused. Or perhaps expansion of the T regulatory cells themselves *in vitro* with subsequent reinfusion. Other possibilities would be therapeutic interventions to enhance T regulatory numbers or function. The means to do this is as yet unknown. A third possibility is gene therapy with a transcription factor that drives T regulatory cell development, e.g. Foxp3 which has recently been shown to be crucial for the development of the $CD4^+CD25^+$ subset[24,25]. Lastly, it may be possible to deviate the pathogenic immune response into one that is beneficial by some form of oral immunization of high-risk individuals using immunodominant enteric bacterial antigens, i.e. an 'IBD vaccine'. One of the major problems limiting the translation of these approaches to humans with IBD is the lack of clinical markers that identify T regulatory cells in patients or suitable assays to measure their activity in order to guide development of these novel therapies.

References

1. Elson CO, Weaver CT. Experimental mouse models of inflammatory bowel disease: new insights into pathogenic mechanisms. In: Targan SR, Shanahan F, Karp LC, editors. Inflammatory Bowel Disease: From Bench to Bedside, 2nd edn. Dordrecht: Kluwer, 2003: 67–99.
2. Levings MK, Roncarolo MG. T-regulatory 1 cells: a novel subset of CD4 T cells with immunoregulatory properties. J Allergy Clin Immunol. 2000;106:S109–12.
3. Fukaura H, Kent SC, Pietrusewicz MJ, Khoury SJ, Weiner HL, Hafler DA. Induction of circulating myelin basic protein and proteolipid protein-specific transforming growth factor-beta1-secreting Th3 T cells by oral administration of myelin in multiple sclerosis patients. J Clin Invest. 1996;98:70–7.
4. Asano M, Toda M, Sakaguchi N, Sakaguchi S. Autoimmune disease as a consequence of developmental abnormality of a T cell subpopulation. J Exp Med. 1996;184:387–96.
5. Takahashi T, Tagami T, Yamazaki S et al. Immunologic self-tolerance maintained by CD25 (+)CD4(+) regulatory T cells constitutively expressing cytotoxic T lymphocyte-associated antigen 4. J Exp Med. 2000;192:303–10.

6. Iqbal N, Oliver JR, Wagner FH, Lazenby AS, Elson CO, Weaver CT. T helper 1 and T helper 2 cells are pathogenic in an antigen-specific model of colitis. J Exp Med. 2002;195: 71–84.
7. Groux H, O'Garra A, Bigler M et al. A CD4$^+$ T cell subset inhibits antigen-specific T-cell responses and prevents colitis. Nature. 1997;389:737–42.
8. Cottrez F, Hurst SD, Coffman RL, Groux H. T regulatory cells 1 inhibit a Th2 specific response *in vivo*. J Immunol. 2000;165:4848–53.
9. Kuhn R, Lohler J, Rennick D, Rajewsky K, Muller W. Interleukin-10-deficient mice develop chronic enterocolitis. Cell. 1993;75:263–74.
10. Spencer SD, Di Marco F, Hooley J, Pitts-Meek S, Bauer M, Ryan AM, et al. The orphan receptor CRF2-4 is an essential subunit of the interleukin 10 receptor. J Exp Med. 1998; 187:571–8.
11. Yang X, Letterio JJ, Lechleider RJ et al. Targeted disruption of SMAD3 results in impaired mucosal immunity and diminished T cell responsiveness to TGF-beta. EMBO J. 1999;18(5): 1280–91.
12. Kulkarni AB, Ward JM, Yaswen L et al. Transforming growth factor-beta 1 null mice. An animal model for inflammatory disorders. Am J Pathol. 1995;146:264–75.
13. Gorelik L, Flavell RA. Abrogation of TGFβ signaling in T cells leads to spontaneous T cell differentiation and autoimmune disease. Immunity. 2000;12:171–81.
14. Shevach EM. Certified professionals: CD4(+)CD25(+) suppressor T cells. J Exp Med. 2001;193:F41–6.
15. Apostolou I, Sarukhan A, Klein L, von Boehmer H. Origin of regulatory T cells with known specificity for antigen. Nat Immunol. 2002;3:756–63.
16. Wakkach A, Fournier N, Brun V, Breittmayer JP, Cottrez F, Groux H. Characterization of dendritic cells that induce tolerance and T regulatory 1 cell differentiation *in vivo*. Immunity. 2003;18:605–17.
17. Khoo UY, Proctor IE, Macpherson AJ. CD4+ T cell down-regulation in human intestinal mucosa: evidence for intestinal tolerance to luminal bacterial antigens. J Immunol. 1997; 158:3626–34.
18. Cong Y, Weaver CT, Lazenby A, Elson CO. Bacterial-reactive T regulatory cells inhibit pathogenic immune responses to the enteric flora. J Immunol. 2002;169:6112–19.
19. Mottet C, Uhlig HH, Powrie F. Cutting edge: cure of colitis by CD4(+)CD25(+) regulatory T cells. J Immunol. 2003;170:3939–43.
20. Nakamura K, Kitani A, Strober W. Cell contact-dependent immunosuppression by CD4 (+)CD25(+) regulatory T cells is mediated by cell surface-bound transforming growth factor beta. J Exp Med. 2001;194:629–44.
21. Asseman C, Mauze S, Leach MW, Coffman RL, Powrie F. An essential role for interleukin 10 in the function of regulatory T cells that inhibit intestinal inflammation. J Exp Med. 1999;190:995–1004.
22. Cong Y, Weaver CT, Lazenby A, Elson CO. T-regulatory-1 (Tr1) cells that prevent CD4+ T cell colitis inhibit the antigen-presenting function and IL-12 production of dendritic cells. Gastroenterology. 2001;120:A38.
23. Fuss IJ, Marth T, Neurath MF, Pearlstein GR, Jain A, Strober W. Anti-interleukin 12 treatment regulates apoptosis of Th1 T cells in experimental colitis in mice. Gastroenterology. 1999;117:1078–88.
24. Fontenot JD, Gavin MA, Rudensky AY. Foxp3 programs the development and function of CD4+CD25+ regulatory T cells. Nat Immunol. 2003;4:330–6.
25. Hori S, Nomura T, Sakaguchi S. Control of regulatory T cell development by the transcription factor Foxp3. Science. 2003;299:1057–61.

26
Imaging of the small and large bowel – from ultrasound to virtual endoscopy

J. F. RIEMANN and U. DAMIAN

INTRODUCTION

The history of gastroenterology has been marked by advances in the imaging of the gastrointestinal tract. During recent years non-invasive methods have become more important for the diagnosis of gastrointestinal diseases. The discovery of X-rays in the nineteenth century introduced a new era of imaging procedures, which resulted in the development and establishment of abdominal ultrasonography and endoscopy. Small bowel disorders are especially difficult to evaluate endoscopically, because of the organ's length and mobility. The evolution from rigid to flexible instruments has allowed us to peer even more deeply into the lumen of the gut. However, inspection of the complete small bowel is in most cases still correlated with difficult and complex procedures such as intraoperative enteroscopy.

In the diagnostic management of bowel diseases the focus is now on some new developments providing more comfort and lower risks for patients. Examples are magnetic resonance imaging (MRI), wireless capsule endoscopy and double-balloon enteroscopy. MRI, which was initially in the focus of neuroradiology, has become a diagnostic procedure used in nearly all parts of the body. The use of new hardware and software has made it possible to improve the quality of the abdominal image.

Wireless capsule endoscopy is also a new approach in the diagnosis of small bowel diseases, and studies suggest a good outcome in the further management of individuals because of pathological findings in the small bowel.

SONOGRAPHY/ENDOSONOGRAPHY

Conventional abdominal sonography is a well-established diagnostic tool in diseases of the gastrointestinal tract. It plays a major role in the follow-up and assessment of the complications of inflammatory bowel diseases (IBD). It has been reported that this method is useful in supporting the diagnosis of Crohn's disease, in the differential diagnosis of ulcerative colitis and in the determination of the extent of disease. Vessel density in affected bowel loops and bowel wall thickness (>5 mm) are especially good sonographic markers. Parente et al. (2002) described a sensitivity of 93.4% and a specificity of 97% in detecting Crohn's disease, based on radiographic and/or endoscopic findings[1]. These data differ from the findings in a prospective study under routine conditions at a university hospital. The sensitivities in detecting Crohn's disease and ulcerative colitis were 84% and 66%, respectively. For the detection of intestinal complications such as strictures, fistulas and abscesses, Gasche et al. were able to demonstrate a high sensitivity[2].

In regard to tumour diagnosis a prospective study was conducted which showed a sensitivity of 77% and a specificity of 99.1% for gastroduodenal cancer. Further it was possible to show a sensitivity of 46% in the evaluation of large bowel tumours, 67% in appendicitis, 65% in unspecific colitis and 60% in the diagnosis of diverticulitis, but it is important to note that sonography depends greatly on the experience of the physician and the technical condition. In a recent study sonography showed a 97% sensitivity and specificity in the management of sigma diverticulitis for reaching an accurate and clinical plausible diagnosis. The authors concluded that sonography can compete with the more complex computed tomography (CT) examination, and therefore represents the recommended primary diagnostic procedure[3].

Doppler sonography is able to estimate the results of abdomen imaging. Spalinger et al. investigated 92 paediatric patients with Crohn's disease with a 7.5–10 MHz or 8–12 MHz transducer, the lowest possible pulse repetition frequency without aliasing, a low wall filter and high Doppler gain setting[4]. In conclusion affected bowel loops were thicker and had a higher vessel density than during remission, but it must be noted that there is no general correlation between wall thickening and disease activity[5]. These promising results were validated in a few studies, so bowel ultrasound (US) examination associated with IBD, and in particular US contrast medium injection, can be used to detect Crohn's disease activity and modulate therapy and follow-up[6].

As a new development during recent years endoscopic ultrasound (EUS) is considered to be the most accurate means currently available for tumour and locoregional nodal staging of the upper gastrointestinal tract (especially the oesophagus and stomach). The overall accuracy for tumour staging using EUS (compared to pathology) is about 85%, and the overall accuracy in predicting resectability in the upper gastrointestinal tract is between 75% and 100%. EUS is also very effective in the diagnosis of pathological changes in the biliary system. The use of EUS in the small and large bowel is focused on the evaluation and management of patients with rectal cancer, on the diagnosis of chronic inflammatory diseases and anal sphincter injury. In published studies the accuracy of EUS in the determination of the depth of invasion of rectal carcinoma ranges from 80% to 95% compared with 75% to 85% for CT and MRI[7].

Perianal fistulas are a frequent manifestation of Crohn's disease that can result in a significant morbidity, including scarring, faecal incontinence and even proctectomy in 10–18% of patients. Several studies have reported excellent accuracy for rectal US in the evaluation of Crohn's perianal fistulas. A recent prospective blind study compared rectal US with MRI and examination under anaesthesia (EAA) in 34 patients. All three methods demonstrated a good accuracy (EUS, 91%; MRI, 87%; EAA, 91%)[7]. In addition a combination of any of the imaging modalities with EAA showed 100% accuracy in these patients. As described above, transrectal EUS has also emerged as an important imaging modality for pretreatment staging of rectal cancer. In the largest study to evaluate the sensitivity of EUS for detecting anal sphincter defects ($n = 44$) the findings compared with operative findings were nearly 100%. EUS has also been shown to be helpful in predicting outcomes of sphincteroplasty[8]; however, the limitation of EUS is the small depth of insertion.

ENTEROSCOPY

Small bowel enteroscopy (SBE) is another possibility to evaluate patients with suspected small bowel lesions. The first report concerning sonde endoscopy appeared in 1986. Difficulties of introducing the sonde, patient discomfort and the length of investigation time initially led to non-acceptance of this method[9]. With technical advancements during recent years, and the possibility of using modern forms of narcosis (i.e. propofol), this technique has become more useful, and is now of important value in small bowel diagnosis. The diagnostic yield varies from 13% to 78%, but the results are dependent on the diagnosis. Gastrointestinal bleeding is the most common finding, and enteroscopy is well established in the management of patients with unclear bleeding episodes. With an average depth of insertion of 70–150 cm push-enteroscopy can investigate only the first part of the small bowel. Using this method a source of bleeding could be proven in 30–50% in prospective studies with patients suffering from chronic gastrointestinal bleeding and negative upper and lower gastrointestinal endoscopy. To improve the depth of insertion it is possible to use an overtube. Taylor et al. investigated 19 patients who underwent enteroscopy with, and 19 patients without, an overtube. The use of an overtube resulted in a deeper insertion, but it is difficult to determine the length of the visible small intestine[10]. In a large study with 80 patients Benz et al. showed the same result; further, the authors were able to show that the length of the enteroscopy seems uncorrelated with deeper insertion[11].

During the past 6 years or so the usefulness of intraoperative enteroscopy (IOE) has been recognized once again, since it offers the possibility of a complete small bowel examination – a promise that conventional sonde enteroscopy fails to fulfil. It offers the facility of immediate treatment of pathological findings by endoscopic or surgical intervention.

Esaki et al. investigated the clinical value of IOE for Crohn's disease. In this study 27 patients requiring surgery were examined by both preoperative radiography and IOE. Eventually IOE was superior in demonstrating small intestinal lesions in detail compared with double-contrast radiography (74% vs. 37%), but there was no prediction of postoperative recurrence in Crohn's disease. However, examination of the small bowel with IOE is invasive, and the correct indication is mandatory[12].

A new approach is the development of the double-balloon enteroscope, which indicates the facility to evaluate the small bowel completely. In preliminary experience in patients with obscure bleeding all earlier capsule endoscopy results could be confirmed. In two patients with multiple angiodysplasia it was possible to examine the whole small bowel and to treat the angiodysplasias. No complications occurred. The authors concluded that the double-balloon technique promises to become a standard method for diagnostic and therapeutic endoscopy of the small bowel surgical laparotomy[13].

However, enteroscopy – especially intraoperative and double-balloon enteroscopy – is available only in specialized endoscopic centres, and is associated with greater risks compared with standard upper gastrointestinal endoscopy, particulary if deep sedation or narcosis is necessary.

WIRELESS CAPSULE ENDOSCOPY

Capsule endoscopy (CE) is a new method enabling non-invasive diagnostic endoscopy of the entire small intestine. It has attracted enormous interest in recent years, and a large number of indications have been discussed, ranging from the original indication of suspected small-bowel bleeding (SSBB) to possible indications in Crohn's disease (CD) and other small-bowel diseases. It seems to be fairly well established that CE is becoming the method of choice after upper and lower gastrointestinal endoscopy (including ileoscopy) in the evaluation of patients with obscure and occult gastrointestinal bleeding – also known as SSSB. The results of studies dealing with CE in SSSB vary from 53% to 88% in identifying pathological lesions. In an important study wireless CE was significantly superior compared to push-enteroscopy[14]. Mata et al. showed similar results in 44 patients: 74% of patients who underwent CE showed signs of bleeding compared with push-enteroscopy (19%). The most common finding was angiodysplasia; however, positive findings were associated with significant management changes ($p<0.0001$)[15].

In CD affecting the small bowel barium radiology has been the technique most widely used to date. Sometimes it is difficult to evaluate a pathological value, and in this case CE is a useful technique. Herrerias et al. observed pathological findings in 43% of patients in whom there was a clinical suspicion of small-bowel CD that could not be confirmed by using traditional techniques, indicating that in these cases CE could be a valuable diagnostic tool[16]. However, large prospective studies are still incomplete.

Primary small bowel tumours are relatively rare, but the need for endoscopic examination of the small bowel, especially for screening of polyposis syndromes, is well established. Schulman et al. showed polyps in the small intestine in 9 of 10 patients with Peutz–Jeghers syndrome, and in 16 of 21 with familial adenomatous polyposis (FAP). Further outcome studies are only slowly beginning to appear, and the use of CE in clinical situations (abdominal pain, diarrhoea), rather than in more or less well-defined diseases or 'disease suspicion' situations has yet to be analysed properly[17].

Though wireless CE is a safe diagnostic tool with a low rate of complications, there are some difficulties: one problem is the imaging of the whole small intestine because of preparation and premedication[18]. It has been demonstrated that complete imaging from stomach to caecum has been achieved in only two-thirds of patients as a result of functionally delayed gastric or small intestinal transit[19]. Erythromycin speeded up gastric emptying but prolonged intestinal passage[20]. CE should also not be used if pregnancy, gastrointestinal obstruction, strictures or fistulas are present. Pacemakers, defibrillators or other implanted electromedical devices are also contraindications.

RADIOGRAPHIC IMAGING TECHNIQUES

There are a few important radiographic techniques in use for the diagnostic management of small and large bowel diseases.

For the assessment of the small bowel, mainly two radiological techniques are presently applied: the classic conventional enteroclysis (CEC) initially described by Sellink and the detailed per-oral small bowel examination ('small bowel follow-through'). The sensitivity and specificity of enteroclysis or small bowel follow-through examination are comparable (sensitivity 85–95%, specificity 89–94%), but this procedure strongly depends on the individual examiner's experience. The problem using conventional enteroclysm is the quite high exposure to radiation (6800–7200 cGy/cm^2). Especially in the diagnosis of IBD sectional imaging techniques (CT, MRI) are able to describe local wall thickening, fistulas, stenotic processes, abscesses, prestenotic dilation or extraluminal lesions, but a complete distension of the bowel is often not possible, so these methods are less sensitive in showing intraluminal changes compared with CEC. The combination of conventional enteroclysm and MRI (MR–Sellink) seems to be most promising. It was possible to show that MR–Sellink is a safe and effective procedure in the diagnosis of Crohn's disease (CD). In patients with a high activity of CD it was possible to find 98.2% of the affected segments, 97.5% of the stenoses and 100% of the fistulas compared with CEC. Additionally it was possible to focus on extraluminal changes such as abscesses, ileosigmoidal adhesions and pseudotumours[20]. There are many different techniques of contrast medium (CM) insertion. One practicable method is the Hydro-MRI; 81 MRI studies in 25 patients conducted within a period of 3 weeks to 4 years were evaluated retrospectively. It was possible to detect the morphological substrate of CD in the Hydro-MRI images reliably, and the imaging of extraluminal changes was superior to endoscopy and enteroclysis[21].

MRI has been continuously developed and is now a standard method in diagnostic procedures in the biliopancreatic system (magnetic resonance cholangiopancretography; MRCP). During recent years the focus of MRI has been on the evaluation of the small and large bowel. MRI enteroclysm provides adequate image quality and sufficient distension of the entire small bowel. In contrast to conventional radiographic enteroclysm there is no need for a duodenal catheter or exposure to radiation. Recent advances in gadolinium-enhanced MRI (G-MRI) have been developed to enhance the resolution of the intestinal mucosa and facilitate the diagnosis of inflammatory or neoplastic processes and their complications (fistula, abscess and stricture), but at present G-MRI is not a routine diagnostic tool.

Since its description in 1994 virtual colonoscopy has emerged as a promising method of colorectal evaluation[22]. Initial studies using CT colonography revealed a sensitivity of 91% relative to conventional colonoscopy for polyps larger than 10 mm[23,24]. However, exposure to ionizing radiation may limit the future applicability of CT as a screening method. The typical X-ray load per examination is up to 10 mSV using CT colonography which may not be acceptable given the high number of healthy subjects undergoing screening.

For this reason efforts have been focused on MRI colonography (MRC). To date most approaches to MRC have been based on administration of a rectal enema containing paramagnetic contrast[25,26]. This method, called 'bright lumen' MRC, has been shown to be accurate in detecting polyps larger than 8 mm in size. On three-dimensional (3D) gradient echo data sets only the contrast-containing colonic lumen is bright, whereas the surrounding tissues (including colonic wall and polyps) remain low in signal intensity. Polypoid masses appear as dark filling defects within the bright colonic lumen – an appearance which is difficult to differentiate from residual faecal material and small pockets of air. To avoid false-positive findings, and to compensate for the presence of residual air, the 3D acquisition is performed in both the prone and supine positions. Turning the patient during examination prolongs the examination, and requires a new landmark to localize the sequence in order to ensure full coverage of the colon in the subsequent 3D acquisition. Although most authors[25] suggest a Gd/water dilution of 1:100, some studies have recommended the use of a 1:50 dilution[26]. Assuming a colonic volume of 3000 ml, between 30 and 60 ml of costly paramagnetic contrast are needed for the rectal enema alone. In addition, most 'bright lumen' MRC protocols call for the additional intravenous administration of paramagnetic contrast at a dose of 0.1 mmol/kg[25,26].

A newly developed, simplified and less costly variation on MRC is dark-lumen MRI colonography[27]. The technique is based on the acquisition of a heavily T1-weighted 3D gradient echo sequence collected after administration of a rectal water enema and an intravenous injection of paramagnetic contrast. Dark-lumen MRC overcomes the limitations inherent to bright-lumen MRC. Intravenous application of the paramagnetic contrast allows for direct depiction of the colorectal wall. Occasionally the presence of residual stool or air bubbles may require direct comparison with the 3D data set collected prior to the administration of paramagnetic contrast. To date only limited data exist comparing dark-lumen MRI colonography with conventional colonoscopy[27]. In a study comparing MRC with conventional colonoscopy in 92 patients the sensitivity of MRC for adenomatous polyps on a per-polyp analysis was 100% for polyps at least 10 mm in diameter, and 84.2% for polyps 6–9 mm in diameter.

In conclusion, the objective is not to compete with conventional colonoscopy as the diagnostic gold standard, but to offer patients an alternative diagnostic option. In our opinion a sufficient evaluation of MRC and goal-oriented additional developments of the magnetic resonance procedure mandates close cooperation between radiologist and gastroenterologist.

References

1. Parente F, Maconi G, Bianchi Porro G. Bowel ultrasound in Crohn disease: current role and future applications. Scand J Gastroenterol. 2002;37:871–6.
2. Gasche C, Moser G, Turetschek K, Schober E, Moeschl P, Oberhuber G. Transabdominal bowel sonography for the detection of intestinal complications in Crohn's disease. Gut. 1999;44:112–17.
3. Soliman M, Wüstner M, Sturm J et al. Primary diagnostics of acute diverticulitis of the sigmoid. Sonography versus CT: a prospective study. Ultraschall Med. 2004;25:342–7.
4. Spalinger J, Patriquin H, Miron MC. Doppler US in patients with crohn disease: vessel density in the diseased bowel reflects disease activity. Radiology. 2000;217:787–91.
5. Mayer D, Reinshagen M, Mason RA et al. Sonographic measurement of thickened bowel wall segments as a quantitative parameter for activity in inflammatory bowel disease. Z Gastroenterol. 2000;38:295–300.
6. Robotti D, Cammarota T, Debani P, Sarno A, Astegiano M. Activity of Crohn disease: value of color-power-Doppler and contrast-enhanced ultrasonography. Abdom Imaging. 2004;27:29.
7. Schwartz DA, Wiersema MJ, Dudiak KM et al. A comparison of endoscopic ultrasound, magnetic resonance imaging, and exam under anesthesia for evaluation of Crohn's perianal fistulas. Gastroenterology. 2001;121:1064–72.
8. Felt-Bersma RJ, Cuesta MA, Koorevaar M. Anal sphincter repair improves anorectal function and endosonographic image. A prospective clinical study. Dis Colon Rectum. 1996;39:878–85.
9. Waye JD. Small-bowel endoscopy. Endoscopy. 2003;35:15–21.
10. Taylor AC, Chen RY, Desmond PV. Use of an overtube for enteroscopy – does it increase depth of insertion? A prospective study of enteroscopy with and without an overtube. Endoscopy. 2001;33:227–30.
11. Benz C, Jakobs R, Riemann JF. Does the insertion depth in push enteroscopy depend on the working length of the enteroscope? Endoscopy. 2002;34:543–5.
12. Esaki M, Matsumoto T, Hizawa K et al. Intraoperative enteroscopy detects more lesions but is not predictive of postoperative recurrence in Crohn's disease. Surg Endosc. 2001;15:455–9.
13. May A, Nachbar L, Wardak A, Yamamoto H, Ell C. Double balloon enteroscopy: preliminary experience in patients with obscure GI bleeding or chronic abdominal pain Endo Heute. 2004;17:28–34.
14. Ell C, Remke S, May A, Helou L, Henrich R, Mayer G. The first prospective controlled trial comparing wireless capsule endoscopy with push enteroscopy in chronic gastrointestinal bleeding Endoscopy. 2002;34:685–9.
15. Mata A, Bordas JM, Feu F et al. Wireless capsule endoscopy in patients with obscure gastrointestinal bleeding: a comparative study with push enteroscopy. Aliment Pharmacol Ther. 2004;20:189–94.
16. Herrerias JM, Caunedo A, Rodriguez-Tellez M, Pellicer F, Herrerias JM Jr. Capsule endoscopy in patients with suspected Crohn's disease and negative endoscopy. Endoscopy. 2003;35:564–8.
17. Schulmann K., Hollerbach S, Kraus K. Value of capsule endoscopy for the detection of small bowel polyps in patients with heriditary polyposis syndromes (FAP, PJS, FJP). Gastroenterology. 2003;124:A550 (abstract).
18. Rosch T, Ell C. Position paper on capsule endoscopy for the diagnosis of small bowel disorders. Z Gastroenterol. 2004;42:247–59.
19. Fireman Z, Mahajna E, Broide E et al. Diagnosing small bowel Crohn's disease with wireless capsule endoscopy. Gut. 2003;52:390–2.
20. Holzknecht N, Helmberger T, Herrmann K, Ochsenkuhn T, Goke B, Reiser M. [MRI in Crohn's disease after transduodenal contrast administration using negative oral MRI contrast media]. Radiologie. 2003;43:43–50 [In German].
21. Ganten M, Encke J, Flosdorff P, Gruber-Hoffmann B, Erb G, Hansmann J. [Follow up of Crohn's disease under therapy with hydro-MRI]. Radiologie. 2003;43:26–33 [In German].
22. Vining DJ, Gelfand DW, Bechthold RE, Scharling ES, Grishaw EK, Shiffrin RY. Technical feasibility of colon imaging with helical CT and virtual reality. Am J Roentgenol. 1994;162 (Suppl. 104) (abstract).

23. Fenlon HM, Nunes DP, Schroy PC 3rd, Barish MA, Clarke PD, Ferrucci JT. A comparison of virtual and conventional colonoscopy for the detection of colorectal polyps. N Engl J Med. 1999;341:1496–503.
24. Yee J, Akerkar GA, Hung RK, Steinauer-Gebauer AM, Wall SD, McQuaid KR. Colorectal neoplasia: performance characteristics of CT colonography for detection in 300 patients. Radiology. 2001;219:685–92.
25. Pappalardo G, Polettini E, Frattaroli FM et al. Magnetic resonance colonography versus conventional colonoscopy for the detection of colonic endoluminal lesions. Gastroenterology. 2000;119:300–4.
26. Luboldt W, Steiner P, Bauerfeind P, Pelkonen P, Debatin JF. Detection of mass lesions with MR colonography: preliminary report. Radiology. 1998;207:59–65.
27. Ajaj W, Pelster G, Treichel U et al. Dark lumen magnetic resonance colonography: comparison with conventional colonoscopy for the detection of colorectal pathology. Gut. 2003;52:1738–43.

27
Colorectal carcinoma – primary prevention and screening

C. POX and W. SCHMIEGEL

INTRODUCTION

Colorectal cancer (CRC) is a major medical burden in industrialized countries. The life-time risk is about 6%. In Germany around 30 000 people die from CRC each year, making it the second most common cancer-related death cause in that country. The long-term survival rate is strongly influenced by the tumour stage at the time of diagnosis. Currently the majority of patients when diagnosed already have local or distant metastases (UICC III and IV) and thus have a poor prognosis. Strategies for either detecting the disease at an early stage with a better prognosis or ideally preventing CRC from developing are thus warranted.

Currently the most effective method for preventing CRC is the detection and endoscopic removal of adenomatous polyps. This has been shown to reduce the incidence of CRC by 66–90%[1,2]. The faecal occult blood test (FOBT) is easy to perform but has a low sensitivity for adenomas. Endoscopic methods have a high sensitivity for adenomas but are invasive and require bowel cleansing. Other methods such as genetic stool testing or CT/MRT colonography are still being investigated and are not available for routine use. Furthermore the high recurrence rate of adenomas after polypectomy makes regular endoscopic follow-up examinations necessary.

Alternative approaches for CRC prevention using dietary supplements or oral medications are therefore desirable. The aim should be preventing the reoccurrence of colorectal adenomas (secondary prevention) in order to reduce the incidence of CRC (primary prevention).

EFFECT OF DIET ON CRC

Cancers develop because of a combination of inherited and acquired factors. The importance of acquired factors is stressed by migratory studies. The risk of CRC greatly increases for people who migrate from an area with a low incidence of CRC to one with a high incidence[3]. A major acquired risk factor for CRC development is life style. Industrialized countries with a Western lifestyle have the highest CRC incidence rates.

Both obesity and low physical activity are known risk factors for the development of CRC[4-8]. Avoiding obesity and regular performance of physical activity are therefore recommended.

Several studies have shown red meat to be a risk factor for CRC development[6,9]. It could be shown in a rat model that the haem molecule from meat can have cytotoxic and hyperproliferative effects on the colonic mucosa[10]. Other explanations for the increased CRC risk include the high-temperature cooking of meat, which can result in the production of carcinogens[11].

An increased intake of fruit and vegetables has been shown to have a protective effect on CRC development[12], with stronger evidence for fruit than for vegetables[13]. It is not clear, however, which constituents (fibre, flavonoids, phyto-oestrogens, etc.) are responsible for the protective effect.

Epidemiological studies have shown an inverse correlation between daily fibre intake and CRC risk[14]. The protective effect of fibre is thought to be partly due to decreased bowel transit time, adsorption of potential carcinogens and positive effects on bile acid composition. The positive effect of fibre was confirmed by two recent studies[15,16]. A European multicentre prospective observational study (EPIC) examined the association between dietary fibre intake and incidence of CRC in 520 000 individuals[15]. The authors found a significant 42% lower CRC incidence for the group with the highest compared to the group with the lowest fibre intake. The US study (PLCO) compared the dietary fibre intake of 33 971 people who showed no polyps on sigmoidoscopy with 3591 people who had at least one adenoma in the distal part of the large bowel[16]. This study showed an adenoma reduction of 27% for the group with the highest compared to the lowest fibre intake. The protective effect was strongest for fibre from grains, cereals and from fruits. These two studies are in contrast to earlier studies that had not been able to show a protective effect[12,17], as well as two randomized intervention studies in which no reduction in adenoma recurrence rate by an increased fibre intake was found[18,19]. The reasons for these different results are not entirely clear. However, the average dietary-fibre intake of the group with the highest fibre intake in the EPIC study was significantly higher compared to the group with the highest fibre intake in the earlier studies such as the US Nurses' studies[20]. The same is true for both intervention studies. It thus seems as if the dietary-fibre intake needs to be increased to about 30 g a day before protection can be demonstrated.

A pooled analysis of eight cohort studies with a single determination of alcohol intake found a modest relative elevation in CRC rate, mainly at the highest level of alcohol intake (relative risk 1.16 for 30 to <45 g alcohol/day, relative risk 1.41 for >45 g/day)[21]. The risk was independent of the kind of alcoholic beverage consumed. The effect of alcohol seems to be pronounced in people with a low folate intake[22]. The suggested mechanisms for the effect of alcohol on the risk of CRC include increased acetaldehyde production which may be responsible for colorectal carcinogenesis, as well as antagonism of methyl-group metabolism which may contribute to abnormal DNA methylation[21].

EFFECT OF MICRONUTRIENTS ON CRC RISK

Calcium is able to form insoluble compounds with bile and fatty acids. It has also been shown to have an inhibitory effect on the proliferation of colonic epithelial cells[23]. In a study analysing data from two prospective cohort studies an increased calcium intake was associated with a reduced incidence of distal colon cancer[24]. One prospective randomized intervention study using 2 g of calcium for secondary adenoma prevention found a modest non-significant effect on adenoma recurrence (risk ratio 0.66, $p = 0.16$)[25]. Another prospective randomized double-blind study found a modest but significant reduction of adenoma recurrence by 1.2 g of calcium (risk ratio 0.85, $p = 0.03$)[26]. The protective effect was observed as early as 1 year after supplementation began, suggesting that calcium acts very early in the pathway of colorectal carcinogenesis.

Folate metabolites play an essential role in DNA methylation, synthesis and repair. Folate has been shown to reduce proliferation of colorectal mucosa[27] and reduce DNA hypomethylation in the rectal mucosa[28]. Several epidemiological studies have suggested a protective effect of folate on CRC development[29-31]. However, in some of these studies the protective effect was either not significant, limited to males or females only or limited to a certain part of the large bowel. The results of prospective intervention trials have to be awaited before firm recommendations concerning folate supplementation can be made.

The data on other vitamins and CRC prevention are either insufficient or have mostly not been able to show a preventive effect[32,33]. A secondary analysis of one study that examined the effect of selenium supplementation on skin cancer found an over 50% reduced incidence of CRC in the selenium-supplemented group[34]. This result has to be confirmed by other studies before recommendations can be made.

EFFECT OF CHEMOPREVENTIVE DRUGS

Non-steroidal anti-inflammatory drugs (NSAID)

The effect of NSAID such as aspirin is known to be a result of their inhibition of cyclooxygenases. Whereas cyclooxygenase-1 (COX-1) is constitutively expressed in most tissues, and has a cytoprotective effect, cyclooxygenase-2 (COX-2) is induced by inflammatory processes or cellular proliferation. It could be shown that in the vast majority of CRC and about half of the adenomas COX-2 was up-regulated, whereas levels were low or undetectable in normal mucosa[35]. Most NSAID such as aspirin or sulindac inhibit both COX-1 and COX-2. The gastrointestinal side-effects, including ulcer formation and gastrointestinal bleeding and platelet dysfunction are caused by COX-1 inhibition. The chemopreventive effect of NSAR on colorectal cancer, however, is a result mainly of COX-2 inhibition. This could be shown elegantly using an intestinal polyposis mouse model. COX-2 inhibition by either knocking-out the gene or using a selective inhibitor greatly decreased the polyp burden[36]. The exact mechanism by which COX-2 inhibition results in CRC prevention is still unknown. It is thought that induction of apoptosis and regulation of angiogenesis play a central role[23]. Some studies also show that NSAID may act by COX-independent mechanisms including induction of apoptosis.

Clinical trials

First clinical data showing a protective effect of NSAID were collected from patients with familial adenomatous polyposis (FAP). This rare disease (<1% of all CRC) is caused by germline mutations in the APC gene and characterized by the development of hundreds of colorectal adenomas as well as CRC at an average age of 36 years. Randomized placebo-controlled studies were able to show a significant decrease in the mean number and size of polyps in patients treated with the non-selective COX-inhibitor sulindac[37,38]. However, a study looking at the efficacy of sulindac in the primary prevention of polyps in FAP found no significant effect[39]. This could imply that the effect of sulindac on tumour initiation is less pronounced than on tumour progression. A study with the selective COX-2 inhibitor celecoxib also found a significant effect on polyp size and number of FAP patients after a follow-up of 6 months[40].

However, up to now no medical therapy has been able to prevent the need for early proctocolectomy in FAP patients. It remains to be seen if NSAID, especially COX-2 inhibitors, will allow later proctocolectomy in patients with very early onset of polyposis who would otherwise require surgery during puberty.

Most patients with CRC do not have a hereditary predisposition but have a so-called sporadic cancer. A series of case–control and cohort studies demonstrated a reduced incidence of colorectal adenomas and carcinomas for patients who took aspirin[23]. Two randomized placebo-controlled prospective trials looking at the effect of aspirin on adenoma recurrence have recently been published[41,42]. In one study 1121 patients with a recent history of removed adenomas were randomized to receive either placebo, 81 mg or 325 mg of aspirin[41]. The recurrence rate was reduced by 11% by the use of aspirin when the results of both aspirin groups were combined (17% for 81 mg and 5% for 325 mg of aspirin). This moderate effect was only significant for the 81 mg aspirin group. For advanced lesions the reduction was 30% for both groups combined (42% for 81 mg, 17% for 325 mg of aspirin) and again only significant for the 81 mg aspirin group. It is unclear why the higher dose of aspirin had less of a protective effect. In a second study 635 patients with a history of CRC were randomized to either placebo or 325 mg of aspirin[42]. After a median of 13 months the recurrent adenoma rate was 35% lower, and the time to the detection of a first adenoma significantly longer, in the aspirin group.

In summary, although there are data to suggest that modification of diet, intake of certain micronutrients and NSAID may be of some benefit in preventing CRC these factors are currently no substitute for screening the general population or surveillance of risk groups.

Screening

It is generally accepted that screening should begin at age 50 for persons who do not belong to one of the known risk groups. More than 90% of cancers arise after this age, and a recent prospective colonoscopy study showed a low detection rate (3.5%) of advanced neoplasia (adenomas $\geqslant 1$ cm, villous histology or high-grade dysplasia) between 40 and 49[43]. No recommendations can be made regarding the age at which screening should stop. This requires an individual decision taking into account comorbidities.

There are several different screening options for the general population: (a) faecal occult blood testing (FOBT), (b) sigmoidoscopy $\pm$ FOBT, (c) colonoscopy, (d) double-contrast barium enema (DCBE), (e) CT/MRT colonography, (f) molecular stool tests.

FOBT

This test method, which detects blood in the stool, relies on the fact that colorectal neoplasms tend to bleed more often than normal mucosa. Most widely used are guaiac-based tests such as the Hemoccult II. If blood is present in the stool the haemoglobin with its pseudoperoxidase activity will result in a blue colour change of the test field in the presence of hydrogen peroxide. The test slides typically contain two fields to which different parts of the stool are applied. Because some colorectal neoplasms will only bleed intermittingly testing several stool samples increases the yield. It has become standard to test three consecutive stools, i.e. use three test slides for screening purposes. A test is positive if one or more of the six test fields turns blue. A positive test has to be followed up by a complete colonoscopy.

The sensitivity of a one-time FOBT for detecting CRC is about 40%, the specificity 96–98%[44]. In studies with repeated biennial testing the sensitivity was between 46% and 64%[45,46]. The sensitivity for detecting adenomas is lower (20–40%). Sensitivity can be improved by rehydrating the test fields; this, however, decreases specificity and is therefore not recommended. False-positive results may be caused by non-neoplastic bleeding sources such as angiodysplasia.

There have been five large prospective randomized studies addressing the effectiveness of FOBT. For four of these studies mortality data have been published[45–48] (Table 1). The three European studies, from Great Britain (Nottingham), Denmark (Funen) and France (Burgundy), used biennial testing without rehydrating test fields. CRC-related mortality was reduced by 13% in the Nottingham study (11 years follow-up), 18% in the Funen study (13 years follow-up) and 16% in the Burgundy study (11 years follow-up)[47,49,50]. The importance of repeated testing was stressed by data from the Funen trial. For persons who took part in every screening round of the study mortality reduction was 30% compared to 18% for the whole screening group[50].

A US study (Minnesota study) compared annual and biennial testing and used rehydrated Hemoccult II tests[48]. Unlike the European studies this trial was performed on volunteers. The positive predictive value for CRC was 2.2%, significantly lower than in the other three studies (8.4–17.7%). This is explained

Table 1 Randomized studies, FOBT screening

Study	Minnesota	Nottingham	Funen	Burgundy
Screening group	Annual test 15 570; biennial test 15 587	76 466	30 967	45 642
Control group	15 394	76 384	30 966	45 557
Rehydration of test fields	Yes	No	No	No
Follow-up (years)	18	11	13	11
Compliance				
With any screening round	>90%	60%	67%	70%
With every screening round	46–60%	38%	46%	38%
Sensitivity for CRC (%)	92	64	46	Not stated
Positive predictive value for CRC	2.2	9.9–11.9	8.4–17.7	8.2–14.7
Relative mortality reduction (%)	Annual test 33; biennial test 21	13	18	16

by the rehydration of the Hemoccult slides, which is known to increase sensitivity but reduces specificity. After 13 years follow-up the CRC-related mortality reduction was 33% for the annual group and 6% for the biennial group. After 18 years follow-up the mortality reduction remained at 33% for the annual group compared to a now 21% reduction for the biennial screening group[51].

The risk reduction by FOBT is due to CRC detection at an earlier stage with a better prognosis. For the Minnesota study, which has the longest follow-up (18 years), it could also be shown that the CRC incidence in the screening group was lower compared to the control group[52]. This decrease is thought to be due to the removal of adenomas; however, it has to be kept in mind that nearly a third of the FOBT group had a colonoscopy performed during the trial compared to 2–5% for the European trials. The reduction of adenoma incidence could therefore be interpreted as a result of adenoma detection and removal by colonoscopy.

Compliance rates for taking part in at least one screening round in the studies have varied between >90% for the Minnesota study and between 60% and 70% in the European studies.

In summary there is currently strong evidence for supporting the use of FOBT as a screening test for the general population, as several randomized studies have shown a reduction of CRC-related mortality. The main disadvantage of FOBT is the moderate sensitivity for detecting CRC and the low sensitivity for adenomas. This has been the rationale for looking at endoscopic methods for screening.

Sigmoidoscopy

The advantage of using sigmoidoscopy as a screening method is that, unlike FOBT, non-bleeding carcinomas and adenomas of the rectum and sigmoid can also be detected. About 40–60% of all adenomas and carcinomas are located within reach of the sigmoidoscope. The sensitivity of detecting neoplasms is >90%, the perforation rate is low with only one perforation occurring in more than 40 000 examinations in a recently published study[53].

Three case–control studies looking at effectiveness have been published[54–56]. In one study the screening histories of people who died of CRC were compared with age- and sex-matched controls. It was found that sigmoidoscopy was associated with a 59% reduction in mortality from cancers in the part of the colon reached by the sigmoidoscope[56]. Another study reported an 80% reduction in the risk of death from rectosigmoid cancer in patients who had undergone one or more sigmoidoscopies compared to a control group that had never done so[55]. The third study again found a 59% CRC mortality reduction[54]. In this study the benefit of endoscopy was shown to last for at least 6 years. In the study by Selby et al. the effectiveness of sigmoidoscopy was similar for people who had undergone the procedure up to 10 years earlier[56]. After an initial negative sigmoidoscopy a control sigmoidoscopy on average 3.4 years after the first examination found an adenoma in 6% but no carcinomas or large adenomas[57]. In a recently published study, however, 0.8% of patients were found to have an advanced adenoma or carcinoma in the rectum or distal colon 3 years after a negative examination[58].

In order to further assess the effectiveness of sigmoidoscopy as a screening method in the general population prospective randomized studies in the UK and the US have been undertaken. In the US trial a 5-year screening interval is currently being assessed[59]. The UK trial is comparing the efficacy of a one-time sigmoidoscopy at age 60 compared to a control group without any screening. The baseline findings of this study, which has recruited 170 000 participants, have recently been published[53]. Compliance with sigmoidoscopy was 71%. Rectosigmoid cancers were detected in 0.3%, distal adenomas in 12.1%. First mortality data should be available in a few years.

It is well known that patients in whom distal adenomas are found during sigmoidoscopy have an increased risk of additional proximal neoplasms. It is therefore generally recommended to perform a complete colonoscopy on patients with distal adenomas >1 cm[60]. It is controversial, however, whether every patient with a small adenoma found during sigmoidoscopy has to be followed up by complete colonoscopy. The guidelines either recommend colonoscopy follow-up for every adenoma found during sigmoidoscopy independent of size, number and histology[61,62], or recommend considering this approach depending on the patient[60]. One study found proximal neoplasias in 29% of patients with a distal adenoma <5 mm[63], in another study 6.4% of patients with a distal tubular adenoma <10 mm had an advanced proximal neoplasia[64]. It thus seems reasonable to offer a complete colonoscopy to anyone with an adenoma found during sigmoidoscopy independent of adenoma characteristics.

Even if every adenoma found during sigmoidoscopy is followed up by a complete colonoscopy a significant number of patients with isolated proximal neoplasms will be missed. In a recently published study with asymptomatic persons aged between 50 and 75 years, 5.4% of patients had an advanced neoplasm proximal to the sigmoid[64]; 52% of these patients had no distal adenomas and would thus not have been diagnosed by sigmoidoscopy. In order to be able to detect isolated proximal neoplasms the combination of sigmoidoscopy every 5 years and annual FOBT has been advocated[60,61]. There is only one study which prospectively compares sigmoidoscopy with the combination of sigmoidoscopy and FOBT[65]. In this study patients were randomized to an annual sigmoidoscopy with or without an additional annual FOBT. Compliance was poor, and although a greater reduction of CRC-related mortality was found for the combination screening group, this was of borderline significance. In a recently published study 2885 asymptomatic subjects (age range 50–75 years) had a FOBT performed[66]. They then underwent a one-time colonoscopy. Defining sigmoidoscopy as examination of the rectum and sigmoid colon during colonoscopy sigmoidoscopy would have identified 70% of subjects with advanced neoplasia, assuming that every distal adenoma would have resulted in a complete colonoscopy. FOBT had a sensitivity of 24% and the combination of sigmoidoscopy and FOBT was slightly more sensitive at detecting advanced neoplasms (76% vs. 70%) without reaching statitistical significance. However, only 19% of isolated proximal advanced neoplasms would have been detected by FOBT. Even though it is unclear how much additional benefit the annual instead of the one-time FOBT would have, this study clearly shows that even the combination of a one-time sigmoidoscopy and FOBT does not greatly improve detection rates for proximal neoplasms.

Colonoscopy

In order to be able to detect isolated proximal neoplasms colonoscopy is an alternative screening method. It has a proven high sensitivity for detecting carcinomas and adenomas of the whole colon. Tandem colonoscopies have shown miss rates between 15% and 24% for adenomas; however, larger adenomas ≥ 1 cm were rarely missed (0–6%)[67,68]. The caecum is reached in 93–99% of all procedures, depending on the skill of the endoscopist and the quality of bowel preparation[69,70]. A colonoscopy on average takes 22 min if no polyps are found; if a polypectomy is performed the examination time increases to 30 min[69]. One disadvantage of colonoscopy is the necessary bowel cleansing before the procedure. Morbidity of the procedure is also higher compared to sigmoidoscopy. One meta-analysis found perforation rates between 0.06% and 0.2% for diagnostic colonoscopies and 0.04% and 0.5% if polypectomies are performed. Mortality varies between 0% and 0.06%[71]. Although no randomized trials evaluating the use of colonoscopy for screening of the general population have been performed, several guidelines have included colonoscopy as a screening option[60,62]. Two recent guidelines have even recommended colonoscopy as the preferred screening strategy[61,72]. Reasons for this recommendation have included the data on isolated proximal neoplasia and the logical thought that data concerning the effectiveness of sigmoidoscocopy should also apply to colonoscopy, i.e. mortality reduction of up to 60%. It is estimated that a negative screening colonoscopy would not have to be repeated for 10 years. After an interval of 5.5 years no cancers were detected, and the incidence of adenomas with advanced pathology was $< 1\%$[73]. In a recently published case–control study the CRC risk reduction by endoscopy was 77% after a median of 7 years and seemed to last for more than 10 years with a risk reduction of 59% after a median of 19 years[74]. However, whereas the protective effect after 7 years was valid for cancers independent of their localization, the protective effect after 19 years was significant only for cancers of the rectosigmoid. Another case–control study also showed that endoscopy seemed to protect from rectosigmoid cancer for at least 10 years[56].

OTHER POSSIBLE SCREENING METHODS
Double-contrast barium enema

Double-contrast barium enemas are infrequently used for screening purposes nowadays. They have been found to be less sensitive for the detection of colorectal neoplasms compared to colonoscopies[75,76]. Like colonoscopy the procedure requires a thorough bowel preparation and if a polyp or neoplasm is suspected an additional colonoscopy has to be performed.

CT/MRT colonography

Virtual colonoscopy using either CT or MRT have also been evaluated as possible CRC-screening methods. In one study comparing CT colonography and conventional colonoscopy in a group at high risk for colorectal neoplasia the sensitivity for detecting large polyps $\geqslant 1$ cm was found to be 91% compared to 82% for medium-sized poyps (6–9 mm) and 55% for small polyps ($\leqslant 5$ mm)[77]. Other studies have reported much lower sensitivities[78,79]. However, in a recent study with 1233 average-risk persons the sensitivity for adenomas >5 mm was reported to be comparable to colonoscopy[80]. One major disadvantage of CT colonography is the high radiation exposure. This is not a problem if MRI is used. In one study the results of colonoscopy and MRI colonography was compared in 132 patients with a possible colonic mass. MRI was found to have a sensitivity of 96% for detecting large polyps (>10 mm), 61% for medium polyps (6–10 mm) but only 6% for detecting polyps <6 mm[81]. Another study with 70 patients found sensitivities of 100% for large polyps, 96% for medium polyps and 33% for small polyps[82]. It therefore looks as if colonography has a fairly high sensitivity for detecting large polyps, but is not able to detect a high proportion of the smaller as well as no flat polyps. It also has be considered that, like conventional colonoscopy, colonography requires a thorough bowel preparation. At this time the use of colonography outside of studies cannot be recommended.

Genetic stool testing

Ahlquist et al. used a panel of five genetic markers for the detection of stool alteraltions in patients with known CRC, adenomas >1 cm or endoscopically normal colons. The sensitivity was found to be 91% for cancers and 82% for adenomas, with a specificity of 93%[83].

Table 2 Summary of guidelines

	Gastrointestinal Consortium	American College of Gastroenterology	US Preventive Services Task Force	Deutsche Gesellschaft für Verdauungs- und Stoffwechselkrankheiten
Year of publication	2003	2000	2002	2004
FOBT	Annually after age 50	Annually after age 50	Annually after age 50	Annually after age 50
Sigmoidoscopy	Every 5 years ± annual FOBT after age 50	Every 5 years ± annual FOBT after age 50	Every 5 years ± annual FOBT after age 50	Every 5 years ± annual FOBT after age 50
Colonoscopy	Every 10 years after age 50	Every 10 years after age 50	Not enough evidence for recommendation	Every 10 years after age 50

Traverso et al. were able to detect 61% of CRC and 50% of adenomas by using a digital Protein Truncation Test applied to stool samples[84]. In a recently published decision analysis faecal DNA testing every 5 years was considered to be effective and cost-effective compared to no screening, but inferior to other strategies such as FOBT or colonoscopy[85]; however, more research is needed before genetic testing can be recommended for screening purposes.

Guidelines

Several guidelines with recommendations on the use of the screening methods described above have been published[61,62,86,87] (Table 2), two of which have recently been updated[60,72].

CURRENT NATIONAL CRC SCREENING PROGRAMME IN GERMANY

In Germany, up to 2002, CRC screening consisted of an annual FOBT beginning at age 45 as part of the recommended cancer screening. Compliance with this cancer screening programme was poor, with only 14% of eligible men and 34% of eligible women taking part[88]. In 2002 a new CRC screening programme was implemented covered by the health insurance companies. It includes an annual FOBT from age 50 to 54 and a colonoscopy at 55 that, if negative, can be repeated after 10 years. For anyone unwilling to undergo colonoscopy a biennial FOBT can be performed after age 55. In the first year around 300 000 screening colonoscopies were performed, 126 000 of which have been evaluated to date. Carcinomas were found in 0.67%, adenomas in 18.1% of examinations. The next few years will give us more information about the efficacy and safety of the implemented screening colonoscopy programme in Germany.

CONCLUSIONS

Ideally CRC could be prevented by diet or medication; however, although several risk factors for CRC development are known the effect of interventions with diet or medication have either been disappointing or been only modest. To significantly reduce CRC-related mortality screening currently seems to be the best method. For any CRC screening programme to be effective the general population has to be included. There are several large prospective randomized trials clearly showing that FOBT is an effective screening method; however, its sensitivity for detecting CRC is moderate, and low for detecting adenomas, the removal of which has been shown to be a very effective way of preventing CRC. Sigmoidoscopy has also been shown to be effective. In case–control studies it was able to reduce CRC-related mortality by at least 60%, making it likely to be more effective than FOBT for reducing mortality of rectosigmoid cancers. Although there is no prospective study assessing the efficacy of colonoscopy for CRC screening the fact that it has a proven high sensitivity for detecting adenomas and CRC of the whole colon, and the data from sigmoidoscopy, as well as cost-effectiveness studies, seem to justify recommending its use for CRC screening and prevention. No matter which screening method is used its impact will be greatly influenced by the compliance it is able to achieve in the general population. Even if one considers colonoscopy to be the most effective method of preventing CRC, if a patient is only willing to perform a FOBT this is certainly much better than performing no screening. Every effort should be made to improve compliance with the existing screening recommendations in the general population.

References

1. Citarda F, Tomaselli G, Capocaccia R et al. Efficacy in standard clinical practice of colonoscopic polypectomy in reducing colorectal cancer incidence. Gut. 2001;48:812–15.
2. Winawer SJ, Zauber AG, Ho MN et al. Prevention of colorectal cancer by colonoscopic polypectomy. The National Polyp Study Workgroup. N Engl J Med. 1993;329:1977–81.
3. McMichael AJ, Giles GG. Cancer in migrants to Australia: extending the descriptive epidemiological data. Cancer Res. 1988;48:751–6.
4. Giacosa A, Franceschi S, La Vecchia C et al. Energy intake, overweight, physical exercise and colorectal cancer risk. Eur J Cancer Prev. 1999;8(Suppl. 1):S53–60.
5. Martinez ME, Heddens D, Earnest DL et al. Physical activity, body mass index, and prostaglandin E2 levels in rectal mucosa. J Natl Cancer Inst. 1999;91:950–3.
6. Giovannucci E. Diet, body weight, and colorectal cancer: a summary of the epidemiologic evidence. J Womens Health (Larchmt). 2003;12:173–82.
7. Lee IM. Physical activity and cancer prevention – data from epidemiologic studies. Med Sci Sports Exerc. 2003;35:1823–7.
8. Calle EE, Rodriguez C, Walker-Thurmond K, Thun MJ. Overweight, obesity, and mortality from cancer in a prospectively studied cohort of U.S. adults. N Engl J Med. 2003;348:1625–38.
9. Zhang B, Li X, Nakama H et al. A case–control study on risk of changing food consumption for colorectal cancer. Cancer Invest. 2002;20:458–63.
10. Sesink AL, Termont DS, Kleibeuker JH, Van der Meer R. Red meat and colon cancer: the cytotoxic and hyperproliferative effects of dietary heme. Cancer Res. 1999;59:5704–9.
11. Pisani P, Mitton N. Cooking methods, metabolic polymorphisms and colorectal cancer. Eur J Cancer Prev. 2002;11:75–84.
12. Terry P, Giovannucci E, Michels KB et al. Fruit, vegetables, dietary fiber, and risk of colorectal cancer. J Natl Cancer Inst. 2001;93:525–33.
13. World Cancer Research Fund AIfCR. Food, nutrition and the prevention of cancer: a global perspective. London, Washington: World Cancer Research Fund/American Institute for Cancer Research 1997.
14. Howe GR, Benito E, Castelleto R et al. Dietary intake of fiber and decreased risk of cancers of the colon and rectum: evidence from the combined analysis of 13 case–control studies. J Natl Cancer Inst. 1992;84:1887–96.
15. Bingham SA, Day NE, Luben R et al. Dietary fibre in food and protection against colorectal cancer in the European Prospective Investigation into Cancer and Nutrition (EPIC): an observational study. Lancet. 2003;361:1496–501.
16. Peters U, Sinha R, Chatterjee N et al. Dietary fibre and colorectal adenoma in a colorectal cancer early detection programme. Lancet. 2003;361:1491–5.
17. Fuchs CS, Giovannuci EL, Colditz GA et al. Dietary fiber and the risk of colorectal cancer and adenoma in women. N Engl J Med. 1999;340:169–76.
18. Schatzkin A, Lanza E, Corle D et al. Lack of effect of a low-fat, high-fiber diet on the recurrence of colorectal adenomas. N Engl J Med. 2000;16:1149–55.
19. Alberts DS, Martinez ME, Roe DJ et al. Lack of effect of a high-fiber cereal supplement on the recurrence of colorectal adenomas. N Engl J Med. 2000;342:1156–62.
20. Fuchs CS, Giovannucci EL, Colditz GA et al. A prospective study of family history and the risk of colorectal cancer. N Engl J Med. 1994;331:1669–74.

21. Cho E, Smith-Warner SA, Ritz J et al. Alcohol intake and colorectal cancer: a pooled analysis of 8 cohort studies. Ann Intern Med. 2004;140:603-13.
22. Giovannucci E, Rimm EB, Ascherio A et al. Alcohol, low-methionine-low-folate diets, and risk of colon cancer in men. J Natl Cancer Inst. 1995;87:265-73.
23. Janne PA, Mayer RJ. Chemoprevention of colorectal cancer. N Engl J Med. 2000;342: 1960-8.
24. Wu K, Willett WC, Fuchs CS et al. Calcium intake and risk of colon cancer in women and men. J Natl Cancer Inst. 2002;94:437-46.
25. Bonithon-Kopp C, Kronborg O, Giacosa A et al. Calcium and fibre supplementation in prevention of colorectal adenoma recurrence: a randomised intervention trial. European Cancer Prevention Organisation Study Group. Lancet. 2000;356:1300-6.
26. Baron JA, Beach M, Mandel JS et al. Calcium supplements for the prevention of colorectal adenomas. Calcium Polyp Prevention Study Group. N Engl J Med. 1999;340:101-7.
27. Biasco G, Zannoni U, Paganelli GM et al. Folic acid supplementation and cell kinetics of rectal mucosa in patients with ulcerative colitis. Cancer Epidemiol Biomarkers Prev. 1997; 6:469-71.
28. Cravo ML, Pinto AG, Chaves P et al. Effect of folate supplementation on DNA methylation of rectal mucosa in patients with colonic adenomas: correlation with nutrient intake. Clin Nutr. 1998;17:45-9.
29. La Vecchia C, Negri E, Pelucchi C, Franceschi S. Dietary folate and colorectal cancer. Int J Cancer. 2002;102:545-7.
30. Konings EJ, Goldbohm RA, Brants HA et al. Intake of dietary folate vitamers and risk of colorectal carcinoma: results from the Netherlands Cohort Study. Cancer. 2002;95:1421-33.
31. Giovannucci E. Epidemiologic studies of folate and colorectal neoplasia: a review. J Nutr. 2002;132:2350-5S.
32. Greenberg ER, Baron JA, Tosteson TD et al. A clinical trial of antioxidant vitamins to prevent colorectal adenoma. Polyp Prevention Study Group. N Engl J Med. 1994;331:141-7.
33. Fairfield KM, Fletcher RH. Vitamins for chronic disease prevention in adults: scientific review. J Am Med Assoc. 2002;287:3116-26.
34. Duffield-Lillico AJ, Reid ME, Turnbull BW et al. Baseline characteristics and the effect of selenium supplementation on cancer incidence in a randomized clinical trial: a summary report of the Nutritional Prevention of Cancer Trial. Cancer Epidemiol Biomarkers Prev. 2002;11:630-9.
35. Eberhart CE, Coffey RJ, Radhika A et al. Up-regulation of cyclooxygenase 2 gene expression in human colorectal adenomas and adenocarcinomas. Gastroenterology. 1994; 107:1183-8.
36. Oshima M, Dinchuk JE, Kargman SL et al. Suppression of intestinal polyposis in Apc delta716 knockout mice by inhibition of cyclooxygenase 2 (COX-2). Cell. 1996;87:803-9.
37. Giardiello FM, Hamilton SR, Krush AJ et al. Treatment of colonic and rectal adenomas with sulindac in familial adenomatous polyposis. N Engl J Med. 1993;328:1313-16.
38. Nugent KP, Farmer KC, Spigelman AD et al. Randomized controlled trial of the effect of sulindac on duodenal and rectal polyposis and cell proliferation in patients with familial adenomatous polyposis. Br J Surg. 1993;80:1618-19.
39. Giardiello FM, Yang VW, Hylind LM et al. Primary chemoprevention of familial adenomatous polyposis with sulindac. N Engl J Med. 2002;346:1054-9.
40. Steinbach G, Lynch PM, Phillips RK et al. The effect of celecoxib, a cyclooxygenase-2 inhibitor, in familial adenomatous polyposis. N Engl J Med. 2000;342:1946-52.
41. Baron JA, Cole BF, Sandler RS et al. A randomized trial of aspirin to prevent colorectal adenomas. N Engl J Med. 2003;348:891-9.
42. Sandler RS, Halabi S, Baron JA et al. A randomized trial of aspirin to prevent colorectal adenomas in patients with previous colorectal cancer. N Engl J Med. 2003;348:883-90.
43. Imperiale TF, Wagner DR, Lin CY et al. Results of screening colonoscopy among persons 40 to 49 years of age. N Engl J Med. 2002;346:1781-5.
44. Ransohoff DF, Sandler RS. Clinical practice. Screening for colorectal cancer. N Engl J Med. 2002;346:40-4.
45. Hardcastle JD, Chamberlain JO, Robinson MH et al. Randomised controlled trial of faecal-occult-blood screening for colorectal cancer. Lancet. 1996;348:1472-7.

46. Kronborg O, Fenger C, Olsen J et al. Randomised study of screening for colorectal cancer with faecal-occult-blood test. Lancet. 1996;348:1467–71.
47. Faivre J, Dancourt V, Lejeune C et al. Reduction in colorectal cancer mortality by fecal occult blood screening in a French controlled study. Gastroenterology. 2004;126:1674–80.
48. Mandel JS, Bond JH, Church TR et al. Reducing mortality from colorectal cancer by screening for fecal occult blood. Minnesota Colon Cancer Control Study. N Engl J Med. 1993;328:1365–71.
49. Scholefield JH, Moss S, Sufi F et al. Effect of faecal occult blood screening on mortality from colorectal cancer: results from a randomised controlled trial. Gut. 2002;50:840–4.
50. Jorgensen OD, Kronborg O, Fenger C. A randomised study of screening for colorectal cancer using faecal occult blood testing: results after 13 years and seven biennial screening rounds. Gut. 2002;50:29–32.
51. Mandel JS, Church TR, Ederer F, Bond JH. Colorectal cancer mortality: effectiveness of biennial screening for fecal occult blood. J Natl Cancer Inst. 1999;91:434–7.
52. Mandel JS, Church TR, Bond JH et al. The effect of fecal occult-blood screening on the incidence of colorectal cancer. N Engl J Med. 2000;343:1603–7.
53. Atkin W, Cook C, Cuzick J et al. Single flexible sigmoidoscopy screening to prevent colorectal cancer: baseline findings of a UK multicentre randomised trial. Lancet. 2002; 359:1291–300.
54. Muller AD, Sonnenberg A. Protection by endoscopy against death from colorectal cancer. A case–control study among veterans. Arch Intern Med. 1995;155:1741–8.
55. Newcomb PA, Norfleet RG, Storer BE et al. Screening sigmoidoscopy and colorectal cancer mortality. J Natl Cancer Inst. 1992;84:1572–5.
56. Selby JV, Friedman GD, Quesenberry CP, Jr., Weiss NS. A case-control study of screening sigmoidoscopy and mortality from colorectal cancer. N Engl J Med. 1992;326:653–7.
57. Rex DK, Lehman GA, Ulbright TM et al. The yield of a second screening flexible sigmoidoscopy in average-risk persons after one negative examination. Gastroenterology. 1994;106:593–5.
58. Schoen RE, Pinsky PF, Weissfeld JL et al. Results of repeat sigmoidoscopy 3 years after a negative examination. J Am Med Assoc. 2003;290:41–8.
59. Prorok PC, Andriole GL, Bresalier RS et al. Design of the Prostate, Lung, Colorectal and Ovarian (PLCO) Cancer Screening Trial. Control Clin Trials. 2000;21:273–309S.
60. Winawer S, Fletcher R, Rex D et al. Colorectal cancer screening and surveillance: clinical guidelines and rationale-Update based on new evidence. Gastroenterology. 2003;124:544–60.
61. Rex DK, Johnson DA, Lieberman DA et al. Colorectal cancer prevention 2000: screening recommendations of the American College of Gastroenterology. Am J Gastroenterol. 2000; 95:868–77.
62. Schmiegel W, Adler G, Frühmorgen P et al. Kolorektales Karzinom: Prävention und Früherkennung in der asynmptomatischen Bevölkerung – Vorsorge bei Risikopatienten – Endoskopische Diagnostik, Therapie und Nachsorge von Polypen und Karzinomen. Z Gastroenterol. 2000;38:49–76.
63. Read TE, Read JD, Butterly LF. Importance of adenomas 5 mm or less in diameter that are detected by sigmoidoscopy. N Engl J Med. 1997;336:8–12.
64. Lieberman DA, Weiss DG, Bond JH et al. Use of colonoscopy to screen asymptomatic adults for colorectal cancer. Veterans Affairs Cooperative Study Group 380. N Engl J Med. 2000;343:162–8.
65. Winawer SJ, Flehinger BJ, Schottenfeld D, Miller DG. Screening for colorectal cancer with fecal occult blood testing and sigmoidoscopy. J Natl Cancer Inst. 1993;85:1311–18.
66. Lieberman DA, Weiss DG. One-time screening for colorectal cancer with combined fecal occult-blood testing and examination of the distal colon. N Engl J Med. 2001;345:555–60.
67. Hixson LJ, Fennerty MB, Sampliner RE et al. Prospective study of the frequency and size distribution of polyps missed by colonoscopy. J Natl Cancer Inst. 1990;82:1769–72.
68. Rex DK, Cutler CS, Lemmel GT et al. Colonoscopic miss rates of adenomas determined by back-to-back colonoscopies. Gastroenterology. 1997;112:24–8.
69. Lieberman DA, Smith FW. Screening for colon malignancy with colonoscopy. Am J Gastroenterol. 1991;86:946–51.
70. Rogge JD, Elmore MF, Mahoney SJ et al. Low-cost, office-based, screening colonoscopy. Am J Gastroenterol. 1994;86:946–51.

71. Froehlich F, Gonvers J-J, Vader J-P et al. Appropriateness of gastrointestinal endoscopy: risk of complications. Endoscopy. 1999;31:684–6.
72. Schmiegel W, Pox C, Adler G et al. [S-3–Guidelines Conference 'Colorectal Carcinoma' 2004]. Z Gastroenterol. 2004;42:1129–77 [In German].
73. Rex DK, Cummings OW, Helper DJ et al. 5-year incidence of adenomas after negative colonoscopy in asymptomatic average-risk persons [see comment]. Gastroenterology. 1996; 111:1178–81.
74. Brenner H, Arndt V, Sturmer T et al. Long-lasting reduction of risk of colorectal cancer following screening endoscopy. Br J Cancer. 2001;85:972–6.
75. Winawer SJ, Stewart ET, Zauber AG et al. A comparison of colonoscopy and double-contrast barium enema for surveillance after polypectomy. National Polyp Study Work Group. N Engl J Med. 2000;342:1766–72.
76. Rex DK, Rahmani EY, Haseman JH et al. Relative sensitivity of colonoscopy and barium enema for detection of colorectal cancer in clinical practice. Gastroenterology. 1997;112: 17–23.
77. Fenlon HM, Nunes DP, Schroy III PC et al. A comparison of virtual and conventional colonoscopy for the detection of colorectal polyps. N Engl J Med. 1999;341:1496–503.
78. Pescatore P, Glücker T, Delarive J et al. Diagnostic accuracy and interobserver agreement of CT colonography (virtual colonoscopy). Gut. 2000;47:126–30.
79. Spinzi G, Belloni G, Martegani A et al. Computed tomographic colonography and conventional colonoscopy for colon diseases: a prospective blinded study. Am J Gastroenterol. 2001;96:394–400.
80. Pickhardt PJ, Choi JR, Hwang I et al. Computed tomographic virtual colonoscopy to screen for colorectal neoplasia in asymptomatic adults. N Engl J Med. 2003;349:2191–200.
81. Luboldt W, Bauerfeind P, Wildermuth S et al. Colonic masses: detection with MR colonography. Radiology. 2000;216:383–8.
82. Pappalardo G, Polettini E, Frattaroli FM et al. Magnetic resonance colonography versus conventional colonoscopy for the detection of colonic endoluminal lesions. Gastroenterology. 2000;119:300–4.
83. Ahlquist DA, Skoletsky JE, Boynton KA et al. Colorectal cancer screening by detection of altered human DNA in stool: feasibility of a multitarget assay panel. Gastroenterology. 2000;119:1219–27.
84. Traverso G, Shuber A, Levin B et al. Detection of APC mutations in fecal DNA from patients with colorectal tumors. N Engl J Med. 2002;346:311–20.
85. Song K, Fendrick AM, Ladabaum U. Fecal DNA testing compared with conventional colorectal cancer screening methods: a decision analysis. Gastroenterology. 2004;126:1270–9.
86. Winawer SJ, Fletcher RH, Miller L et al. Colorectal cancer screening: clinical guidelines and rationale. Gastroenterology. 1997;112:594–642.
87. Screening for colorectal cancer: recommendation and rationale. Ann Intern Med. 2002; 137:129–31.
88. Gesetzliche Krankheitsfrüherkennungsmassnahmen. Dokumentation der Untersuchungsergebnisse – Männer und Frauen – Krebs 1989 und 1990. Kassenärztliche Bundesvereinigung und Spitzenverbände der Krankenkassen.

28
Treatment of inflammatory bowel disease: 'early hit' or stepwise escalation

W. J. SANDBORN

INTRODUCTION

This chapter will review the natural history of Crohn's disease (CD) and ulcerative colitis under the current treatment paradigm of stepwise escalation, and the rationale for changing to a future treatment paradigm of an 'early hit' with immunosuppressive and/or biological therapies in an attempt to change the natural history of these diseases.

CROHN'S DISEASE

Current treatment paradigm

At the present time, patients with CD are treated in a therapeutic pyramid of stepwise escalation of therapy beginning with agents that have low efficacy and low toxicity, and ending with agents that have greater efficacy and greater toxicity[1]. The first tier of the treatment pyramid for patients with CD has typically consisted of sulphasalazine and mesalamine, antibiotics, and more recently enteric-release budesonide. Patients who fail this first tier of therapy typically receive second-tier therapy with conventional corticosteroids, azathioprine or 6-mercaptopurine, and methotrexate. The third tier of the pyramid includes infliximab, cyclosporin and tacrolimus, and surgical resection.

Natural history

Patients with CD have evolution in disease behaviour over time. Approximately 90% of patients presenting with a new diagnosis of CD have a luminal inflammatory disease behaviour pattern. A minority of patients will present initially with stricturing disease or penetrating disease with fistulas or abscesses[2]. During long-term follow-up the proportion of patients with luminal inflammatory disease behaviour decreases to less than 20% by 20 years and, conversely, the proportion of patients who develop penetrating or stricturing disease behaviour steadily rises over time[2]. Thus, the typical patient has a progression over time in disease behaviour from luminal inflammatory disease to the development of disease complications including strictures and intestinal penetration. As a result of the development of disease complications, the cumulative probability of surgical resection rises over time. By 20 years of disease approximately 80% of patients with CD will have required at least one surgical resection[3]. The natural history of CD following surgical resection is to reoccur. By 1 year after operation approximately 70% of patients will already have endoscopic evidence of recurrence in the neoterminal ileum[4]. By 3 years following operation the percentage of patients with endoscopic recurrence approaches 90%. Following behind after the endoscopic recurrence will be inevitable increases in the percentages of patients with laboratory recurrence, clinical recurrence, and eventually the need for repeat operation[4]. In Copenhagen County, Denmark, by 15 years after diagnosis 30% of patients will have had no surgery, 34% of patients will have had one surgery, 14% of patients will have had two surgeries, and 22% of patients will have had three or more surgeries[3]. Thus, by 15 years, one-third of patients will have already had two or more operations.

During the first year following the diagnosis of CD over 90% of patients will have active disease[5]. This is not surprising, since it is active symptoms that typically lead to diagnostic evaluation to establish the diagnosis of CD. For all years after the first year, in any given year, approximately 50% of patients will be in symptomatic remission, and 50% of patients will have active CD over the course of the year[5]. If the window of observation is widened from 1 year to 5 years, then 22% of patients will have continuously inactive CD over a 5-year period, 25% of patients will have continuously active CD, and the remaining 53% of patients will alternate between periods of inactivity and periods of relapse[5]. Thus, over a 5-year period, 78% of patients will have either intermittent or continuous disease activity.

Lack of long-term efficacy with current first-line therapies

The traditional first-line medical therapies for CD are of only modest and short-term benefit. In the National Cooperative Crohn's Disease Trial, sulphasalazine at an average dose of 4.7 g per day resulted in clinical remission in 43% of patients, compared to 30% of placebo-treated patients[6]. Three large trials have been performed with oral mesalamine (Pentasa) at doses of 4 g per day[7,8]. One trial involving 155 patients showed a significant benefit for mesalamine[7]. Two subsequent trials, involving 150 patients and 310 patients respectively, failed to demonstrate any benefit of oral mesalamine for CD[8]. Maintenance of remission studies with sulphasalazine at an average dose of 2.3 g/day have been uniformly negative[6]. Likewise, studies evaluating oral mesalamine for maintenance of medically induced remission have, for the most part, not shown any maintenance benefit[9]. A recent meta-analysis published by the Cochrane Collaboration showed an odds ratio of 1.0 for maintenance of medically induced remission with oral mesalamine[10]. Prednisone and prednisolone are highly effective for inducing remission over the short term in patients with CD. In the National Cooperative Crohn's Disease Trial, by 16 weeks, 60% of patients treated with prednisone had entered clinical remission compared to only 30% of placebo-treated patients[6]. However, when patients receive maintenance therapy with a lower dose of prednisone (approximately 20 mg/day) over 2 years, no maintenance benefit was demonstrated[6]. Nevertheless, in clinical practice, we recognize that some patients do appear to derive symptomatic benefit from maintenance therapy with corticosteroids. These patients are classified as being steroid-dependent. In one population-based study from Olmsted County, Minnesota, 84% of patients experienced short-term response to corticosteroids[11]. By 1 year 32% of patients were steroid-dependent, 38% of patients had undergone surgical resection either for failure to respond to corticosteroids or for steroid dependency, and only 28% of patients were in symptomatic remission off steroids[11].

To summarize, the consequences of stepwise escalation therapy in patients with CD include progression over time from luminal inflammatory disease behaviour to complications of stricturing and penetrating disease, progression over time to surgical resection, endoscopic recurrence of disease after operation ultimately leading to clinical recurrence and need for repeat operation, and the frequent occurrence of steroid dependency, which in turns leads to steroid-associated osteopenia and osteoporosis.

Potential future first-line therapies that could provide long-term efficacy and possibly alter the natural history of CD

There are several candidate therapies which have the potential to alter the natural history of CD. The first candidates to be considered are the thiopurine drugs azathioprine and 6-mercaptopurine. In one study, patients with active CD were treated with a tapering course of corticosteroids over 3 months and randomized to azathioprine 2.5 mg/kg per day or placebo and followed for 15 months. By month 15 approximately 40% of azathioprine-treated patients were in remission off corticosteroids compared to less than 10% of placebo-treated patients[12]. In a similar study, children with newly diagnosed CD were treated with a tapering course of corticosteroids over 6 months and randomized to therapy with 6-mercaptopurine 1.5 mg/kg per day or placebo, and followed for 1 year. At 1 year 85% of patients who had received 6-mercaptopurine were in remission and off corticosteroids, compared to 54% of placebo-treated patients[13]. The cumulative steroid exposure in the 6-mercaptopurine-treated patients was approximately half of the steroid exposure in placebo-treated patients.

The second candidate drug which has potential to modify the natural history of CD is methotrexate. Feagan and colleagues randomized patients with active CD despite treatment with corticosteroids to methotrexate 25 mg per week intramuscularly or placebo. At week 16, 39% of methotrexate-treated patients were in remission and off corticosteroids compared to 19% of placebo-treated patients[14]. In a subsequent follow-up study, patients who responded to induction therapy with methotrexate 25 mg/week were randomized to continued methotrexate at a reduced dose of 15 mg/week or placebo and followed for 40 weeks. At the end of 40 weeks of maintenance therapy over 60% of patients who continued methotrexate therapy were in remission and off corticosteroids compared to approximately 40% of placebo-treated patients[15].

The final candidate drug which has the potential to modify the natural history of CD is the anti-tumour necrosis factor antibody infliximab. In a study by Hanauer, patients with moderate to severely active CD unresponsive to conventional therapy were treated with a single dose of infliximab 5 mg/kg. Patients who responded were then randomized to maintenance therapy with placebo or maintenance therapy with infliximab 5 mg/kg or 10 mg/kg at weeks 2 and 6 and then every 8 weeks through week 46, and were followed until week 54. The median time to loss of response through week 54 was 19 weeks for placebo-treated patients, 38 weeks for infliximab 5 mg/kg-treated patients, and greater than 54 weeks for infliximab 10 mg/kg-treated patients[16]. Clinical remission at week 54 was observed in 13% of placebo-treated patients, 28% of infliximab 5 mg/kg-treated patients, and 38% of infliximab 10 mg/kg-treated patients[16].

ULCERATIVE COLITIS

Current treatment paradigm

At the present time patients with ulcerative colitis are treated in a treatment pyramid of stepwise escalation of therapy beginning with agents that have moderate efficacy and low toxicity, and ending with agents that have greater efficacy and greater toxicity[17]. The first tier of the treatment pyramid for patients with ulcerative colitis is sulphasalazine and mesalamine. Patients who fail this first tier of therapy typically receive second-tier therapy with conventional corticosteroids and azathioprine or 6-mercaptopurine. The third tier of the pyramid includes cyclosporin and colectomy with ileoanal pouch.

Natural history

The cumulative probability of undergoing colectomy for ulcerative colitis over 25 years is approximately 30%[18]. If the risk of colectomy is stratified by the extent of disease, then it can be appreciated that approximately 30% of patients with left-sided ulcerative colitis and 40% of patients with pancolitis will undergo operation, usually by 5 years, and in contrast that only 10–15% of patients with distal ulcerative proctosigmoiditis will undergo colectomy[18]. For patients who undergo colectomy, disease recurrence in the form of pouchitis is common. The cumulative rate of pouchitis 5 years after colectomy with ileoanal pouch approaches 50%[19]. For patients with ileoanal pouches the median 24-h stool frequency 1 year after operation is eight stools per day[20].

Among patients with ulcerative colitis over 90% of patients have symptoms of active disease during the first year following diagnosis[21]. In subsequent years approximately 50% of patients will be in symptomatic remission in any given year, with the remainder of patients either having active disease or having undergone colectomy[21]. If the window of observation is widened from 1 year to 5 years, then the data demonstrate that 25% of patients will have disease continuously in remission over a 5-year period, 18% of patients will have continuously active disease, and the remaining 57% of patients will alternate between symptomatic remission and relapse[21], For patients who require corticosteroids, 84% of patients will respond acutely[11]. However, when patients requiring corticosteroids are followed out to 1 year, then 22% of patients will be steroid-dependent, 29% of patients will have come to colectomy, and only 49% of patients will be in symptomatic remission off corticosteroids at 1 year[11].

To summarize the consequences of stepwise escalation therapy for left-sided ulcerative colitis and pancolitis, approximately 30–40% of patients will come to colectomy, often within 5 years. Pouchitis occurs after operation in up to 50% of patients by 5 years, and the median stool frequency over 24 h at 1 year after ileoanal pouch is eight stools per day. Steroids are used frequently in this patient population, and steroid dependency occurs often. Steroid dependency in turn frequently leads to steroid-associated osteopenia and osteoporosis.

Potential future first-line therapies that could provide long-term efficacy and possibly alter the natural history of ulcerative colitis

Candidate therapies to alter the natural history of ulcerative colitis include azathioprine and 6-mercaptopurine, and potentially in the near future, infliximab. To date these therapies have not been sufficiently studied in patients with ulcerative colitis to advocate their earlier introduction in the treatment paradigm. Additional studies are needed to address this issue.

CONCLUSIONS

In conclusion, current treatment guidelines for CD and ulcerative colitis advocate a stepwise escalation approach to therapy. This stepwise approach begins with sulphasalazine and mesalamine, progresses through corticosteroids, and finally arrives at immunosuppressive and biological therapy. In patients with CD randomized, controlled trials have not demonstrated that mesalamine induces or maintains remission. For both ulcerative colitis and CD corticosteroids are effective in the short term but do not result in durable remission for a majority of patients. Because of toxicity, corticosteroids should not be used for maintenance of remission. The natural history of patients with CD and patients with left-sided and pancolonic ulcerative colitis who are treated in a stepwise fashion with mesalamine and corticosteroids is to progress to operation. The natural history of patients undergoing surgery is for the disease to recur. In patients with CD mesalamine administered after operation does not have a meaningful impact on disease recurrence. Current treatment paradigms do not modify the natural course of CD and left-sided and pancolonic ulcerative colitis, which is to progress to surgery. New treatment approaches, such as the earlier introduction of azathioprine, methotrexate, and infliximab, are needed to alter the natural history of these diseases and to prevent operation.

References

1. Hanauer SB, Sandborn W. The Practice Parameters Committee of the American College of Gastroenterology. Management of Crohn's disease in adults. Am J Gastroenterol. 2001;96:635-43.
2. Cosnes J, Cattan S, Blain A et al. Long-term evolution of disease behavior of Crohn's disease. Inflamm Bowel Dis. 2002;8:244-50.
3. Munkholm P, Langholz E, Davidsen M, Binder V. Intestinal cancer risk and mortality in patients with Crohn's disease. Gastroenterology. 1993;105:1716-23.
4. Rutgeerts P, Geboes K, Vantrappen G, Beyls J, Kerremans R, Hiele M. Predictability of the postoperative course of Crohn's disease. Gastroenterology. 1990;99:956-63.
5. Munkholm P, Langholz E, Davidsen M, Binder V. Disease activity courses in a regional cohort of Crohn's disease patients. Scand J Gastroenterol. 1995;30:699-706.
6. Summers RW, Switz DM, Sessions JT Jr et al. National Cooperative Crohn's Disease Study: results of drug treatment. Gastroenterology. 1979;77:847-69.
7. Singleton JW, Hanauer SB, Gitnick GL et al. Mesalamine capsules for the treatment of active Crohn's disease: results of a 16-week trial. Pentasa Crohn's Disease Study Group. Gastroenterology. 1993;104:1293-301.
8. Hanauer SB, Stromberg U. Oral Pentasa in the treatment of active Crohn's disease: a meta-analysis of double-blind, placebo-controlled trials [see comment]. Clin Gastroenterol Hepatol. 2004;2:379-88.
9. Camma C, Giunta M, Rosselli M, Cottone M. Mesalamine in the maintenance treatment of Crohn's disease: a meta-analysis adjusted for confounding variables. Gastroenterology. 1997;113:1465-73.
10. Akobeng AK, Gardener E. Oral 5-aminosalicylic acid for maintenance of medically-induced remission in Crohn's disease (review). Cochrane Database Syst Rev. 2005;1: CD003715.
11. Faubion WJ, Loftus EJ, Harmsen WS, Zinsmeister AR, Sandborn WJ. The natural history of corticosteroid therapy for inflammatory bowel disease: a population-based study. Gastroenterology. 2001;121:255-60.
12. Candy S, Wright J, Gerber M, Adams G, Gerig M, Goodman R. A controlled double blind study of azathioprine in the management of Crohn's disease. Gut. 1995;37:674-8.
13. Markowitz J, Grancher K, Kohn N, Lesser M, Daum F. A multicenter trial of 6-mercaptopurine and prednisone in children with newly diagnosed Crohn's disease. Gastroenterology. 2000;119:895-902.
14. Feagan BG, Rochon J, Fedorak RN et al. Methotrexate for the treatment of Crohn's disease. North American Crohn's Study Group Investigators. N Engl J Med. 1995;332:292-7.
15. Feagan BG, Fedorak RN, Irvine EJ et al. A comparison of methotrexate with placebo for the maintenance of remission in Crohn's disease. North American Crohn's Study Group Investigators. N Engl J Med. 2000;342:1627-32.
16. Hanauer SB, Feagan BG, Lichtenstein GR et al. Maintenance infliximab for Crohn's disease: the ACCENT I randomised trial. Lancet. 2002;359:1541-9.
17. Kornbluth A, Sachar DB, Practice Parameters Committee of the American College of Gastroenterology. Ulcerative colitis practice guidelines in adults (update): American College of Gastroenterology, Practice Parameters Committee. Am J Gastroenterol. 2004; 99:1371-85.
18. Langholz E, Munkholm P, Davidsen M, Binder V. Colorectal cancer risk and mortality in patients with ulcerative colitis. Gastroenterology. 1992;103:1444-51.
19. Penna C, Dozois R, Tremaine W et al. Pouchitis after ileal pouch–anal anastomosis for ulcerative colitis occurs with increased frequency in patients with associated primary sclerosing cholangitis. Gut. 1996;38:234-9.
20. Gionchetti P, Rizzello F, Helwig U et al. Prophylaxis of pouchitis onset with probiotic therapy: a double-blind, placebo-controlled trial. Gastroenterology. 2003;124:1202-9.

29
Clinical impact of mesalazine for research and therapy in inflammatory bowel diseases

U. KLOTZ

INTRODUCTION

Mesalazine (5-aminosalicylic acid; 5-ASA) was indirectly introduced as prodrug sulphasalazine (consisting of 5-ASA and sulphapyridine; see Figure 1) as early as 1942 for the treatment of ulcerative colitits[1]. Many years later controlled clinical trials were performed to determine whether the therapeutic potential for chronic inflammatory bowel disease (IBD) resides in the parent drug or in the primary metabolites sulphapyridine and/or 5-ASA. Thereby 5-ASA was administered in the form of enemas or suppositories, mainly to patients with ulcerative colitis. As 5-ASA was at least as effective as sulphasalazine (SZ), this metabolite was regarded as the active therapeutic moiety of the azo-prodrug[2-4].

The favourable clinical results initiated the development of various 5-ASA preparations (e.g. slow/controlled-release formulations; suppositories, enemas, foam) for direct oral and rectal administration in the treatment of Crohn's disease or ulcerative colitis, and in 1984 the first 5-ASA product (Salofalk®) was marketed[5].

Many comparative studies using 5-ASA in different dosages and formulations, either for inducing or maintaining remission in patients with IBD, were performed. It was also noted that most of the observed side-effects of SZ could be attributed to sulphapyridine[6,7], whereas 5-ASA was well tolerated, allowing even higher dosage than initially selected. These considerations also resulted in the development of other azo-prodrugs[8] by replacing the 'toxic' sulphapyridine by an inert carrier (e.g. balsalazide) or forming a double molecule (dimer) of 5-ASA in the case of olsalazine (see Figure 1).

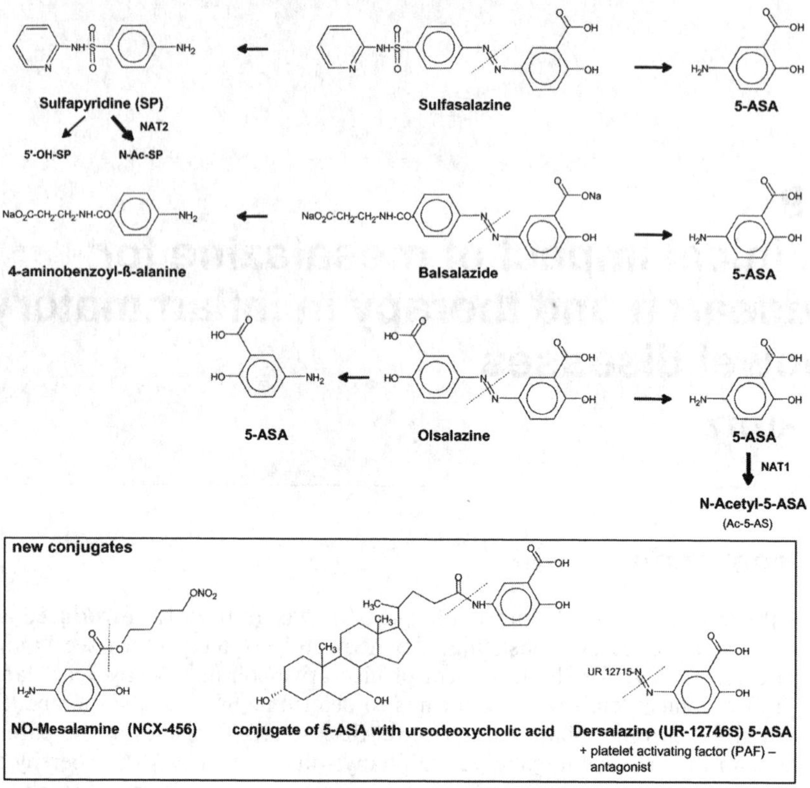

Figure 1 Structures of various azo-prodrugs of 5-aminosalicylic acid (5-ASA) and corresponding metabolic steps; three potential new agents are given in the lower part of the figure

(PATHO)PHYSIOLOGICAL AND CLINICAL CONSIDERATIONS

Crohn's disease and ulcerative colitis represent distinct entities of IBD, and within both disorders different subgroups have to be assumed[9]. Various genetic and environmental susceptibility or risk factors have been delineated for IBD[10,11]. The exact aetiopathogenesis still remains elusive, and most often a defective intestinal barrier function and an uncontrolled and inappropriate activation of the mucosal immune system, driven by yet-unknown (external) stimuli, have been assumed (see Figure 2). So far such dysregulated processes with subsequent inflammatory reactions can be treated only symptomatically, and 5-ASA represents an important option in IBD, especially ulcerative colitis[12-16].

As IBD represents a local inflammation of the (sub-)mucosa in the small and/or large bowel it would be ideal to target 5-ASA directly to the affected areas. By acting from the luminal site effective mucosal drug concentrations

MESALAZINE AND IBD

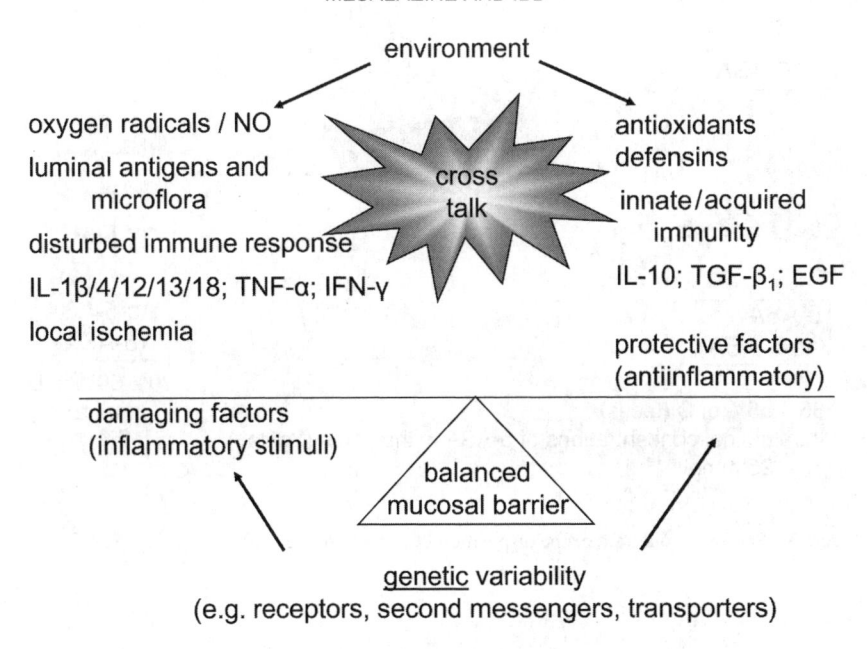

Figure 2 Pathophysiological background of IBD and factors affecting the activity of the chronic disorders

must be achieved and systemic availability should be limited to reduce the potential for adverse effects. Apparently the local (mucosal) concentrations of 5-ASA are determinants of its clinical response. All postoperative IBD patients with mucosal 5-ASA concentrations lower than 20 ng/mg showed recurrences at the neo-ileal site, whereas no patient had a recurrence when the levels were above 100 ng/mg of tissue[17]. Similarly, in patients with ulcerative colitis significant inverse correlations were found between the mucosal concentrations of 5-ASA and inflammatory signs[18] or between a disease activity index and 5-ASA levels in the rectum[19].

DELIVERY OPTIONS AND DISPOSITION OF 5-ASA

5-ASA is available either in the form of inactive prodrugs (e.g. SZ, balsalazide, olsalazine) or as special slow/controlled-release formulations (tablets, sachets), suppositories, enemas and foam. The prodrugs have to be split by reductive cleavage by bacteria to deliver 5-ASA into the colon, and to become effective in patients with ulcerative colitis, whereas the various oral 5-ASA preparations were designed to deliver the active agents directly to its target sites in the lower intestinal tract[5,8,20].

Following oral or rectal administration of 5-ASA the released active drug is taken up by the epithelial cells in the small and large bowel (see Figure 3).

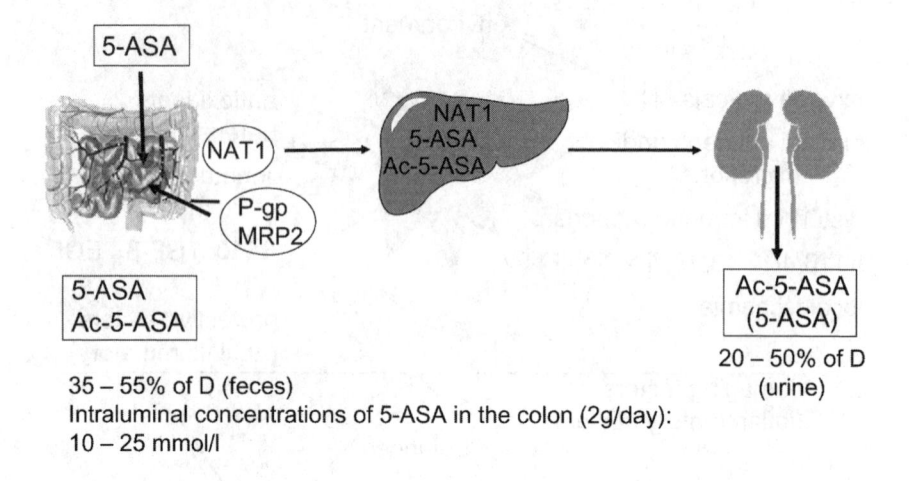

```
           5-ASA
            |
    ┌───┐  ↓
    │   │(NAT1) ──→   NAT1        ──→    [kidneys]
    │   │             5-ASA
    │   │(P-gp        Ac-5-ASA
    │   │ MRP2)
    └───┘
   5-ASA                                 Ac-5-ASA
   Ac-5-ASA                              (5-ASA)

                                         20 – 50% of D
   35 – 55% of D (feces)                 (urine)
   Intraluminal concentrations of 5-ASA in the colon (2g/day):
   10 – 25 mmol/l
```

Figure 3   Schematic diagram of the disposition of 5-ASA (see ref. 28)

During absorption capacity-limited intestinal acetylation occurs[5,21]. 5-ASA and its inactive major metabolite Ac-5-ASA are partly secreted back into the intestinal lumen[22,23]. Active transport of the two compounds from the basolateral to the apical site of epithelial cells is probably accomplished by membrane-bound drug transporters such as P-glycoprotein and MRP2[24,25]. During its first pass through the liver the absorbed part of 5-ASA is rapidly ($t_{\frac{1}{2}}$: 1.0–2.4 h) acetylated – like in the intestinal wall – by N-acetyltransferase 1 (NAT1). Subsequently Ac-5-ASA is renally eliminated ($t_{\frac{1}{2}}$: 1.3–11 h) by glomerular filtration and active tubular secretion[5,8]. Thus, the interindividual variability in the expression and activity of both NAT1 and drug efflux pumps will affect mucosal concentrations of 5-ASA and consequently drug response[26].

Ideally, selection among the various oral or rectal preparations should be guided by the location of the disease. Scintigraphic monitoring has demonstrated that enemas distributed the labelled 5-ASA within 0.5–2 h from the rectum and sigma up to the transverse colon, and partly even to the ascending colon. 5-ASA from foam will reach the proximal sigmoid colon. When given as suppositories 5-ASA will be consistently delivered only to the rectosigmoid region[26].

According to the different release patterns of the available oral preparations of 5-ASA some therapeutic efficacy can also be seen in Crohn's disease, e.g. with Salofalk® and Pentasa® tablets there is release of 5-ASA from the duodenum to the ileum[22,23]. Based on a review of extensive disposition and recovery data local availability of 5-ASA can be regarded as quite similar for the various oral formulations[27]. In general, peak plasma levels of 5-ASA range between 3 and 13 μmol/L, and concentrations between 10 and 25 mmol/L have been observed in the lumen of the colon when 2 g of 5-ASA are administered[28].

As already mentioned, these concentrations, as well as the intestinal mucosal tissue levels of 5-ASA (40–2080 μmol/L), depend on the extent/rate of uptake and elimination. Absorption and tissue uptake of 5-ASA seems to be affected by P-glycoprotein. The expression and activity of this drug efflux pump can be altered in IBD[29–31], which might have consequences both for the intestinal barrier function and the topical efficacy of 5-ASA.

SAFETY PROFILE OF 5-ASA

The development of sulpha-free 5-ASA has enabled physicians to increase its dosage. Whereas treatment with SZ has to be stopped in at least 10–20% of patients because of dose-dependent side-effects or unwanted drug reactions, the 5-ASA preparations are well tolerated by most patients. 5-ASA is safe to use during pregnancy and for nursing mothers[20,32,33]. Male fertility is very often affected in patients on SZ but not with 5-ASA[34]. In contrast to the azo-prodrug olsalazine 5-ASA does not induce diarrhoea[20].

In an unusual approach to relate spontaneously reported serious adverse reactions to the number of prescriptions[35] a greater overall number (odds ratio 1.31; 95% CI 1.22–1.40) was recorded for SZ compared with mesalazine[36]. In a recent systematic review of fully published randomized controlled trials it was concluded that frequencies of adverse events or withdrawal due to adverse events of patients treated with 5-ASA, olsalazine or balsalazide were comparable with those in placebo-treated patients and lower than those in SZ-treated patients[37].

There is still some debate as to whether the occurrence of proteinuria in patients with IBD is an extraintestinal manifestation of the disease or a toxic reaction to 5-ASA. In the first systematic study, performed in 1984, no evidence of nephrotoxic lesions induced by 5-ASA was noted in a small group of patients with Crohn's disease[38]. In more extensive studies proteinuria of renal marker proteins sometimes observed in patients with IBD was attributed to disease activity rather than to treatment with 5-ASA[20,39–42]. In the most recent study data from the UK General Practice Research Database were used to estimate incidences of renal disease in adult patients. In IBD patients using 5-ASA an incidence rate of 0.17 cases per 100 patients per year was calculated. The incidence among patients with IBD but without 5-ASA use was 0.25, among patients without IBD incidence was 0.08, and in patients with active rheumatoid arthritis taking SZ it was 0.29. Thus, users of 5-ASA (and SZ) have a low but increased risk of renal disease which is partly due to the underlying disease[43].

Case reports of acute pancreatitis during treatment with 5-ASA have been reported. In a large population-based case–control study a nearly four-fold increased risk of acute pancreatitis in patients with Crohn's disease and a 1.5-fold increased risk for ulcerative colitis has been found. However, the use of 5-ASA (or SZ) was not associated with an increased risk for this adverse event[44].

Finally, in contrast to other salicylates, 5-ASA has no effect on platelet aggregation and fibrinolytic activity; the risk of drug-induced gastrointestinal bleeding was estimated as much lower (1% vs. 18%) for 5-ASA than for aspirin[45].

MODE OF ACTION OF 5-ASA

Whereas the topical action of 5-ASA in the inflamed mucosa is generally accepted, its exact mode of action remains obscure. Because 5-ASA exerts several biochemical actions *in vitro* and *in vivo* it is regarded as a poly-potent ('dirty') drug. Similar to other NSAID, 5-ASA interferes with inflammation, immune regulation, proliferation and/or apoptosis by reversible COX-(in)dependent mechanisms and by scavenging reactive oxygen species. 5-ASA can block the production and/or release of proinflammatory prostanoids, leukotrienes, interleukin 1 and TNF-α[20,46]. One key effect is apparently the inhibition of the activation of the nuclear transcription factor (NF) kappa B[47]. COX-inhibition and suppression of NF-κB are accomplished *in vitro* by 5-ASA concentrations in the range 0.1–1 mM and 2–20 mM, respectively[46].

5-ASA is able to inhibit production of reactive oxygen metabolites by scavenging superoxide and hydroxyl radicals in a dose-dependent fashion: 5 mM 5-ASA decreased the production of damaging products by 90%[46,48]. The antioxidant properties of 5-ASA, and its potential to disrupt several critical transduction signals in inflammatory processes and to interfere in gene transcription, have placed 5-ASA in a position of a valuable therapeutic agent for IBD and a useful tool in biomedical research.

FUTURE PERSPECTIVES

There is accumulating evidence from experimental work and clinical studies that 5-ASA is an effective chemopreventive agent for colorectal cancer in patients with ulcerative colitis[45,46]. A recent meta-analysis of six previously published studies calculated a pooled odds ratio of 0.25 (95% CI 0.15–0.40) for cancer and of 0.47 (95% CI 0.24–0.92) for cancer or dysplasia, indicating significant chemoprotective effects of 5-ASA[49]. This new indication of 5-ASA is based on its multiple actions, such as inhibition of cell proliferation, activation of apoptotic processes, inhibition of NF-κB activation, inhibition of DNA hydroxylation which impairs DNA repair and scavenging DNA-damaging free radicals[45,46].

The poly-potency of 5-ASA could be modified by creating new conjugates of 5-ASA (see Figure 1). Coupling of 5-ASA with NO-donators[50], ursodeoxycholic acid[51] or the platelet-activating factor (PAF)-antagonist UR 12715[52] might even expand the therapeutic potential of 5-ASA. Thus, one can assume that, even after many years of extensive clinical investigations with 5-ASA, there are still chances for further progress in the treatment of IBD.

In the past, when working with 5-ASA we have gained new insights in drug- and patient-specific factors which will affect therapeutic (non-)response, such as drug delivery/targeting, drug uptake and elimination, mechanisms of action, compliance and side-effects, genetic polymorphisms or new targets. In the near future it can be anticipated that subgroups of drug (non-)responders can be (pre-)defined, and combining supplementary therapeutic principles might also provide new therapeutic options. We have also learnt that 'dirty' drugs (e.g. 5-ASA) are not inferior to highly selective agents as IBD are very complex disorders. Therefore a completely new approach with another 'dirty cocktail' (parasitic worm eggs) – similar to 5-ASA – might again attract the interest of clinical pharmacologists and gastroenterologists[53].

Acknowledgements

This work was supported by the Robert Bosch Foundations, Stuttgart (Germany). The secretarial help of Mrs U. Hengemühle is greatly appreciated.

References

1. Svartz N. Salazopyrin – a new sulfanilamide preparation. A: Therapeutic results in rheumatoid arthritis. B: Therapeutic results in ulcerative colitis. C: Toxic manifestations on treatment with sulfanilamide preparations. Acta Med Scand. 1942;110:577–90.
2. Azad Khan AK, Piris J, Truelove SC. An experiment to determine the active therapeutic moiety of sulphasalazine. Lancet. 1977;II:892–5.
3. Van Hees PAM, Bakker JH, Van Tongeren JHM. Effect of sulphapyridine, 5-aminosalicylic acid, and placebo in patients with idiopathic proctitis: a study to determine the active therapeutic moiety of sulphasalazine. Gut. 1980;21:632–5.
4. Klotz U, Maier K, Fischer C, Heinkel K. Therapeutic efficacy of sulfasalazine and its metabolites in patients with ulcerative colitis and Crohn's disease. N Engl J Med. 1980;303:1499–502.
5. Schwab M, Klotz U. Pharmacokinetic considerations in the treatment of inflammatory bowel disease. Clin Pharmacokinet. 2001;40:723–51.
6. Das KM, Eastwood MA, McManus JPA et al. Adverse reactions during salicylazosulfapyridine therapy and the relation with drug metabolism and acetylator phenotype. N Engl J Med. 1973;289:491–5.
7. Fischer C, Klotz U. Is plasma level monitoring of sulfasalazine indicated in the treatment of Crohn's disease or ulcerative colitis? Ther Drug Monit. 1980;2:153–8.
8. Klotz U. Clinical pharmacokinetics of sulphasalazine, its metabolites and other prodrugs of 5-aminosalicylic acid. Clin Pharmacokinet. 1985;10:285–302.
9. Podolsky D. Inflammatory bowel disease. N Engl J Med. 2002;347:417–29.
10. Ahmad T, Tamboli CP, Jewell D, Colombel J-F. Clinical relevance of advances in genetics and pharmacogenetics of IBD. Gastroenterology. 2004;126:533–49.
11. Loftus Jr EV. Clinical epidemiology of inflammatory bowel disease: incidence, prevalence and environmental influences. Gastroenterology. 2004;126:1504–17.
12. Rizzello F, Gionchetti P, Venturi A et al. Review article: medical treatment of severe ulcerative colitis. Aliment Pharmacol Ther 2003;17(Suppl. 2):7–10.
13. Sandborn WJ. Rational selection of oral 5-aminosalicylate formulations and prodrugs for the treatment of ulcerative colitis. Am J Gastroenterol. 2002;97:2939–41.
14. Hanauer SB. Medical therapy for ulcerative colitis 2004. Gastroenterology. 2004;126:1582–92.
15. Egan LF, Sandborn WF. Advances in the treatment of Crohn's disease. Gastroenterology. 2004;126:1574–81.
16. Bebb JR, Scott BB. Systematic review: how effective are the usual treatments for Crohn's disease? Aliment Pharmacol Ther. 2004;20:151–9.
17. Frieri G, Pimpo MT, Andreoli A et al. Prevention of postoperative recurrence of Crohn's disease requires adequate mucosal concentrations of mesalazine. Aliment Pharmacol Ther. 1999;13:557–82.
18. Frieri G, Giacomelli G, Pimpo M et al. Mucosal 5-aminosalicylic acid concentrations inversely correlate with severity of colonic inflammation in patients with ulcerative colitis. Gut. 2000;47:410–14.
19. Naganuma M, Iwao Y, Ogata H et al. Measurement of colonic mucosal concentrations of 5-aminosalicylic acid is useful for estimating its therapeutic efficacy in distal ulcerative colitis: comparison of orally administered mesalamine and sulfasalazine. Inflamm Bowel Dis. 2001;7:221–5.

20. Klotz U. The role of aminosalicylates at the beginning of the new millenium in the treatment of chronic inflammatory bowel disease. Eur J Clin Pharmacol. 2000;56:353–62.
21. Vree TB, Dammers E, Exler PS et al. Liver and gut mucosa acetylation of mesalazine in healthy volunteers. Int J Clin Pharmacol Ther. 2000;38:514–22.
22. Goebell H, Klotz U, Nehlsen B, Layer P. Oroileal transit of slow release 5-aminosalicylic acid. Gut. 1993;34:669–75.
23. Layer PH, Goebell H, Keller J, Dignass A, Klotz U. Delivery and fate of oral mesalamine microgranules within the human small intestine. Gastroenterology. 1995;108:1427–33.
24. Zhou SY, Fleisher D, Pao LH et al. Intestinal metabolism and transport of 5-aminosalicylate. Drug Metab Dispos. 1999;27:479–85.
25. Proudfoot LE, Yacyshyn BR. Mechanisms of transport and structure – permeability relationship of sulfasalazine and its analogs in Caco-2 cell monolayers. Pharm Res. 2000; 17:1168–74.
26. Klotz U, Schwab B. Topical delivery of therapeutic agents in the treatment of inflammatory bowel disease (IBD). Adv Drug Delivery Rev. 2005;57:267–79.
27. Sandborn WJ, Hanauer SB. Systematic review: the pharmacokinetic profiles of oral mesalazine formulations and mesalazine pro-drugs used in the management of ulcerative colitis. Aliment Pharmacol Ther. 2003;17:29–42.
28. Laursen LS, Stokholm M, Bukhave J et al. Disposition of 5-aminosalicylic acid by olsalazine and three mesalazine preparations in patients with ulcerative colitis: comparison of intraluminal colonic concentrations, serum values, and urinary excretion. Gut. 1990;31:1271–6.
29. Yacyshyn B, Maksymowych W, Bowen-Yacyshyn MB. Differences in P-glycoprotein-170 expression and activity between Crohn's disease and ulcerative colitis. Hum Immunol. 1999;60:677–87.
30. Farrell RJ, Murphy A, Long A et al. High multidrug resistance (P-glycoprotein 170) expression in inflammatory bowel disease patients who fail medical therapy. Gastroenterology. 2000;118:279–88.
31. Schwab M, Schaeffeler E, Marx C et al. Association between the C3435T MDR1 gene polymorphism and susceptibility for ulcerative colitis. Gastroenterology. 2003;124:26–33.
32. Schroeder KW. Role of mesalazine in acute and long-term treatment of ulcerative colitis and its complications. Scand J Gastroenterol. 2002;37(Suppl. 236):42–7.
33. Nørgård, Fonager K, Pedersen L, Jacobsen BA, Sørensen HT. Birth outcome in women exposed to 5-aminosalicylic acid during pregnancy: a Danish cohort study. Gut. 2003;52:243–7.
34. Di Paolo MC, Paoluzi OA, Pica R et al. Sulphasalazine and 5-aminosalicylic acid in long-term treatment of ulcerative colitis: report on tolerance and side-effects. Dig Liver Dis. 2001;33:563–9.
35. D'Haens G, van Bodegraven AA. Mesalazine is safe for the treatment of IBD. Gut. 2004; 53:155.
36. Ransford RAJ, Langman MJS. Sulphasalazine and mesalazine: serious adverse reactions re-evaluated on the basis of suspected adverse reaction reports to the Committee on Safety of Medicines. Gut. 2002;51:536–9.
37. Loftus Jr EV, Kane SV, Bjorkman D. Systematic review: Short-term adverse effects of 5-aminosalicylic acid agents in the treatment of ulcerative colitis. Aliment Pharmacol Ther. 2004;19:179–89.
38. Diener U, Tuczek H-V, Fischer C, Maier K, Klotz U. Renal function was not impaired by treatment with 5-aminosalicylic acid in rats and man. Naunyn-Schmiedeberg's Arch Pharmacol. 1984;326:278–82.
39. Herrlinger KR, Noftz MK, Fellermann K et al. Minimal renal dysfunction in inflammatory bowel disease is related to disease activity but not to 5-ASA use. Aliment Pharmacol Ther. 2003;15:363–9.
40. Fraser JS, Muller AF, Smith DJ, Newman DJ, Lamb EJ. Renal tubular injury is present in acute inflammatory bowel disease prior to the introduction of drug therapy. Aliment Pharmacol Ther. 2001;15:1131–7.
41. Mahmud N, O'Toole D, O'Hae N et al. Evaluation of renal function following treatment with 5-aminosalicylic acid derivatives in patients with ulcerative colitis. Aliment Pharmacol Ther. 2002;16:207–15.

42. Dehmer C, Greinwald R, Löffler J et al. No dose-dependent tubulotoxicity of 5-aminosalicylic acid: a prospective study in patients with inflammatory bowel diseases. Int J Colorect Dis. 2003;18:406–12.
43. Van Staa TP, Travis S, Leutkens HGM, Logan RF. 5-Aminosalicylic acid and the risk of renal disease: a large British epidemiologic study. Gastroenterology. 2004;126:1733–9.
44. Munk EM, Pedersen L, Floyd A et al. Inflammatory bowel diseases, 5-aminosalicylic acid and sulfalsalazine treatment and risk of acute pancreatitis: a population-based case-control study. Am J Gastroenterol. 2004;99:884–8.
45. Eaden J. Review article: The data supporting a role for aminosalicylates in the chemoprevention of colorectal cancer in patients with inflammatory bowel disease. Aliment Pharmacol Ther. 2003;18(Suppl 2):15–21.
46. Allgayer H. Review article: Mechanisms of action of mesalazine in preventing carcinoma in inflammatory bowel disease. Aliment Pharamcol Ther. 2003;18(Suppl 2):10–14.
47. Bantel H, Berg C, Vieth M et al. Mesalazine inhibits activation of transcription factor NF kappa B in inflamed mucosa of patients with ulcerative colitis. Am J Gastroenterol. 2000; 95:3452–7.
48. Allgayer H, Rang S, Klotz U et al. Superoxide inhibition following different stimuli of respiratory burst and metabolism of aminosalicylates in neutrophils. Dig Dig Sci. 1994;39: 145–51.
49. Velayos FS, Walsh JME, Terdiman JP. Effect of 5-aminosalicylic acid use on colorectal cancer and dysplasia risk in ulcerative colitis. Gastroenterology. 2004;126(Suppl 2):A-20, abstract 138.
50. Wallace JL. Nitric oxid-releasing mesalamine: potential utility for treatment of inflammatory bowel disease. Dig Liver Dis. 2003;35(Suppl 2):S35–40.
51. Batta AK, Tint GS, Xu G, Shefer S, Salen G. Synthesis and intestinal metabolism of ursodeoxycholic acid conjugate with an anti-inflammatory agent, 5-aminosalicylic acid. J Lipid Res. 1998;39:1641–6.
52. Gálvez J, Garrido M, Rodriguez-Cabezas ME et al. The intestinal anti-inflammatory activity of UR-12746S on reactivated experimental colitis is mediated through downregulation of cytokine production. Inflamm Bowel Dis. 2003;9:363–71.
53. Wickelgren I. Can worms tame the immune system? Science. 2004;305:170–1.

30
Gastroenterology: history of the future

D. K. PODOLSKY

As Nobel Prize-winning physicist Niels Bohr first said, 'Prediction is difficult, especially when it concerns the future.' Anticipating where trends in clinical gastroenterology and research may lead in the new millennium is therefore fraught with self-evident dangers. However, it is at least apparent that a number of different forces will result in significant changes to the field of gastroenterology.

Predicting the future is best begun with an appreciation of past advances. In the very early years progress was based on the sciences of anatomy, pathology, histology, and physiology. Additional progress was made through the identification of infectious agents which were responsible for many of the major disorders that affect the gastrointestinal (GI) tract. Progress has begun to provide even more fundamental understanding of the basis of GI disease. Thus, the genes responsible for many disorders have now been identified. These are well illustrated by the several genes which confer risk for the polyposis syndromes (e.g. 'APC'), the gene for haemochromatosis ('HFE'), and the gene responsible for cystic fibrosis, 'CFTR' – admittedly, a more systemic disorder, but one which nonetheless affects the GI tract.

In addition to this impressive set of accomplishments, developments in technology have helped define the practice of modern gastroenterology. Of course foremost is the rapid evolution of endoscopy, which now provides expanding therapeutic modalities. Advances in endoscopy have been complemented by other imaging modalities, which are essential for the daily practice of gastroenterology and contribute to more precise diagnosis and treatment. These include conventional forms of radiology, CT scanning and, more recently, MRI and related techniques. Finally, 100 years after the emergence of gastroenterology, effective therapeutics are now available for many disorders. Many of these therapeutic agents are truly impressive in their effectiveness, including the proton pump inhibitors, antibiotics for the treatment of specific infections, a variety of anti-inflammatory drugs, and hepatitis vaccines which have changed the landscape for the future because of their ability to prevent disease.

Notwithstanding these many developments, considerable challenges remain to meet the needs of patients. Understanding has still not been reduced to its most fundamental, i.e. the nature of the genes responsible for GI tract function. Understanding of the fundamental basis of function can make possible understanding of basic aetiology of disease and the basis of dysfunction for the many disorders which remain enigmas, e.g. the aetiology and pathogenesis of inflammatory bowel disease remain uncertain. Similarly, there is no definitive understanding of the causes of the most common forms of GI malignancy, which now dominate – and will continue to dominate – the clinical arena of gastroenterology.

Indeed, even if definitive therapies that could reliably treat the full range of GI diseases were available, that would still really have achieved only half the goal of medicine, and it would be of paramount importance to develop the means to prevent disease rather than treat its aftermath.

Thus, very large unmet needs persist, prompting the question: What are the future possibilities of meeting these needs? Before attempting to answer that question it is useful to consider how the very nature of the clinical problems which preoccupy gastroenterologists will change. A number of factors are causing very significant changes in the spectrum of diseases with which the gastroenterologist contends. While the past 30–40 years have been dominated by the very important, ongoing problems related to viral hepatitis, in the distant future that may no longer be the case, because of the eventual impact of widespread vaccination leading to decreases in the frequency of hepatitis B and, hopefully, hepatitis A, in conjunction with better hygiene and overall socioeconomic development. Thus chronic hepatitis and its consequent cirrhosis and hepatocellular carcinoma, which are very common today, may become much less common. In addition to the import of specific developments such as vaccines, there are the more general effects of what hopefully will be improving socioeconomic conditions throughout most of the world. The impact of the latter is difficult to exaggerate, because many GI conditions have a basis of risk related to socioeconomic conditions; e.g. the quality of water supply and the quality of food supply. In developed countries, improving sanitation has certainly already had an impact on the frequency of hepatitis A. It is reasonable to expect that the same will be true for *Helicobacter pylori*-related disease. Thus, remarkable changes in the frequency of a hugely prevalent disorder can be anticipated.

Unfortunately, decreases in disorders which are generally associated with lower socioeconomic development will likely be offset by increases in the problems associated with development. Inflammatory bowel disease, GERD and, most importantly, colon cancer, offer just a few examples of problems which will loom larger in the future. Finally, demographic trends will have a significant impact on the prevalence of GI disorders. The population, in association with improving socioeconomic conditions, is ageing. As a consequence the problems associated with ageing will be more common for the gastroenterologist. Furthermore, the growing worldwide epidemic of obesity will have a significant impact on gastroenterology practice: both in treating the complications of obesity (e.g. NAFLD) and perhaps an important role in treatment of the obesity itself through endoluminal intervention, and eventually more effective pharmacological therapy.

Thus, the clinical landscape of gastroenterology will be different. How, then, will the practice of gastroenterology change? It is likely that four forces will determine the further evolution of the field. These four defining forces are: (1) the impact of the full elucidation of the human genome; (2) the ability ultimately to cross the immune identity barrier without toxic drugs; (3) development of increasingly more sophisticated tools which will allow new approaches to bioengineering and micro-devices; and (4) development of the capacity for high-throughput screening, which will allow more powerful approaches to drug development.

The complete determination of the human genome has resulted in an almost immediate important impact, most obviously through identification of disease-associated genes. It is reasonable to assume that identification of the genes associated with diseases will enable better understanding of disease mechanism for those disorders which have remained a puzzle, such as inflammatory bowel disease. In addition, gene identification will almost immediately allow subclassification of patients on the basis of genetic profiles. Most important, full delineation of the genetic basis of disease will result in a profound change for medicine generally. Definition of the association between specific genes and later disease development will permit diagnosis before individuals are actually patients: presymptomatic diagnosis. In the future the time spent treating disease may be equally balanced by the time treating people before they have disease, resulting in a fundamentally different type of medicine.

The challenges for gastroenterology in benefiting from this genomic revolution are considerable, because most GI disorders do have some genetic component. However, most are not simple monogenic disorders like haemochromatosis. Rather, most of the common problems of gastroenterology result from the interactions of the products of many different genes. The future ability to realize the promise of the identification of disease genes will also depend on a more sophisticated understanding of the mechanisms through which multiple genes interact to eventually cause one disease in a given individual. Thus, perhaps as many as 20% of individuals with idiopathic chronic pancreatitis may have mutations of the CFTR gene without other signs of cystic fibrosis. It is possible that a background mutation of this gene may contribute to the development of chronic pancreatitis secondary to alcohol intake in some individuals while others consuming equivalent amounts of alcohol do not develop this condition, reflecting the determining interaction between an environmental agent and an underlying genetic susceptibility. Indeed, many other disorders, which we never suspected clinically, may also be associated with this gene now that we can study its mutations in different patient groups.

What can be expected in the reasonably near future from knowing the various components of the human genome? Within the next few years it may be possible to identify the genes associated with IBD, coeliac disease and GI cancer, and therefore understand those at risk before they actually develop the disease. One can guess that this predisposition is, in fact, more broadly important than its role in these purely genetic disorders. For example, there is reasonable evidence to suppose that the nature of the outcome from HCV infection in a given individual will be determined by the nature of the underlining genetically determined host characteristics. It is already apparent that response to a drug, as well as a risk of a toxic reaction to the drug, in most instances are determined by specific genetic loci including those responsible for drug metabolism. Within the very near future, genetic tests may be available to assess the risk of toxicity and the likelihood of drug response prior to administration of the agent, as already exemplified by testing for TPMT prior to using 6-mercaptopurine.

The 'genomic revolution' will place physicians in a position to diagnose illness (actually risk of illness) before individuals have disease. It also means that gastroenterologists will need additional skills and different approaches or perspectives than have been necessary in the past. In particular, greater sophistication will be needed to counsel patients about genetic risk, an issue fraught with many potential ethical implications. In addition, if the diseases that we treat have some genetic basis, and we identify genes that confer the likelihood of developing that disease in an index patient, there are also broader implications for involving the entire family in understanding what those genes mean to them.

A second force determining the future of gastroenterology is the eventual ability to circumvent the immune barrier, which has constrained the treatment of many disorders and the entire area of transplantation. With a full understanding of the complexity of the immune system, it is reasonable to expect that highly targeted immunosuppression will become possible, allowing such currently radical notions as xenotransplantation to become a reality. As a result, the future will offer the possibility of treating end-stage GI disease, which is really, at best, imperfect for our patients with end-stage liver disease, pancreatic disease, or even intestinal disease.

Crossing the immune barrier is actually part of a broader set of possibilities, as the molecular and cellular basis of GI tract function and disease are finally understood. There is already evidence of new innovative approaches which will deal with end-stage disease by variations on the theme of transplantation, and without the use of whole organ transplantation as we currently think about it. For example, efforts are under way to fabricate organs through the combined use of specific cell populations and artificial matrices. Further, these organs which can be fabricated, can also be engineered to have specific functional capabilities, e.g. to express a protein which would be therapeutically important in a given patient, so that patients no longer have to take a therapeutic substance on an intermittent basis in the usual way that a drug is administered to a patient. A whole host of exciting possibilities will emerge once the immune barrier, which prevents easy transplantation across individuals and across species, has been breached. These will include the development of cloned organs and extracorporeal, liver-assist devices which are truly practical. Which of these will turn out to be the most powerful approach(es) remains to be seen, but broadly they will offer the opportunity to treat patients with end-stage diseases, that are currently at best managed with palliative and empirical measures.

The third factor which will transform our future is engineering and technology innovation. This should be viewed in the context of the present applications of endoscopy, which currently dominates the field. If the development of endoscopy continues on its current, natural path, what can be expected? Already new technologies build on conventional endoscopy for refined diagnosis. These include optical coherence tomography (OCT) and confocal endoscopy, which approach single cell layer resolution to permit '*in-vivo* histology'. In addition, endoscopy will be coupled to some of the other specific capabilities already mentioned for even more precise diagnosis, either *in vivo*, through special spectroscopic and other means of metabolic scanning, or through more sophisticated analysis of mucosal and organ biopsies obtained through the endoscope. It is also reasonable to assume that the therapeutic uses of endoscopy itself will continue to expand. Although there are already an impressive variety of interventions in use, imminent progress in endoluminal and trans-gastric surgery will make it possible that many procedures that are now the purviews of the general GI surgeon will soon be amenable to techniques that will become commonplace in GI practice.

Thus, there is certainly room for further sophistication in endoscopy – and, with the kind of innovation and creativity that is being displayed currently by members of our field, their development is inevitable. However, it is still reasonable to ask: Is there no other transforming event which could, in fact, change the landscape for endoscopy in a more fundamental way? Already CT colonography (also known as virtual colonography) is beginning to offer a potential alternative to conventional practices for diagnostic evaluation of the colon.

In general terms, technology advances will result in remote sensing diagnostics, remote disease monitoring and regulation of drug administration. Real prototypes already exist for each now, so that in the next few years it is reasonable to expect the availability of microdiagnostics; small capsules which can traverse the GI tract and transmit physiological data: pressures, sampling of luminal contents, to a remote – that is to say, outside the body – receiver. As the engineering challenges are resolved, and these techniques become widely available, this could have a transforming effect on the need to do endoscopy, at least as conventionally defined. This will also be coupled with the enablement of continuous monitoring of disease and drug levels, by subcutaneous, small sensors which will transmit the data regarding current drug level (e.g. the level of insulin and blood glucose in the diabetic) to a remote station, while the patient is going about his/her daily activities. Taken one step further, it should be possible to transmit instructions to a subcutaneous drug delivery depot vehicle to release more or less insulin or, in a patient with GI dysmotility, more or less of a drug to regulate motility on a real-time basis while the patient is going about his/her daily activities.

Although these modalities may seem like science fiction, each exists at least in experimental demonstration. The future offers the potential for convergence of engineering with medicine, and specifically gastroenterology. Telemetry and the ability to measure motility on an ongoing basis may finally provide insight into the alterations present in patients with irritable bowel syndrome. In the short term, engineering should facilitate more precise use of endoscopy as better and better scopes are made. The same kind of micro-capsulization that can make telemetry possible, will also allow *in-vivo* 'metabolic biopsy', e.g. current status of hepatic or mucosal oxygenation to assess potential ischaemia.

These possibilities prompt the question: Is it possible that, 20 years from now, endoscopy will be something that fellows will read about as a historical footnote in a textbook? While that is unlikely, because of the overall power of the technique, it is likely that the curve of increasing usage may not continue in the same exponential fashion, because newer technologies will supersede many current uses of endoscopy.

Finally, though perhaps not as obvious, a fourth transforming factor that will determine the future of gastroenterology is the ability already available to carry out high-throughput screening. Pharmaceutical companies can now evaluate many hundreds of thousands of compounds for their ability to interact with a receptor in a matter of a few days. This capability suggests that, just as soon as all human genes have been identified, it will be possible to apply this incredible power to develop or identify new agents which might be useful in a treatment of disease rather than the slow trial-and-error that was possible when only one drug candidate could be tested at a time. As much as this may be looked at as a simple, technical footnote to drug development, this capability should accelerate development of the medications that will be available to provide to patients. Thus, the process of drug development itself will be a major determining factor in the future of gastroenterology. As a result better treatments should be available for many of the disorders which are treated essentially empirically today. Treatment is largely empirical because at present the causes of disease are mostly unknown, and because current drug development, which has depended on evaluation of one compound at a time, is remarkably tedious. The convergence of molecular biology, identification of target genes, and the ability to develop new drugs is already leading to new effective therapies which are specific for a given type of receptor, e.g. irritable bowel syndrome. Potent ways to develop better chemotherapeutic agents for GI cancers, and specific agents to treat some of the more important aspects of liver disease for which currently there is no effective treatment, such as fibrosis in the patient with chronic hepatitis, will become therapeutically accessible.

Having summarized four areas which may result in a very different type of gastroenterology, it is worth noting some more general ways in which the experiences of the future will differ. Not only will there be change in clinical care, but there will also be very important changes in GI research and training. Research is likely to evolve through a number of phases. For the most part research in the past has been accomplished by relatively small groups of individuals: a senior scientist or physician scientist working with a group of students and fellows. However, increasingly, the tools which are described briefly above require an intensive use of resources and large amounts of money, equipment and space. As a result, small research group efforts will, in part, be overtaken by larger and larger research consortiums which can bring together all these resources. Investigators working in groups of three, five, or ten, or even twenty, may soon be superseded by much larger collaborative interrelated groups. Many of these will involve further collaborations between academic and commercial interests with academic investigators partnering with industry scientists. Thus, in the future, science will be carried out on a bigger scale.

Interesting and paradoxical new challenges will also emerge in the clinical investigation arena. The aggregate effect of powerful high-throughput screening, the identification of genes related to most of the GI diseases, and an eventual better understanding of the mechanisms of diseases, will present a challenge for clinical investigators: to select those agents which deserve a priority for clinical trials. It is easy to list several dozen different potential targets for pharmacological intervention in inflammatory bowel diseases, and even today it is possible that, for each one of those targets, there may be ten different drugs which could be used to get a pharmacological effect. However, it would be impractical to simultaneously launch 500 different clinical trials in IBD patients. So selection of the best drug candidates to actually commit to treating patients will be a central challenge for GI clinical research. They will also conspire to promote movement to larger networks of collaboration, particularly international collaboration for drug development, in a way which have only begun in the past 10 years.

Finally, all these changes will have a major impact on the training of fellows. If fellows will be seeing a different spectrum of patients, and if they are going to use different sets of tools, they are going to need to learn different skills than needed for medicine in the 1990s. First, there will be a larger foundation of science to understand in order to be an effective clinician. There will, at least in the short term, be a broader spectrum of endoscopic skills that will require expertise if an individual is going to offer the patient everything that is possible in modern gastroenterology. Finally, because gastroenterology will expand into new territory in terms of some of the effects of the genomic revolution, and the other factors discussed above, trainees will need to have experience in things which have not traditionally been a part of GI training. These will include the skills to interpret genetic tests, and provide genetic counselling.

Some of these changes will also come with new challenges of a different sort: ethical issues which will need to be met in a very thoughtful way. The impact of a genetic diagnosis is profound. If we are making it, or have the ability to make it, while a child is still developing, particularly if definitive treatment is not yet available for that disorder (e.g. polyposis), the possibility of genetic discrimination is especially worrisome. Once you can identify someone who is at risk of a disease, will she/he still be given equal opportunity for jobs? These advances will also challenge the notion of the essence of the very uniqueness of human life. With this resource-intensive development of medicine, the ethics of access to care will be increasingly at the forefront of society's dilemmas. The treatment of end-stage disease becomes more and more sophisticated at the very time when society is confronting the difficult problem of determining when intervention is no longer appropriate in an ageing population.

All of these considerations highlight a certain irony. If you accept even part of the described vision for future gastroenterology, it is reasonable to expect 'smarter,' or at least more precise diagnosis and knowledge of causes of GI, and more sophisticated equipment for diagnosis and treatment. As more and more sophisticated telemetry and other tools are available that permit almost automatic management by computers, what is the role for the gastroenterologist? The paradox is that the true value of the physician will increasingly return to the historical value of the physician: the ability to care for the patient, to advise patients as someone interested in their humanity and their well-being, not simply in the management of a specific problem. The role of the physician historically was as much counsellor as healer in the very broad sense.

The gastroenterologist should be at the centre of that interaction by virtue of his/her ability to provide something irreplaceable: the physician can actually talk to patients and ask them how they are feeling. With ultimate progress in diagnostic technology and self-correcting automated therapy, the primary value of the gastroenterologist will be the intangible value of the physician as humanist caring for the patient – the same as that at the threshold of modern scientific medicine. Although any one of these predictions or assumptions may prove mistaken, one thing is clear: Gastroenterology won't be the same – the future is not what it once was.

Index

abdominal collateral circulation   100
abdominal radiography   216
absorption disorders   229
achlorhydria   61, 86
acid reflux, non-erosive reflux disease (NERD)   6
acid regurgitation, gastro-oesophageal reflux disease   4
acinar cell mass   215
acute gastrointestinal bleeding   105
adefovir dipivoxil resistance   120, 121
agnoprotein   250
albumin
   expression   161
   portal hypertension   100
alcohol
   chronic pancreatitis   217, 222
   colorectal cancer   285
   haemochromatosis   138
alcoholic pancreatitis   227
allelic deletions   247
ammonium tetrathiolmolybdate   155
amylase, pancreatic   227
anaemia   112
aneuploidy   251
antibiotics   299
   Helicobacter pylori   67, 78
antidepressants   206–7
antireflux surgery, gastro-oesophageal reflux disease   14
antiviral therapy   111–12
antral cancer   62
APC *see* argon plasma coagulation
apoptosis   180–1
appendicitis   277
argon plasma coagulation (APC), Barrett's oesophagus   28
arthritis, HHC   136
5-ASA *see* mesalazine
ascites, portal hypertension   100
aspirin   39–40

ataxia, WND   148
atrophic gastritis   88
autofluorescence   93
autoimmune hepatitis   189
azathioprine   190, 301

B lymphocytes, *Helicobacter pylori*   70
baclofen   7
bacterial cholangitis   197
bacterial infections   176
bacterial lipase   229
Barrett's oesophagus   22–34
   cancer risk   22–3
   endoscopy   23–6, 93
   treatment   27–30
basal cell nevus syndrome   237
benign recurrent intrahepatic cholestasis (BRIC)   175
β-adrenergic antagonists   104
β-blockers   106
bile duct carcinoma   197–8
bile ducts, stenoses   197
bile salt export pump (BSEP)   175, 176
bile salt transporters, adaptive regulation   186–7
biliary pancreatitis   222
bioendoscopy   91, 93, 94
bleeding, gastro-oesophageal reflux disease   5, 15
bosentan   176
breath tests   261
BRIC *see* benign recurrent intrahepatic cholestasis
bright lumen MRI colongraphy   281
bronze pigmentation, HHC   136
brush cytology   93
BSEP *see* bile salt export pump
budesonide   193
butorphanol   207

calcification   224

INDEX

calcium, colorectal cancer 286
calprotectin 259
CAM *see* cell adhesion molecule
cancer, Barrett's oesophagus 22–3
capsule endoscopy (CE) 279
CAR *see* constitutive adrostane receptor
cardiomyopathy, HHC 136
CBDL *see* common bile duct ligation
CD *see* Crohn's disease
CE *see* capsule endoscopy
celecoxib 46
cell adhesion molecule (CAM) 161
cell differentiation 163
chemopreventive drugs, colorectal cancer 286–8, 310
cholestasis
   bile salt transporters 186–7
   pathomechanisms 175–83
   pruritus 203–7
cholestyramine 204
chromoendoscopy, Barrett's oesophagus 23–5
chromoscopy 94
chromosomal instability (CIN) 247
chronic graft-versus-host disease (GVHD) 182
chronic hepatitis C, treatment 111–12
chronic pancreatitis (CP) 213–24
   enzyme replacement therapy 226–30
CIN *see* chromosomal instability
cirrhosis
   endoscopy 104
   HHC 136
CK *see* cytokeratin
colchicine 193
colectomy 302
coliform bacteria 261
colitis 271–2, 277
collaterals 103
colonic carcinoma 198
colonoscopy 291–2
colorectal cancer (CRC) 284, 315
   chemopreventive drugs 286–8, 310
   diet 284–5
   JC virus 247–52
   micronutrients 286
   screening 288–94
common bile duct ligation (CBDL) 186
complicated reflux disease (CRD) 3
computed tomography (CT) 277
   portal hypertension 103
conjugate export pump 176
constitutive adrostane receptor (CAR) 186

conventional enteroclysis (CE) 280
copper toxicosis 154
copper transport pathway 148–9
   MURR1 154–5
corticosteroids 193
COX-2 inhibitors 43–4, 286
CP *see* chronic pancreatitis
CRC *see* colorectal cancer
CRD *see* complicated reflux disease
creatorrhoea 228
Crohn's disease (CD)
   capsule endoscopy 279
   sonography 277
   treatment 299–304
   see also inflammatory bowel disease
CT *see* computed tomography
cyclosporin 190
cyclosporin A 176
cystic fibrosis 175, 176, 182, 314
cytokeratin (CK)-19, expression 161
cytokines 127
cytopenia 112

dark-lumen MRI colongraphy 281
DCA *see* deoxycholic acid
death-inducing signalling complex (DISC) 180
deoxycholic acid (DCA) 180
diabetes, HHC 136
diet
   colorectal cancer 284–5
   gastric cancer 85
dietary fibre, colorectal cancer 285
digital processing 91
DISC *see* death-inducing signalling complex
distal gastric cancer, pathogenesis 57–65
divalent metal transporter (DMT1) 135
diverticulitis 271–2, 277
DMT *see* divalent metal transporter
doppler sonography
   collaterals 103
   portal vein 102
   splanchnic veins 102–3
double-balloon enteroscopy 276
double-contrast barium enema 292
dronabinol 206
drug resistance
   hepatitis B virus 120–1
   hepatitis C virus 121–2
   viral mutations 120
   viral quasispecies 119
drugs, nociception 206
Dubin Johnson syndrome 176

INDEX

duodenal ulcer 59–60, 63
dysphagia, gastro-oesophageal reflux disease 5, 15
dysplasia
   argon plasma coagulation 32
   Barrett's oesophagus 23
   colonic 198
   fluorescence spectroscopy 93
   gastric cancer 86
   laser therapy 33
   photodynamic therapy 32
   surgery 30, 33

E-cadherin gene 84
EAA *see* examination under anaesthesis
early viral response (EVR) 110
embryonic signalling pathways 234
EMR *see* endoscopic mucosal resection
endocytoscopy 92
endoscopic antireflux procedures, gastro-oesophageal reflux disease 15
endoscopic mucosal resection (EMR) 31
endoscopic retrograde cholangiopancreatography (ERCP) 197
endoscopic sonography 101
endoscopic ultrasound (EUS) 78–9, 277
endoscopy 91–5, 318
   Barrett's oesophagus 23–6
   cirrhosis 104
   erosive reflux disease 9
   gastric lymphoma 78–9
   gastro-oesophageal reflux disease 5, 16
   portal hypertension 101
endosonography 276–8
entecavir resistance 121
enteric coating 228
enzyme replacement therapy 226–30
ERCP *see* endoscopic retrograde cholangiopancreatography
erosive reflux disease (ERD) 3
   treatment 9–14
erythromycin 280
erythropoietin 112, 145
esomeprazole 7
esophagogastroendoscopy 101
EUS *see* endoscopic ultrasound
EVR *see* early viral response
examination under anaesthesia (EAA) 278
exocrine insufficiency 227–8

faecal chymotrypsin 215
faecal markers 259

faecal occult blood test (FOBT) 284, 288
familial adenomatous polyposis (FAP) 279, 287
familial gastric cancer 84
FAP *see* familial adenomatous polyposis
farnesoid X receptor (FXR) 177, 186
fat malabsorption 228
ferritin 135, 140
ferroportin 135
fetal human liver cells 164–5
α-fetoprotein, expression 161
fibre, colorectal cancer 285
fibrosis 100
   inhibition 181
   pancreatic dysfunction 216
fluorescence detection, Barrett's oesophagus 26
fluorescence spectroscopy 93, 94
fluorophores 93
FOBT *see* faecal occult blood test
folate, colorectal cancer 286
free radicals 86, 88
fruit, colorectal cancer 285
FXR *see* farnesoid X receptor

gabapentin 206
gallstones 222
gastric acid 63–4
gastric cancer 60–3
   familial 84
   gender 87
   genetics 86–7
   sporadic 85–9
gastric lymphoma
   endoscopy 78–9
   therapy 80–1
gastric ulcer 58–9, 63
gastritis
   Helicobacter pylori 58
   IL-10 71
gastro-oesophageal reflux disease (GORD) 3–4
   management 4–6
   uninvestigated 15–16
gastroduodenal cancer 277
gastrointestinal lymphomas 77
gender, gastric cancer 87
genetic stool testing 292
genetics, gastric cancer 86–7
Giardia lamblia 229
glibenclamid 176
3-*O*-D-*glucose* 255
glycyrrhizin 112

INDEX

GORD *see* gastro-oesophageal reflux disease
Gorlin syndrome 237
green fluorescence protein 94
gut function testing 253–64
GVHD *see* chronic graft-versus-host disease

HAART *see* highly active antiretroviral therapy
haemochromatosis 135–45, 314
haemojuvelin 144
HBV *see* hepatitis B virus
HCV *see* hepatitis C virus
heartburn
  gastro-oesophageal reflux disease 4
  non-erosive reflux disease 6
hedgehog signalling, pancreatic cancer 234–41
Helicobacter pylori
  distal gastric cancer 57
  duodenal ulcer 59–60
  gastro-oesophageal reflux disease 14
  sporadic gastric cancer 85
  vaccination 67–72
hepatic stem cells 158–68
hepatic venous pressure 101–2
hepatitic episodes 189
hepatitis B virus (HBV)
  clinical course 116
  drug resistance 120–1
  global prevalence 116
  pathogenesis 115
  viral quasispecies 118–19
  viral replication strategies 117
hepatitis C virus (HCV)
  antiviral therapy 109
  chronic 111–12
  clinical course 116
  combination therapy 109–10
  drug resistance 121–2
  global prevalence 116
  non-nucleoside inhibitors 122–3
  NS3/4A protease 124
  NS5B polymerase 122–3
  pathogenesis 115
  viral quasispecies 118–19
  viral replication strategies 117–18
hepatoblasts 160
hepatocyte transplantation 158–68
hepcidin 144
hephaestin 135
hereditary haemochromatosis (HHC) 136
  diagnosis 139–42
  family screening 143–4

genetics 138–9
heterozygosity 144
prevalence 137–8
screening 142–3
screening age 144
treatment 142
hereditary pancreatitis 222
HFE protein 135, 136
HHC *see* hereditary haemochromatosis
high-resolution endoscopy 91–2, 94
highly active antiretroviral therapy (HAART) 120
HIV AIDS
  ileal function 259
  intestinal absorption 256–8
  intestinal disaccharidase activities 261
  intestinal inflammation 259
  intestinal permeability 258–9
  small bowel bacterial overgrowth 261
  transit tests 259–61
HLA *see* human lymphocyte antigen
host susceptibility 126
human lymphocyte antigen (HLA), immune response 127
hydrophilic-lipophobic markers 255
hypercholesterolaemia 204
hypertension
  COX-2 inhibitors 44–6
  NSAIDs 42
hypogonadism, HHC 136

IBD *see* inflammatory bowel disease
IFN *see* interferon
IL *see* interleukin
ileal function, HIV AIDS 259
ileocolonoscopy 259
immune escape, viral quasispecies 119
immune response
  bacterial microbiota 269
  Helicobacter pylori 68
  NS3/4A protease 124–5
immune suppression, intestinal permeability 258
immunization, *Helicobacter pylori* 68–9
infection, host susceptibility 126
inflammatory bowel disease (IBD) 270, 273, 315
  mesalazine 305–11
  sonography 276
  treatment 299–303
infliximab 302
cis-inhibition 176
insulin 236

INDEX

integral membrane protein (IREG1)   135
interferon (IFN)   109, 125
   resistance   125-6
interferon (IFN)-γ
   HBV infection   127
   Helicobacter pylori   70
interleukin (IL)-1B   87
interleukin (IL)-2   127
interleukin (IL)-4, *Helicobacter pylori*   70
interleukin (IL)-10   270, 272
intestinal absorption   254-6
   HIV AIDS   256-8
intestinal disaccharidase activities   261
intestinal inflammation, HIV AIDS   259
intestinal metaplasia   61, 86
intestinal permeability, HIV AIDS   258-9
intraoperative enteroscopy (IOE)   278
IREG1 *see* integral membrane protein
iron homeostasis, regulation   135-6
isosorbide-5-mononitrate   105

JC virus (JCV)   248-52
jejunal feeds   256

kappa agonists   7
Kayser-Fleischer rings   148
KTP *see* potassium titanyl phosphate laser

lactoferrin   259
lamivudine resistance   120-1
laser-scanning confocal microscopy (LCM)   92, 94
LCM *see* laser-scanning confocal microscopy
light therapy   207
lipase, pancreatic   227
liver
   iron storage   135
   regenerative capacity   160
liver biopsy, HHC   140, 142
liver transplantation   156
liver-directed cell therapy   164, 165
LOH *see* loss of heterozygosity
loss of heterozygosity (LOH)   247
lower bowel, NSAID   55
lumiracoxib   48-50

magnetic resonance imaging (MRI)   276, 280
   portal hypertension   103
magnification endoscopy, Barrett's oesophagus   25
malabsorption, HIV AIDS   256
male fertility   309

malnutrition   226
MALT *see* mucosa-associated lymphoid tissue
MAPC *see* multipotent adult progenitor cells
medical training   320
Menkes disease   149
6-mercaptopurine   302
mesalamine   299, 300
mesalazine (5-ASA)   305-11
metallothionein   155
methotrexate   193, 301
micronutrients, colorectal cancer   286
miniprobe endoscopy, Barrett's oesophagus   25-6
morphine, pruritus   204, 207
MRI *see* magnetic resonance imaging
mucosa-associated lymphoid tissue (MALT) lymphoma   76-81
multipotent adult progenitor cells (MAPC)   163
mutation   119
mycophenolate   193
myocardial infarction, NSAID   42

NABT *see* nocturnal acid breakthrough
nadolol   104
nalmefene   205
naloxone   205
naltrexone   205
naproxen   43
narrow-band imaging (NBI)   92, 94
necrosis, pancreatitis   216
NERD *see* non-erosive reflux disease
nitrate administration   105
nitrogen metabolism   62
nitroglycerine   105
nociception, drugs   206
nocturnal acid breakthrough (NABT)   11
non-aspirin NSAIDS   41
non-erosive reflux disease (NERD)   3
   treatment   6-9
non-steroidal anti-inflammatory drugs (NSAID)   41
   colorectal cancer   286-8
NS3/4A protease   124
NS4B, IFN resistance   125-6
NS5A, IFN resistance   125-6
NS5B polymerase   122-3
NSAIDs *see* non-steroidal anti-inflammatory drugs
nuclear receptors   177, 186

obesity   64, 315
   colorectal cancer   285

INDEX

OCT *see* optical coherence tomography
oesophageal carcinoma, Barrett's oesophagus 23
omeprazole 6, 8
optical coherence tomography (OCT) 318
oral immunization, *Helicobacter pylori* 69
organogenesis 161
oval cells 160

pain, chronic pancreatitis 217–21
pancolitis 303
pancreatic cancer 234–41
pancreatic intraepithelial lesions (PanIN) 234
pancreatin 228
PanIN *see* pancreatic intraepithelial lesions
paramagnetic contrast material 281
parenteral immunization, *Helicobacter pylori* 69
PBC *see* primary biliary cirrhosis
PDT *see* photodynamic therapy
penicillamine 155
peptic ulcers 67
  pathogenesis 57–65
perianal fistulas 277
PFIC *see* progressive familial intrahepatic cholestasis
phlebotomy, HHC 142
photodynamic therapy (PDT), Barrett's oesophagus 29–30, 32
pigmentation, HHC 136
platelets 39, 43, 309
polymorphism 119
polyomaviruses 248
portal hypertension
  computed tomography 103
  diagnosis 99–101
  doppler sonography 102–3
  haemodynamic evaluation 101–2
  magnetic resonance imaging 103
  treatment 104–6
portal pressure 101
portal vein 102
potassium titanyl phosphate (KTP) laser, Barrett's oesophagus 30
pouchitis 302
PPI *see* proton pump inhibitor
pregnane X receptor (PXR) 177, 186
primary biliary cirrhosis (PBC) 175, 181–3
  liver transplantation 200
  treatment 189–93
primary sclerosing cholangitis (PSC) 175, 182
  UDCA 196–200
progressive familial intrahepatic cholestasis (PFIC) 175, 182
propranolol 104
prostaglandin synthesis 39
protease, pancreatic 227
prothrombin time, portal hypertension 100
proton pump inhibitor (PPI)
  Barrett's oesophagus 27
  erosive reflux disease 9–11
  non-erosive reflux disease 6
pruritus 203–7
PSC *see* primary sclerosing cholangitis
pseudocysts 219
PXR *see* pregnane X receptor

radiographic imaging techniques 280–1
RBV *see* ribavirin
rectal cancer 277
recurrent gastrointestinal bleeding 106
recurrent pancreatitis 214
red meat, colorectal cancer 285
regulatory T cells 269–74
reporter molecules 93
L-rhamnose 255
ribavirin (RBV) 109
  resistance 123
rifampicin 179, 180, 181, 205
rofecoxib 46
rogue lymphocytes 248

SBE *see* small bowel enteroscopy
screening, colorectal cancer 288–94
selective COX-2 inhibitors 39–51
sepsis 176
serotonin reuptake inhibitors 7
sertraline 206
short bowel syndrome 258
short-segment Barrett's oesophagus (SSBO) 22, 23
sigmoidoscopy 289–91
single-nucleotide polymorphisms (SNP) 127
small bowel barium studies 259
small bowel enteroscopy (SBE) 278–9
smoking, gastric cancer 85
SNP *see* single-nucleotide polymorphisms
somatostatin 105
sonde enteroscopy 259
sonography 276–8
splanchnic veins 102–3
splenomegaly, portal hypertension 99–100
sporadic gastric cancer 85–9
SSBB *see* suspected small-bowel bleeding

INDEX

SSBO *see* short-segment Barrett's oesophagus
stature   64
steatorrhoea   226, 227–8
stem cells   159
stenotic fibrosing colonopathy   229
step-down principle   12
sulphasalazine   299, 300
suspected small-bowel bleeding (SSBB)   279
sustained virologic response (SVR)   109
SVR *see* sustained virologic response
symptoms, gastro-oesophageal reflux disease   4

T lymphocytes, *Helicobacter pylori*   70
taurolithocholic acid (TLCA)   179
terlipressin   105
Th1/Th2 lymphocytes
   Helicobacter pylori   70–1
   regulation   269
thermocoagulation, Barrett's oesophagus   27–8
timolol   104
tissue sampling   94
TLCA *see* taurolithocholic acid
TNF *see* tumour necrosis factor
total parenteral nutrition   256
transaminases   189
transferrin   135, 140
transit tests, HIV AIDS   259–61
tremors, WND   148
trientene   155
troglitazone   176
trypsin, pancreatic   227
tumour diagnosis, sonography   277
tumour necrosis factor (TNF)-α   87, 127
tumour necrosis factor (TNF)-β   270, 272

UDCA *see* ursodeoxycholic acid
ulcerative colitis
   sonography   277
   treatment   302–3

ulcers, NSAID   41
ultrasound (US)   277
ursodeoxycholic acid (UDCA)   180, 181–2, 189, 191–2
   primary sclerosing cholangitis   196–200
US *see* ultrasound

VAK *see* virus-activated kinase
vanishing bile duct syndrome (VBDS)   175
variceal pressure   102
vascular thrombosis, COX-2 inhibitors   46
vasopressin   105
VBDS *see* vanishing bile duct syndrome
vimentin   161
viral hepatitis   176
viral mutations, drug resistance   120
viral quasispecies   118–19
viral replication strategies   117–18
virtual colonoscopy   281, 292
virtual histology   92
virulence factors, *Helicobacter pylori*   68
virus-activated kinase (VAK)   125
vitamin E   156

weight, oesophageal carcinoma   23
weight loss, gastro-oesophageal reflux disease   5, 15
Wilson disease (WND)
   biochemical diagnostic features   150
   copper transport pathway   148–9
   disease-causing mutant   152–3
   mutation analysis   150–2
   sib diagnosis   153
   treatment   155–6
wireless capsule endoscopy   276
WND *see* Wilson disease
Wnt signalling pathway   239

D-xylose   255

zinc   155

Falk Symposium Series

43. Reutter W, Popper H, Arias IM, Heinrich PC, Keppler D, Landmann L, eds.: *Modulation of Liver Cell Expression*. Falk Symposium No. 43. 1987
ISBN: 0-85200-677-2*
44. Boyer JL, Bianchi L, eds.: *Liver Cirrhosis*. Falk Symposium No. 44. 1987
ISBN: 0-85200-993-3*
45. Paumgartner G, Stiehl A, Gerok W, eds.: *Bile Acids and the Liver*. Falk Symposium No. 45. 1987 ISBN: 0-85200-675-6*
46. Goebell H, Peskar BM, Malchow H, eds.: *Inflammatory Bowel Diseases – Basic Research & Clinical Implications*. Falk Symposium No. 46. 1988
ISBN: 0-7462-0067-6*
47. Bianchi L, Holt P, James OFW, Butler RN, eds.: *Aging in Liver and Gastrointestinal Tract*. Falk Symposium No. 47. 1988 ISBN: 0-7462-0066-8*
48. Heilmann C, ed.: *Calcium-Dependent Processes in the Liver*. Falk Symposium No. 48. 1988 ISBN: 0-7462-0075-7*
50. Singer MV, Goebell H, eds.: *Nerves and the Gastrointestinal Tract*. Falk Symposium No. 50. 1989 ISBN: 0-7462-0114-1
51. Bannasch P, Keppler D, Weber G, eds.: *Liver Cell Carcinoma*. Falk Symposium No. 51. 1989 ISBN: 0-7462-0111-7
52. Paumgartner G, Stiehl A, Gerok W, eds.: *Trends in Bile Acid Research*. Falk Symposium No. 52. 1989 ISBN: 0-7462-0112-5
53. Paumgartner G, Stiehl A, Barbara L, Roda E, eds.: *Strategies for the Treatment of Hepatobiliary Diseases*. Falk Symposium No. 53. 1990 ISBN: 0-7923-8903-4
54. Bianchi L, Gerok W, Maier K-P, Deinhardt F, eds.: *Infectious Diseases of the Liver*. Falk Symposium No. 54. 1990 ISBN: 0-7923-8902-6
55. Falk Symposium No. 55 not published
55B. Hadziselimovic F, Herzog B, Bürgin-Wolff A, eds.: *Inflammatory Bowel Disease and Coeliac Disease in Children*. International Falk Symposium. 1990
ISBN 0-7462-0125-7
56. Williams CN, eds.: *Trends in Inflammatory Bowel Disease Therapy*. Falk Symposium No. 56. 1990 ISBN: 0-7923-8952-2
57. Bock KW, Gerok W, Matern S, Schmid R, eds.: *Hepatic Metabolism and Disposition of Endo- and Xenobiotics*. Falk Symposium No. 57. 1991 ISBN: 0-7923-8953-0
58. Paumgartner G, Stiehl A, Gerok W, eds.: *Bile Acids as Therapeutic Agents: From Basic Science to Clinical Practice*. Falk Symposium No. 58. 1991 ISBN: 0-7923-8954-9
59. Halter F, Garner A, Tytgat GNJ, eds.: *Mechanisms of Peptic Ulcer Healing*. Falk Symposium No. 59. 1991 ISBN: 0-7923-8955-7
60. Goebell H, Ewe K, Malchow H, Koelbel Ch, eds.: *Inflammatory Bowel Diseases – Progress in Basic Research and Clinical Implications*. Falk Symposium No. 60. 1991
ISBN: 0-7923-8956-5
61. Falk Symposium No. 61 not published
62. Dowling RH, Folsch UR, Löser Ch, eds.: *Polyamines in the Gastrointestinal Tract*. Falk Symposium No. 62. 1992 ISBN: 0-7923-8976-X
63. Lentze MJ, Reichen J, eds.: *Paediatric Cholestasis: Novel Approaches to Treatment*. Falk Symposium No. 63. 1992 ISBN: 0-7923-8977-8
64. Demling L, Frühmorgen P, eds.: *Non-Neoplastic Diseases of the Anorectum*. Falk Symposium No. 64. 1992 ISBN: 0-7923-8979-4
64B. Gressner AM, Ramadori G, eds.: *Molecular and Cell Biology of Liver Fibrogenesis*. International Falk Symposium. 1992 ISBN: 0-7923-8980-8

*These titles were published under the MTP Press imprint.

Falk Symposium Series

65. Hadziselimovic F, Herzog B, eds.: *Inflammatory Bowel Diseases and Morbus Hirschprung.* Falk Symposium No. 65. 1992   ISBN: 0-7923-8995-6
66. Martin F, McLeod RS, Sutherland LR, Williams CN, eds.: *Trends in Inflammatory Bowel Disease Therapy.* Falk Symposium No. 66. 1993   ISBN: 0-7923-8827-5
67. Schölmerich J, Kruis W, Goebell H, Hohenberger W, Gross V, eds.: *Inflammatory Bowel Diseases – Pathophysiology as Basis of Treatment.* Falk Symposium No. 67. 1993
                                                                                                             ISBN: 0-7923-8996-4
68. Paumgartner G, Stiehl A, Gerok W, eds.: *Bile Acids and The Hepatobiliary System: From Basic Science to Clinical Practice.* Falk Symposium No. 68. 1993
                                                                                                            ISBN: 0-7923-8829-1
69. Schmid R, Bianchi L, Gerok W, Maier K-P, eds.: *Extrahepatic Manifestations in Liver Diseases.* Falk Symposium No. 69. 1993   ISBN: 0-7923-8821-6
70. Meyer zum Büschenfelde K-H, Hoofnagle J, Manns M, eds.: *Immunology and Liver.* Falk Symposium No. 70. 1993   ISBN: 0-7923-8830-5
71. Surrenti C, Casini A, Milani S, Pinzani M, eds.: *Fat-Storing Cells and Liver Fibrosis.* Falk Symposium No. 71. 1994   ISBN: 0-7923-8842-9
72. Rachmilewitz D, ed.: *Inflammatory Bowel Diseases – 1994.* Falk Symposium No. 72. 1994   ISBN: 0-7923-8845-3
73. Binder HJ, Cummings J, Soergel KH, eds.: *Short Chain Fatty Acids.* Falk Symposium No. 73. 1994   ISBN: 0-7923-8849-6
73B. Möllmann HW, May B, eds.: *Glucocorticoid Therapy in Chronic Inflammatory Bowel Disease: from basic principles to rational therapy.* International Falk Workshop. 1996
                                                                                                    ISBN 0-7923-8708-2
74. Keppler D, Jungermann K, eds.: *Transport in the Liver.* Falk Symposium No. 74. 1994
                                                                                               ISBN: 0-7923-8858-5
74B. Stange EF, ed.: *Chronic Inflammatory Bowel Disease.* Falk Symposium. 1995
                                                                                               ISBN: 0-7923-8876-3
75. van Berge Henegouwen GP, van Hoek B, De Groote J, Matern S, Stockbrügger RW, eds.: *Cholestatic Liver Diseases: New Strategies for Prevention and Treatment of Hepatobiliary and Cholestatic Liver Diseases.* Falk Symposium 75. 1994.
                                                                                              ISBN: 0-7923-8867-4
76. Monteiro E, Tavarela Veloso F, eds.: *Inflammatory Bowel Diseases: New Insights into Mechanisms of Inflammation and Challenges in Diagnosis and Treatment.* Falk Symposium 76. 1995.   ISBN 0-7923-8884-4
77. Singer MV, Ziegler R, Rohr G, eds.: *Gastrointestinal Tract and Endocrine System.* Falk Symposium 77. 1995.   ISBN 0-7923-8877-1
78. Decker K, Gerok W, Andus T, Gross V, eds.: *Cytokines and the Liver.* Falk Symposium 78. 1995.   ISBN 0-7923-8878-X
79. Holstege A, Schölmerich J, Hahn EG, eds.: *Portal Hypertension.* Falk Symposium 79. 1995.   ISBN 0-7923-8879-8
80. Hofmann AF, Paumgartner G, Stiehl A, eds.: *Bile Acids in Gastroenterology: Basic and Clinical Aspects.* Falk Symposium 80. 1995   ISBN 0-7923-8880-1
81. Riecken EO, Stallmach A, Zeitz M, Heise W, eds.: *Malignancy and Chronic Inflammation in the Gastrointestinal Tract – New Concepts.* Falk Symposium 81. 1995
ISBN 0-7923-8889-5
82. Fleig WE, ed.: *Inflammatory Bowel Diseases: New Developments and Standards.* Falk Symposium 82. 1995   ISBN 0-7923-8890-6
82B. Paumgartner G, Beuers U, eds.: *Bile Acids in Liver Diseases.* International Falk Workshop. 1995   ISBN 0-7923-8891-7

Falk Symposium Series

83. Dobrilla G, Felder M, de Pretis G, eds.: *Advances in Hepatobiliary and Pancreatic Diseases: Special Clinical Topics.* Falk Symposium 83. 1995. ISBN 0-7923-8892-5
84. Fromm H, Leuschner U, eds.: *Bile Acids – Cholestasis – Gallstones: Advances in Basic and Clinical Bile Acid Research.* Falk Symposium 84. 1995 ISBN 0-7923-8893-3
85. Tytgat GNJ, Bartelsman JFWM, van Deventer SJH, eds.: *Inflammatory Bowel Diseases.* Falk Symposium 85. 1995 ISBN 0-7923-8894-1
86. Berg PA, Leuschner U, eds.: *Bile Acids and Immunology.* Falk Symposium 86. 1996
ISBN 0-7923-8700-7
87. Schmid R, Bianchi L, Blum HE, Gerok W, Maier KP, Stalder GA, eds.: *Acute and Chronic Liver Diseases: Molecular Biology and Clinics.* Falk Symposium 87. 1996
ISBN 0-7923-8701-5
88. Blum HE, Wu GY, Wu CH, eds.: *Molecular Diagnosis and Gene Therapy.* Falk Symposium 88. 1996 ISBN 0-7923-8702-3
88B. Poupon RE, Reichen J, eds.: *Surrogate Markers to Assess Efficacy of TReatment in Chronic Liver Diseases.* International Falk Workshop. 1996 ISBN 0-7923-8705-8
89. Reyes HB, Leuschner U, Arias IM, eds.: *Pregnancy, Sex Hormones and the Liver.* Falk Symposium 89. 1996 ISBN 0-7923-8704-X
89B. Broelsch CE, Burdelski M, Rogiers X, eds.: *Cholestatic Liver Diseases in Children and Adults.* International Falk Workshop. 1996 ISBN 0-7923-8710-4
90. Lam S-K, Paumgartner P, Wang B, eds.: *Update on Hepatobiliary Diseases 1996.* Falk Symposium 90. 1996 ISBN 0-7923-8715-5
91. Hadziselimovic F, Herzog B, eds.: *Inflammatory Bowel Diseases and Chronic Recurrent Abdominal Pain.* Falk Symposium 91. 1996 ISBN 0-7923-8722-8
91B. Alvaro D, Benedetti A, Strazzabosco M, eds.: *Vanishing Bile Duct Syndrome – Pathophysiology and Treatment.* International Falk Workshop. 1996
ISBN 0-7923-8721-X
92. Gerok W, Loginov AS, Pokrowskij VI, eds.: *New Trends in Hepatology 1996.* Falk Symposium 92. 1997 ISBN 0-7923-8723-6
93. Paumgartner G, Stiehl A, Gerok W, eds.: *Bile Acids in Hepatobiliary Diseases – Basic Research and Clinical Application.* Falk Symposium 93. 1997 ISBN 0-7923-8725-2
94. Halter F, Winton D, Wright NA, eds.: *The Gut as a Model in Cell and Molecular Biology.* Falk Symposium 94. 1997 ISBN 0-7923-8726-0
94B. Kruse-Jarres JD, Schölmerich J, eds.: *Zinc and Diseases of the Digestive Tract.* International Falk Workshop. 1997 ISBN 0-7923-8724-4
95. Ewe K, Eckardt VF, Enck P, eds.: *Constipation and Anorectal Insufficiency.* Falk Symposium 95. 1997 ISBN 0-7923-8727-9
96. Andus T, Goebell H, Layer P, Schölmerich J, eds.: *Inflammatory Bowel Disease – from Bench to Bedside.* Falk Symposium 96. 1997 ISBN 0-7923-8728-7
97. Campieri M, Bianchi-Porro G, Fiocchi C, Schölmerich J, eds. *Clinical Challenges in Inflammatory Bowel Diseases: Diagnosis, Prognosis and Treatment.* Falk Symposium 97. 1998 ISBN 0-7923-8733-3
98. Lembcke B, Kruis W, Sartor RB, eds. *Systemic Manifestations of IBD: The Pending Challenge for Subtle Diagnosis and Treatment.* Falk Symposium 98. 1998
ISBN 0-7923-8734-1
99. Goebell H, Holtmann G, Talley NJ, eds. *Functional Dyspepsia and Irritable Bowel Syndrome: Concepts and Controversies.* Falk Symposium 99. 1998
ISBN 0-7923-8735-X
100. Blum HE, Bode Ch, Bode JCh, Sartor RB, eds. *Gut and the Liver.* Falk Symposium 100. 1998 ISBN 0-7923-8736-8

Falk Symposium Series

101. Rachmilewitz D, ed. *V International Symposium on Inflammatory Bowel Diseases.* Falk Symposium 101. 1998 ISBN 0-7923-8743-0
102. Manns MP, Boyer JL, Jansen PLM, Reichen J, eds. *Cholestatic Liver Diseases.* Falk Symposium 102. 1998 ISBN 0-7923-8746-5
102B. Manns MP, Chapman RW, Stiehl A, Wiesner R, eds. *Primary Sclerosing Cholangitis.* International Falk Workshop. 1998. ISBN 0-7923-8745-7
103. Häussinger D, Jungermann K, eds. *Liver and Nervous System.* Falk Symposium 102. 1998 ISBN 0-7924-8742-2
103B. Häussinger D, Heinrich PC, eds. *Signalling in the Liver.* International Falk Workshop. 1998 ISBN 0-7923-8744-9
103C. Fleig W, ed. *Normal and Malignant Liver Cell Growth.* International Falk Workshop. 1998 ISBN 0-7923-8748-1
104. Stallmach A, Zeitz M, Strober W, MacDonald TT, Lochs H, eds. *Induction and Modulation of Gastrointestinal Inflammation.* Falk Symposium 104. 1998 ISBN 0-7923-8747-3
105. Emmrich J, Liebe S, Stange EF, eds. *Innovative Concepts in Inflammatory Bowel Diseases.* Falk Symposium 105. 1999 ISBN 0-7923-8749-X
106. Rutgeerts P, Colombel J-F, Hanauer SB, Schölmerich J, Tytgat GNJ, van Gossum A, eds. *Advances in Inflammatory Bowel Diseases.* Falk Symposium 106. 1999 ISBN 0-7923-8750-3
107. Špičák J, Boyer J, Gilat T, Kotrlik K, Mareček Z, Paumgartner G, eds. *Diseases of the Liver and the Bile Ducts – New Aspects and Clinical Implications.* Falk Symposium 107. 1999 ISBN 0-7923-8751-1
108. Paumgartner G, Stiehl A, Gerok W, Keppler D, Leuschner U, eds. *Bile Acids and Cholestasis.* Falk Symposium 108. 1999 ISBN 0-7923-8752-X
109. Schmiegel W, Schölmerich J, eds. *Colorectal Cancer – Molecular Mechanisms, Premalignant State and its Prevention.* Falk Symposium 109. 1999 ISBN 0-7923-8753-8
110. Domschke W, Stoll R, Brasitus TA, Kagnoff MF, eds. *Intestinal Mucosa and its Diseases – Pathophysiology and Clinics.* Falk Symposium 110. 1999 ISBN 0-7923-8754-6
110B. Northfield TC, Ahmed HA, Jazwari RP, Zentler-Munro PL, eds. *Bile Acids in Hepatobiliary Disease.* Falk Workshop. 2000 ISBN 0-7923-8755-4
111. Rogler G, Kullmann F, Rutgeerts P, Sartor RB, Schölmerich J, eds. *IBD at the End of its First Century.* Falk Symposium 111. 2000 ISBN 0-7923-8756-2
112. Krammer HJ, Singer MV, eds. *Neurogastroenterology: From the Basics to the Clinics.* Falk Symposium 112. 2000 ISBN 0-7923-8757-0
113. Andus T, Rogler G, Schlottmann K, Frick E, Adler G, Schmiegel W, Zeitz M, Schölmerich J, eds. *Cytokines and Cell Homeostasis in the Gastrointestinal Tract.* Falk Symposium 113. 2000 ISBN 0-7923-8758-9
114. Manns MP, Paumgartner G, Leuschner U, eds. *Immunology and Liver.* Falk Symposium 114. 2000 ISBN 0-7923-8759-7
115. Boyer JL, Blum HE, Maier K-P, Sauerbruch T, Stalder GA, eds. *Liver Cirrhosis and its Development.* Falk Symposium 115. 2000 ISBN 0-7923-8760-0
116. Riemann JF, Neuhaus H, eds. *Interventional Endoscopy in Hepatology.* Falk Symposium 116. 2000 ISBN 0-7923-8761-9
116A. Dienes HP, Schirmacher P, Brechot C, Okuda K, eds. *Chronic Hepatitis: New Concepts of Pathogenesis, Diagnosis and Treatment.* Falk Workshop. 2000 ISBN 0-7923-8763-5

Falk Symposium Series

117. Gerbes AL, Beuers U, Jüngst D, Pape GR, Sackmann M, Sauerbruch T, eds. *Hepatology 2000 – Symposium in Honour of Gustav Paumgartner.* Falk Symposium 117. 2000　　　　　　　　　　　　　　　　　　　ISBN 0-7923-8765-1
117A. Acalovschi M, Paumgartner G, eds. *Hepatobiliary Diseases: Cholestasis and Gallstones.* Falk Workshop. 2000　　　　　　　ISBN 0-7923-8770-8
118. Frühmorgen P, Bruch H-P, eds. *Non-Neoplastic Diseases of the Anorectum.* Falk Symposium 118. 2001　　　　　　　　　　　ISBN 0-7923-8766-X
119. Fellermann K, Jewell DP, Sandborn WJ, Schölmerich J, Stange EF, eds. *Immunosuppression in Inflammatory Bowel Diseases – Standards, New Developments, Future Trends.* Falk Symposium 119. 2001　　　　　　　ISBN 0-7923-8767-8
120. van Berge Henegouwen GP, Keppler D, Leuschner U, Paumgartner G, Stiehl A, eds. *Biology of Bile Acids in Health and Disease.* Falk Symposium 120. 2001
　　　　　　　　　　　　　　　　　　　　　　　ISBN 0-7923-8768-6
121. Leuschner U, James OFW, Dancygier H, eds. *Steatohepatitis (NASH and ASH).* Falk Symposium 121. 2001　　　　　　　　　　　ISBN 0-7923-8769-4
121A. Matern S, Boyer JL, Keppler D, Meier-Abt PJ, eds. *Hepatobiliary Transport: From Bench to Bedside.* Falk Workshop. 2001　　　　　ISBN 0-7923-8771-6
122. Campieri M, Fiocchi C, Hanauer SB, Jewell DP, Rachmilewitz R, Schölmerich J, eds. *Inflammatory Bowel Disease – A Clinical Case Approach to Pathophysiology, Diagnosis, and Treatment.* Falk Symposium 122. 2002　　ISBN 0-7923-8772-4
123. Rachmilewitz D, Modigliani R, Podolsky DK, Sachar DB, Tozun N, eds. *VI International Symposium on Inflammatory Bowel Diseases.* Falk Symposium 123. 2002　　　　　　　　　　　　　　　　　　　　　ISBN 0-7923-8773-2
124. Hagenmüller F, Manns MP, Musmann H-G, Riemann JF, eds. *Medical Imaging in Gastroenterology and Hepatology.* Falk Symposium 124. 2002 ISBN 0-7923-8774-0
125. Gressner AM, Heinrich PC, Matern S, eds. *Cytokines in Liver Injury and Repair.* Falk Symposium 125. 2002　　　　　　　　　　　ISBN 0-7923-8775-9
126. Gupta S, Jansen PLM, Klempnauer J, Manns MP, eds. *Hepatocyte Transplantation.* Falk Symposium 126. 2002　　　　　　　　　　　ISBN 0-7923-8776-7
127. Hadziselimovic F, ed. *Autoimmune Diseases in Paediatric Gastroenterology.* Falk Symposium 127. 2002　　　　　　　　　　　　　ISBN 0-7923-8778-3
127A. Berr F, Bruix J, Hauss J, Wands J, Wittekind Ch, eds. *Malignant Liver Tumours: Basic Concepts and Clinical Management.* Falk Workshop. 2002
　　　　　　　　　　　　　　　　　　　　　　　ISBN 0-7923-8779-1
128. Scheppach W, Scheurlen M, eds. *Exogenous Factors in Colonic Carcinogenesis.* Falk Symposium 128. 2002　　　　　　　　　　　ISBN 0-7923-8780-5
129. Paumgartner G, Keppler D, Leuschner U, Stiehl A, eds. *Bile Acids: From Genomics to Disease and Therapy.* Falk Symposium 129. 2002　　ISBN 0-7923-8781-3
129A. Leuschner U, Berg PA, Holtmeier J, eds. *Bile Acids and Pregnancy.* Falk Workshop. 2002　　　　　　　　　　　　　　　　　　　　ISBN 0-7923-8782-1
130. Holtmann G, Talley NJ, eds. *Gastrointestinal Inflammation and Disturbed Gut Function: The Challenge of New Concepts.* Falk Symposium 130. 2003
　　　　　　　　　　　　　　　　　　　　　　　ISBN 0-7923-8783-X
131. Herfarth H, Feagan BJ, Folsch UR, Schölmerich J, Vatn MH, Zeitz M, eds. *Targets of Treatment in Chronic Inflammatory Bowel Diseases.* Falk Symposium 131. 2003
　　　　　　　　　　　　　　　　　　　　　　　ISBN 0-7923-8784-8
132. Galle PR, Gerken G, Schmidt WE, Wiedenmann B, eds. *Disease Progression and Carcinogenesis in the Gastrointestinal Tract.* Falk Symposium 132. 2003
　　　　　　　　　　　　　　　　　　　　　　　ISBN 0-7923-8785-6

Falk Symposium Series

132A. Staritz M, Adler G, Knuth A, Schmiegel W, Schmoll H-J, eds. *Side-effects of Chemotherapy on the Gastrointestinal Tract*. Falk Workshop. 2003
ISBN 0-7923-8791-0

132B. Reutter W, Schuppan D, Tauber R, Zeitz M, eds. *Cell Adhesion Molecules in Health and Disease*. Falk Workshop. 2003 ISBN 0-7923-8786-4

133. Duchmann R, Blumberg R, Neurath M, Schölmerich J, Strober W, Zeitz M. *Mechanisms of Intestinal Inflammation: Implications for Therapeutic Intervention in IBD*. Falk Symposium 133. 2004 ISBN 0-7923-8787-2

134. Dignass A, Lochs H, Stange E. *Trends and Controversies in IBD – Evidence-Based Approach or Individual Management?* Falk Symposium 134. 2004
ISBN 0-7923-8788-0

134A. Dignass A, Gross HJ, Buhr V, James OFW. *Topical Steroids in Gastroenterology and Hepatology*. Falk Workshop. 2004 ISBN 0-7923-8789-9

135. Lukáš M, Manns MP, Špičák J, Stange EF, eds. *Immunological Diseases of Liver and Gut*. Falk Symposium 135. 2004 ISBN 0-7923-8792-9

136. Leuschner U, Broomé U, Stiehl A, eds. *Cholestatic Liver Diseases: Therapeutic Options and Perspectives*. Falk Symposium 136. 2004 ISBN 0-7923-8793-7

137. Blum HE, Maier KP, Rodés J, Sauerbruch T, eds. *Liver Diseases: Advances in Treatment and Prevention*. Falk Symposium 137. 2004 ISBN 0-7923-8794-5

138. Blum HE, Manns MP, eds. *State of the Art of Hepatology: Molecular and Cell Biology*. Falk Symposium 138. 2004 ISBN 0-7923-8795-3

138A. Hayashi N, Manns MP, eds. *Prevention of Progression in Chronic Liver Disease: An Update on SNMC (Stronger Neo-Minophagen C)*. Falk Workshop. 2004
ISBN 0-7923-8796-1

139. Adler G, Blum HE, Fuchs M, Stange EF, eds. *Gallstones: Pathogenesis and Treatment*. Falk Symposium 139. 2004 ISBN 0-7923-8798-8

140. Colombel J-F, Gasché C, Schölmerich J, Vucelic C, eds. *Inflammatory Bowel Disease: Translation from Basic Research to Clinical Practice*. Falk Symposium 140. 2005. ISBN 1-4020-2847-4

141. Paumgartner G, Keppler D, Leuschner U, Stiehl A, eds. *Bile Acid Biology and its Therapeutic Implications*. Falk Symposium 141. 2005 ISBN 1-4020-2893-8

142. Dienes H-P, Leuschner U, Lohse AW, Manns MP, eds. *Autoimmune Liver Disease*. Falk Symposium 142. 2005 ISBN 1-4020-2894-6

143. Ammann RW, Büchler MW, Adler G, DiMagno EP, Sarner M, eds. *Pancreatitis: Advances in Pathobiology, Diagnosis and Treatment*. Falk Symposium 143. 2005
ISBN 1-4020-2895-4

144. Adler G, Blum AL, Blum HE, Leuschner U, Manns MP, Mössner J, Sartor RB, Schölmerich J, eds. *Gastroenterology Yesterday – Today – Tomorrow: A Review and Preview*. Falk Symposium 144. 2005 ISBN 1-4020-2896-2